Weight Loss *and* Good Health— The Atkins Way

This is an updated version of the book I wrote ten years ago to help as many people as I could to lose weight. I felt certain then—and continue to do so—that the widespread dissemination of misinformation about what constitutes a healthy diet has caused that epidemic of weight gain in this country.

The book made a greater impact than anyone might have predicted. Its sales exceeded ten million copies, and it was the number one–selling diet and health book in the United States for nearly five years. In fact, it has been the all-time top seller in its field. Certainly, of the millions of people who've read it, a large percentage followed its precepts, lost weight, kept it off, and decisively improved their health.

What you hold in your hands is a thoroughly rewritten version of that work. Having listened with care to the people who followed my weight-control program, I've clarified and improved the "do-ability" of the practical chapters of this book. I've added many new case histories and a horde of new and improved recipes. Finally, I've incorporated information on the recent upsurge of scientific evidence. We had it right ten years ago, but now we have twice as much research to confirm the nutritional approach championed by *New Diet Revolution*.

—Robert C. Atkins, M.D.

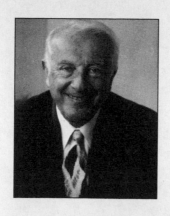

About the Author

ROBERT C. ATKINS, M.D., was the founder and executive medical director of the Atkins Center for Complementary Medicine in New York City. A 1951 graduate of the University of Michigan, Dr. Atkins received his medical degree from Cornell University Medical School in 1955, and went on to specialize in cardiology. In 1972, he published his groundbreaking weight-loss book, *Diet Revolution*—the first major work to prescribe a low-carbohydrate diet—followed in 1992 by the revised and updated *Dr. Atkins' New Diet Revolution*, which spent more than three years on the *New York Times* bestseller list. In addition, he was the author of several books that promote nutritional medicine, including *Dr. Atkins' Quick & Easy New Diet Cookbook* (1997), *Dr. Atkins' Vita-Nutrient Solution: Nature's Answer to Drugs* (1998), *Dr. Atkins' Age-Defying Diet Revolution* (1999), and, most recently, *Atkins for Life* (2003). He appeared or was featured on *The Oprah Winfrey Show*, *20/20*, *Larry King Live*, *CBS Evening News*, *Sally Jessy Raphael*, *Dateline NBC*, *Today*, *Good Morning America*, *CBS This Morning*, *The View*, and *ABC World News*, to name but a few. Dr. and Mrs. Atkins lived in New York City, where he passed away in April 2003.

DR. ATKINS' NEW DIET REVOLUTION

COMPLETELY UPDATED!

Robert C. Atkins, M.D.

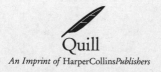

Quill

An Imprint of HarperCollinsPublishers

The advice offered in this book, although based on the author's experience with many thousands of patients, is not intended to be a substitute for the advice and counsel of your personal physician. If you are currently taking diuretics, insulin or oral diabetes medications, consult your physician before starting Atkins. You will need to reduce and then closely monitor your dosage as you lower your blood-sugar level. People with severe kidney disease should not do Atkins. The weight loss phases of the Atkins Nutritional Approach are not appropriate for pregnant women and nursing mothers.

HarperCollins books may be purchased for educational, business, or sales promotional use. For information please write: Special Markets Department, HarperCollins Publishers Inc., 10 East 53rd Street, New York, NY 10022.

First Quill edition published 2002.

Library of Congress Cataloging-in-Publication Data

Atkins, Robert C.
    Dr. Atkins' new diet revolution.
      p. cm.
    Completely updated.
    Originally published: New York, 1992.
    Includes bibliographical references and index.
    ISBN 0-06-008159-7
    1. Reducing diets. 2. Low-carbohydrate diet. I. Title: Doctor Atkins' new diet revolution. II. Title: New diet revolution. III. Title.

RM222.2 .A843 2002
613.2'5—dc21
                                      2001058600

03 04 05 WB/RRD 30 29

*To my loving and lovely wife Veronica,
who has unfailingly provided me with
emotional, intellectual, spiritual,
and controlled carbohydrate nourishment.*

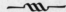

Acknowledgments

The revision of this book was a massive team effort. Michael Bernstein, senior vice president of Atkins Health and Medical Information Services at Atkins Nutritionals, Inc., led the team. Olivia Bell Buehl, the company's information director, coordinated and edited the copy. Contributing writer Bill Fryer reworked much of the manuscript.

A heartfelt thanks goes to the following employees at my companies, all of whom contributed time, energy and expertise to this effort—At Atkins Nutritionals, Inc.: Valerie Berkowitz, MS, RD, CDE; Cynthia Cicchesi; Rebecca Freedman; Stephanie Grozdea; Colette Heimowitz, MS; Richard Hirsch; Kathy Maguire; Dan O'Brien; Tamara Richardson and Matt Spolar. At the Atkins Center for Complementary Medicine: Geri Brewster, RD, MPH, CDN; Jacqueline Eberstein, RN; Patrick Fratellone, MD; Eva Katz, RD, MPH and Aliceson Swigart, CCN, CPT. A special thanks goes to Paul D. Wolff, the chief executive officer of our company, and Scott Kabak, the chief operating officer, both of whom were instrumental in getting this project off the ground.

The book also benefited from the contributions of Lynn Prowitt-Smith and Janet Blake.

Finally, this project would not have occurred had it not been for the contribution of literary agent Mike Cohn and the superb efforts of associate publisher and editor Jennifer Hershey and her team at Avon Books/HarperCollins.

Contents

Preface

This is an updated version of the book I wrote ten years ago to help as many people as I could to lose weight. I felt certain then—and continue to do so—that the widespread dissemination of misinformation about what constitutes a healthy diet had caused that epidemic of weight gain in this country.

The book made a greater impact than anyone might have predicted. Its sales exceeded ten million copies, and it was the number one-selling diet and health book in the U.S. for nearly five years. In fact, it has been the all-time top seller in its field. Certainly of the millions of people who've read it, a large percentage followed its precepts, lost weight, kept it off and decisively improved their health.

But now something even more significant is taking place. The view of the medical world has been changing, and *New Diet Revolution* celebrates its tenth anniversary in a climate that is infinitely more receptive to controlled carbohydrate weight loss. Medical opinion, slowly evolving, is finally catching up with—and beginning to absorb—the vast weight of scientific evidence that supports a controlled carbohydrate nutritional approach.

And what a godsend that is, because when I first wrote

this book, well-meaning but poorly informed organizations were so fat-phobic that people became convinced that so long as food was low in fat it was healthy.

People were taught to regard sugary cereals, which bore the American Heart Association's seal of approval, as health food, along with bread, pasta, bagels and the like. We were taught to shrink in terror from a steak or lamb chops. The low-fat craze—in vogue for two decades—significantly lowered the percentage of fat in the American diet but simultaneously resulted in a massive increase in carbohydrate consumption. Nor did the reduction in fat intake mean people were eating more vegetables; instead, it was refined carbohydrates, sugar and flour. Such quintessential junk foods had become the staple of American cuisine.

I hope you agree with me that if you wanted to create a nation of fat, tired, unhealthy people, this would be the perfect dietary plan. Every year the statistics poured in confirming that the obesity rates were escalating. And even more frightening, the number of diabetics worldwide has escalated. As I will show you, all too often the flipside of the coin of being overweight is having diabetes.

These twin epidemics, obesity and diabetes, were clearly the result of the low-fat, high-carbohydrate diet that was being preached to the public as gospel. The same groups that championed low fat denigrated the controlled carbohydrate nutritional approach—which was the very answer to these epidemics—as exceedingly harmful.

Now that millions of people have switched from the low-fat fiasco to the controlled carbohydrate lifestyle, a growing number of them are learning with certainty the degree to which they have been blatantly misinformed. I'll wager that there has never been another example in modern medicine of propaganda of such magnitude than the statements made by those worshipping the low-fat dogma.

Let me give you a few examples taken from the dozens of untruths designed to keep you from making the health-promoting change to a controlled carbohydrate nutritional approach. First, thousands of these low-fat fanatics have claimed that a high-protein diet would impair kidney function. Yet, I have never seen or heard a single accuser provide a single example of a single case in which that happened. This is one of the many examples of untruths fashioned out of the whole cloth.

Another example is an idea so fixed that not even overwhelming evidence can change some people's minds. I'm speaking of the belief that eating the controlled carbohydrate way will create cholesterol problems. The truth, as you will learn from reading this book, is that every one of a score of studies on eating regimens low enough in carbohydrates to produce the desired shift to stored fat as the primary energy source showed a significant improvement in cholesterol and triglycerides. Yes, there was a single exception, one in which cholesterol levels rose insignificantly after the subjects were told not to take their vitamins. This is one of the many examples of untruths being perpetrated because the accusers don't bother to read the scientific literature.

As you read this book, you will be informed, and, I expect, taken aback by the magnitude of the misinformation that stands behind our society's staggering increase in rates of diabetes and obesity. This propaganda campaign and the severity of the twin epidemics changed my focus on what I wanted this edition of the book to accomplish. I want so many millions of people to succeed in overcoming obesity, diabetes, heart disease, hypertension and all the other medical conditions aggravated by excessive carbohydrates that all the leaders of the medical profession recognize controlled carbohydrate eating as the treatment of choice for optimum health.

I probably will never again have to write a book that was as defiant and controversial as the first edition of this one was. What you hold in your hands is a thoroughly rewritten version of that work. Having listened with care to the people who followed my weight control program, I've clarified and improved the "do-ability" of the practical chapters of this book. I've added many new case histories* and a horde of new and improved recipes. Finally, I've incorporated information on the recent upsurge of scientific evidence. We had it right ten years ago, but now we have twice as much research to confirm the nutritional approach championed by *New Diet Revolution.*

Weight loss? Now you can't avoid it. You've bought this book, haven't you? Health? Don't forget, the carbohydrate controlled nutritional approach is a major part of the teaching of complementary medicine, and this medicine is focused on restoring ideal health, no matter what the cause.

The names of the people within the case histories have been changed to protect their privacy.

DR. ATKINS'
NEW DIET
REVOLUTION

PART ONE

Why Atkins Works

1

The Promise

Lose weight! Increase energy! Look great! This book will show you how it's done.

Not only that, it will show you how to change your life once and for all.

You hold in your hands a book that has sold more than ten million copies since 1992. Probably two to three times that number of people have followed its teachings. Most of you will have heard people say it's the most effective weight loss plan they've tried. It is!

If you're like many people, you've been through the weight loss wars. Name it and you've probably tried it, whether it's a low-fat diet, a food-combining diet, the grapefruit diet, liquid fasts, other fad diets and on and on. You've learned how to count calories, but ultimately with no success. Even if you lost weight, you were often hungry and always felt deprived. Then when you went back to your old way of eating, those pounds crept back, often joined by a few more.

If this scenario sounds all too familiar, I have a solution that will help end the game of yo-yo dieting once and for all. Instead, I'll help you adopt a permanent way of eating that:

- lets you lose weight without counting calories.
- makes you feel and look better.
- naturally re-energizes you.
- keeps lost pounds off forever with a new lifetime nutritional approach that includes rich, delicious foods.

But in addition to weight loss, there is an even more important benefit: The nutritional approach you'll learn about here is also a revolutionary method for living a long, healthy life. I want my readers to say: "I knew I'd lose weight, but I never realized I would feel so much healthier."

The typical modern American diet—or, as I sometimes call it, the high-sugar horrors—makes you fat. In the short term, it's also a sure road to daily misery, making you irritable and tired during the day and sleepless at night. In the long term, it leads grimly on toward heart disease, hypertension, diabetes and a host of other catastrophes.

What I'm going to show you is not just a way to lose weight, but a way to eat for the rest of your life so you can be slim and healthy and stay that way. For too many people, the word *diet* implies not an approach to eating for a lifetime, but a two-months-on, ten-months-off weight loss game that they play with themselves—year after year. *That is not what this book is about!* I believe this so strongly that from now on I'll speak not of the Atkins *Diet*, but of the Atkins Nutritional Approach or "doing Atkins" or even just "Atkins." It's a shorthand that others have been using, so I'm going to start using it, too.

The Atkins Nutritional Approach will make you healthy because it *is* different from the typical American way of eating. Simply put, you avoid the negative consequences of too much carbohydrate intake, all of which can be attributed to too much insulin release in your body.[1]

Would you like to see what I mean? Well, since they say a picture is worth a thousand words, how about two?

The Two Pictures

In the first picture, I am standing behind a huge table heaped with food. My expression is a mixture of pride and anticipation, and no wonder. There are mounds of seeds and nuts, platters of fish, a lobster in drawn butter, well-seasoned fish, turkey and duck and certainly a juicy steak. You'll spy an omelette that would do any breakfast table proud. There's no lack of variety here. I see vegetables in abundance, fresh green salads drenched in healthy olive oil-based dressing overflowing their bowls, and peeking out through the foliage, blueberries, strawberries and raspberries topped with whipped cream. There's a variety of cheeses. And since this is a picture of the food you'll be eating *after* you've lost your extra pounds and have reached the Lifetime Maintenance phase of Atkins, you will also notice a glass of wine, pan-fried sweet potatoes, a platter of melon and slices of peaches and plums. Finally, developments in creating controlled carbohydrate substitute ingredients make it possible to also place a pleasing array of controlled carb bread, cheesecake, ice cream and cookies on the groaning table.

It's a mouthwatering spread, and I'm hovering over it with a hungry eye. To my mind, the food I've just envisioned is quite luxurious. If you believe that weight loss requires self-deprivation, I'm going to insist on teaching you otherwise. I equate healthy eating with gastronomic pleasure and, soon, you will too.

My second picture is of you. I'm very hopeful that it resembles the *future* you.

The you in this picture I'm conjuring up is finally the weight you've always had as your goal, or fairly close. You feel great—full of energy. Your skin is glowing with health. If you've been exercising, your toned muscles show it. The you in this picture isn't worried about weight loss anymore. You no longer need to spend your time planning the stages of a new diet, constantly concerned about your eating, feeling guilty when you break promises you've made to yourself. After all, you've found a nutritional approach that will last you for a healthy and vigorous lifetime, and it's become so natural you hardly have to think about it anymore. It's second nature.

This is an obvious win-win situation. It offers you the pleasure of eating and the promise of being healthier than before. The major reason for turning it down would be skepticism. "How could anything be so perfect?" you might ask. If that's it, here's my answer: Read this book. When it's all boiled down, what I'm going to show you in *New Diet Revolution* is how to eat what's in the first picture and look just like the second.

Delicious eating and lifetime health. Not a bad bargain!

The Two Boasts

I don't make such promises lightly—and if I have to boast to get your attention then here goes.

Atkins is the most successful weight loss—and weight maintenance—program of the last quarter of the twentieth century. The fact is, by methods you're about to learn, it works an astonishing proportion of the time for the vast majority of men and women.

Atkins works because it targets our stored body fat. The fat is not there just to make us overweight but is our body's back-up system for fuel to generate energy. If we take it out of the back-up position and convert our body to using it as a primary fuel source, the result is an extremely efficient weight loss and weight maintenance program. This switch occurs when only an insignificant amount of carbohydrates, our body's primary fuel, is available. And it's an easy switch to control, because very little glycogen (made from carbohydrate) is stored in our bodies; if we eat fewer carbs, we almost immediately trip the switch.

The Atkins Nutritional Approach can positively impact the lives of people facing the risk factors associated with diabetes, heart disease, and hypertension. It can also alleviate gastrointestinal problems, and certain allergies, chronic pain and immune system weaknesses.

In my clinical practice we treat individuals with optimized diets and vitanutrients. Only a small percentage of patients come to us with weight problems alone. Usually nutritional solutions make the difference that medication alone cannot accomplish.

There is a close relationship between the first boast and the second. Making proper nutritional choices is the largest single component of retaining or restoring good health.

My goal is to make you become a healthy and happy person and to show you how to stay that way. *I will certainly also show you how to lose weight and keep it off forever.*

Changing Your Mind Set

Have you bought into the idea that to lose weight and feel good you have to adopt a low-fat diet? If so, the principles and approach I'm about to outline for you might just seem counterintuitive. They certainly do to those who criticize them. But in the ten years since this book was first published, new scientific research has been conducted and published that shows that a controlled carbohydrate nutritional approach is better for you—and for your body—than a low-fat, high-carbohydrate nutritional approach.

But let's cut to the chase. Here are three questions you should be asking yourself right about now:

1. Is this safe?
2. Is this nutritionally sound?
3. Will I keep the weight off once I lose it?

I take these questions, and the misinformation that surrounds the answers, so seriously that I've devoted an entire chapter (Chapter 9) to the myths and misconceptions that have been spread about controlled carbohydrate nutrition. But allow me to tip my hand:

- *Safe?* Yes, and there is plenty of hard science to back that up. In fact, a number of studies conducted in the past two years (which we will refer to in future chapters) show that a controlled carbohydrate nutritional approach helps improve the clinical parameters affecting heart disease and other illnesses while not causing harm to your liver, kidneys or bone structure.
- *Nutritionally sound?* Yes, a person following the typical menu and eating foods containing just 20 grams of carbohydrates meets or exceeds the daily recommended allowance of most vitamins and minerals. As you move through the phases of Atkins, you get even more. And that's not according to me, but to analysis using the leading nutritional software program, the one used by most of the practicing nutritionists in this country.
- *Keep off all the lost weight?* Nothing could be more true. Once you've seen the results and committed yourself to good health you'll realize that it's much easier than you ever thought possible. Because of the types of foods that are part of Atkins, it's actually possible to happily make a change in the way you eat—and look and feel—for good.

The Four Principles of the Atkins Nutritional Approach

By following the Atkins Nutritional Approach for a lifetime, you will achieve four things:

A Typical Success Story

Is it hard to keep the pounds off doing Atkins? Tim Wallerdeine doesn't think so.

Blessed with three young children and a happy marriage, Tim started Atkins because he wanted to live to see those kids grow up. At 35 years old, Tim weighed 335 pounds—far too much even for a strongly built six-footer. His blood pressure was borderline high; his triglycerides (a risk factor for heart disease) were through the roof.

The day after his wife's birthday—they went for a final carbohydrate blowout—Tim started Atkins. Within two weeks, he lost 21 pounds. After four weeks, 34 pounds. "By July 27, 1999, after nine months on the program, I had shed 122 pounds and weighed 213." Without difficulty, enjoying the food and adhering faithfully to the Atkins Lifetime Maintenance phase, Tim has stayed right around that weight for two and a half years.

Tim's blood pressure normalized. His cholesterol, glucose and triglyceride levels went down—and they've stayed down. The back and neck pain he used to suffer is gone. He exercises regularly today. And, as he emphatically believes, "I'm a better dad and husband. My old phrase used to be, 'No, I'm not up for that.' Now I love to play with my children."

Final comments? How about this: "Just the other night, we went out for ice cream to celebrate Ethan's fifth birthday. No, I didn't indulge, and I didn't feel deprived. I felt alive!"

---

1. You *will* lose weight. It's hard not to. Both men and women who follow the Atkins approach to weight loss readily take off pounds and inches. For the small num-

bers who have a truly hardcore metabolic resistance to weight loss, Chapter 20 will go into detail about how to overcome the barriers that prevent a successful outcome. Optimizing body weight is a valuable element of any health-oriented program because, by and large, being significantly overweight is an indicator of potential health problems, now or in the future. When you've taken the pounds off, you'll see the benefits, and they will be far more than merely cosmetic.

2. You *will* maintain your weight loss. This is where the Atkins Nutritional Approach leaves most other diets in the dust. Almost every experienced dieter has gone on a diet, worked hard, lost a lot of pounds and gained them all back in a few months or perhaps a year. This is usually due to the expected consequence of low-fat/low-calorie diets—hunger. Although many people can tolerate hunger for a while, very few can tolerate it for a lifetime. Deprivation is no fun. Once the biological gap between hunger and fulfillment grows too large, the rebound can be amazingly rapid as well as heartbreaking and humiliating. But that's the problem of diets that restrict quantities. The Atkins program refuses to accept hunger as a way of life. The plan includes foods that have enough fat and protein so hunger is not the huge issue it is on other weight loss plans. But it still allows dieters to maintain a healthy weight for a lifetime.

3. You *will* achieve good health. The change is amazing. Doing Atkins, you meet your nutritional needs by eating delicious, healthy, filling foods and avoiding the sugar and carbs that junk food is loaded with. As a result, you become less tired and more energetic, not merely because of the weight loss, but because the physical consequences of a truly dysfunctional blood sugar and insulin metabolism are reversed. Doing Atkins, people start feeling good even before they reach their goal weight. Once they abandon the catastrophic American diet of refined carbohydrates for

whole, unrefined food, they start to *live* again. It's one of the most rewarding experiences I've had the privilege of witnessing with thousands of my patients.

4. You *will* lay the permanent groundwork for disease prevention. You will change your life, which, believe it or not, is even more important than looking good on the beach next summer. By following an individualized controlled carbohydrate nutritional approach that results in lower insulin production, people at high risk for chronic illnesses such as cardiovascular disease, hypertension[2-16] and diabetes[17-25] will see a marked improvement in their clinical parameters. We will explore many of the studies referenced here throughout the later chapters of this book.

Why Is the Atkins Nutritional Approach So Revolutionary and So Right?

The U.S. is the fattest nation in the world. More than sixty percent of Americans are overweight or obese.[26] Yet thirty years ago, it was less than forty percent. Are Americans exceptionally weak-willed? Or could it be that we've developed an extraordinary collective compulsion to become thicker from front to back and wider from side to side than the rest of humanity?

Please don't laugh. You know that isn't the answer. Why are we in the midst of an obesity epidemic?

The obvious answer is that Americans don't eat the types of foods that are consistent with maintaining a normal healthy metabolism. Mankind is not geared to handle an abundance of refined carbohydrates. Losing weight is not a matter of counting calories; it is a matter of eating food your body is able to handle.

Let me place a few facts on the table, all of which we will explore throughout the remainder of this book:

- Most obesity exists when the body's metabolism—the process by which it turns food into fuel—isn't functioning correctly. The more overweight a person is, the more certain is the presence of metabolic disturbance.
- The basis of the metabolic disturbance in obesity doesn't have to do with the fat you eat. It has to do with eating too many carbohydrates, which leads to metabolic problems such as insulin resistance and hyperinsulinism. And these metabolic problems are directly related to your general health picture and your likelihood of being victimized by killers such as diabetes, heart disease and stroke. Moreover, high insulin levels have been associated with a higher incidence of diabetes. (Since Type II diabetics also have high insulin levels, the two epidemics, obesity and diabetes, can quite properly be considered a single epidemic.)
- The metabolic effect resulting from excess insulin production can be circumvented by controlling carbohydrates.[27] When you control your intake of refined carbohydrates, *you avoid the foods that cause you to be fat.*
- This metabolic correction is so striking that some of you will be able to lose weight eating a higher number of calories than you've been eating on diets top-heavy in carbohydrates.[28–29]
- Diets high in carbohydrates are precisely what most overweight people don't need and can't become permanently slim on. Low-fat diets are, by their very nature, almost always high-carbohydrate diets and bring on the very problems that they were intended to protect us from.
- Our epidemics of diabetes, heart disease and high blood pressure are very largely the results of our overconsumption of refined carbohydrates and its connection to hyperinsulinism.
- The Atkins Nutritional Approach can and has corrected these serious risk factors associated with obesity.

There has been sufficient evidence to make
tions for more than thirty years now. But the he
government and such prominent organizations a
States Department of Agriculture blanketed the
messages about low-fat dieting from the 1970s to the present. In fact, U.S. government statistics for this time period
clearly demonstrate that along with the dramatic decrease in
dietary fat intake (from forty percent to thirty-three percent
of our caloric intake) there was also a dramatic increase in
the intake of refined carbohydrates, not only sugar but white
flour.[30] There is no doubt in my mind that this increase in refined carbohydrates has been spurred by the media attention
given to the Food Guide Pyramid, created by the U.S. Department of Agriculture, which made six to eleven daily
servings of these wheat derivatives the basis of the pyramid.
I believe that the Food Guide Pyramid's recommendations
have directly contributed to the twin epidemics of obesity
and diabetes we now face in this country.

There are many examples in history of things we've thought
were true that we eventually realized were wrong. Remember,
we once were *sure* the earth was flat. But we learn, make
progress and *can* correct our missteps. Only during the last few
years has a significant percentage of Americans begun to question what we've been taught about how to eat.

And in just the last year or two, the news media has finally
begun reporting the range of scientific studies showing that
low-fat/high-carbohydrate diets lead to high levels of insulin
and to the number-one risk factor for heart disease, high
triglycerides. These studies also reveal that controlled carbohydrate diets reverse these problems in a very large percentage of the population. Many of these important studies
are referenced throughout this book.

If you've been overweight for very long, it's almost certain you have a blood sugar or a metabolic disorder. This
means that refined carbohydrates—which include sugars,
white flour products and junk foods that are such a whopping proportion of the American diet—are slow poison to

Different Kinds of Food

Protein in the original Greek means "of first importance." The Greeks had it right! Protein—complex
chains of amino acids—is the basic building block of
life and essential to almost every chemical reaction in
the human body. Food rich in protein includes meat,
fish, fowl, eggs—most of which contain almost *no*
carbohydrates—and cheese, nuts, and seeds. Many
vegetables are also well supplied, but unlike animal
foods, don't contain all the essential amino acids.

Fat provides glycerol and essential fatty acids, which
the body cannot make. The thirty-year-long campaign
against dietary fat is as misguided as it is futile. Fat is
found in meat, fish, fowl, dairy products and the oils
derived from nuts and seeds and a few vegetables
such as avocados. Oils extracted from these foods
represent one hundred percent fat and contain no carbohydrates.

Carbohydrate includes sugars and starches that are
chains of sugar molecules. Although carbohydrate
provides the quickest source of energy, we eat much
more of it, by far, than our body needs to be healthy.
Vegetables do contain some carbohydrates, but they
also contain a wide and wondrous variety of vitamins
and minerals. However, you can eat plenty of vegetables with high concentrations of beneficial nutrients
and still control your carbs. On the other hand, carbohydrates such as those in sugar and white flour contain almost nothing that your body needs in large
quantities.

you. Those foods are bad for your health, bad for your energy level, bad for your mental state, bad for your figure. Bad for your career prospects, bad for your sex life, bad for your digestion, bad for your blood chemistry, bad for your heart. What I'm saying is that they're bad.

I believe that most of the overweight people in the world are carbohydrate sensitive. Often they're true carbohydrate addicts. They need a metabolic, controlled carbohydrate solution, not a low-fat one.

When I wrote the first edition of this book in 1992, I was hotly indignant over the dietary guidelines that I felt were ruining people's lives. I was very critical of some of the individuals who proposed low-fat weight loss programs, and I apologize, because many of them were sincere in their efforts to help people.

But that doesn't mean there isn't a more effective, healthy alternative to the low-fat diet. Today there is an ever-increasing number of medical practitioners who recognize the health benefits of controlled carbohydrate nutrition. But I am not satisfied, and neither should you be, with those practitioners who fail to see that the truly deadly component of American eating is the junk food culture in which we're all brought up.

All this discussion about insulin levels, blood sugar and metabolism may seem complicated to you right now. In the next few chapters I'll tell you everything you need to know. Then you'll begin to understand why the Atkins Nutritional Approach produces healthy weight loss. Before we go there, though, let me review what you will gain by reading this book from cover to cover:

- On most diets you'll be hungry a fair percentage of the time. This program includes foods that leave you feeling much more full and satisfied.
- On most diets you'll be counting calories. When you do Atkins there's no need for that.

- On most diets you'll never stop eating addictive high-carbohydrate foods. When you do Atkins, you'll quickly learn how to overcome your addictions.
- On most diets you won't learn how to make a gradual transition to a lifetime maintenance plan. After reading this book, you'll learn how to develop a healthy way to eat that will feel comfortable and natural enough to adopt for good.

You know what I'm going to remind you of next. The Atkins Nutritional Approach is not a "diet." In the limiting sense of a weight loss program that you go on and off, it doesn't deserve to be called a diet at all. *It's a way of eating for the rest of your (healthy) life.*

KEY POINTS!

- The typical American style of eating is grossly mismatched to the normal human metabolism.
- Most obesity is the result of metabolic disturbances, not overconsumption of fat.
- Studies consistently show that sugar, refined white flour and junk foods are bad for your health, your energy level, your mental state and your figure.
- Low-fat diets are in effect high-carbohydrate diets and bring on the very problems that they were intended to protect us from.
- By doing Atkins you will control your weight, achieve good health and help prevent disease.
- The Atkins Nutritional Approach is composed of protein and fat, both essential to the human body, plus controlled quantities of the most nutrient-dense carbohydrates, primarily in the form of vegetables.

2

~m~

Understanding Some Basics

There are a few principles I need you to understand in order to put Atkins into action. Let's start with a couple of definitions. First, a calorie is simply a unit of energy—precisely the amount of heat needed to raise 1 gram of water 1 degree Celsius at sea level.

Second, metabolism is the sum of the physical and chemical processes by which food is transformed into energy.

Now let's move on to some concepts and misconceptions.

Don't Excess Calories Cause Weight Gain?

It is true that gaining weight results from taking in more calories than you expend. But excess calories certainly cause you to pile on the pounds—and this is a gigantic "but"—only when you are eating a lot of carbohydrate along with fat.

So it's time to abandon the assumption that the only way to lose weight is to strictly control your intake of calories. Many people think that only one thing matters: how many calories you take in and use up. It's not that simple.

When you follow a controlled carbohydrate approach,

you get what I call a "metabolic advantage."[1-6] When you control carbohydrate consumption sufficiently, your body will switch from burning glucose derived from carbohydrate to burning primarily fat for energy. This means you could eat, say, 2,000 calories and still begin losing pounds and inches.

In contrast, if you were consuming 2,000 calories on a low-fat diet, you might not lose weight, and you might actually gain weight. The metabolic advantage is that burning fat takes more energy so you expend more calories. And if you eat *fewer* calories—as many Atkins people do because their appetite is usually diminished—you'll likely lose weight even faster. So it's not that calories don't count, it's just that you will burn more of them, with less hunger, when your body is operating on a fat-based metabolism.

When I published the first edition of this book ten years ago, that claim was quite controversial. Today it is galloping into acceptance among scientists who study the human metabolism. Glance through the references listed at the back of this book and you will see the numerous studies and articles published in the past six years. And, we will deal with the metabolic advantage in greater detail in Chapter 7.

Eating the Atkins Way Must Have Special Advantages

You bet it does. Here are six reasons why doing Atkins works:

1. As I've just said, it mobilizes more fat for use as energy than any diet you have ever encountered. In a clinical setting and countless testimonials, Atkins has repeatedly been proven to take off more fat than other programs when an equal number of calories is con-

sumed. This incredible advantage has been researched and validated.[7-14]

2. The controlled carbohydrate nutritional approach is not one of deprivation. Sheer hunger is the main reason for the failure of most weight loss efforts. A lifetime eating plan needs to be palatable, pleasant and filling. You will have to abandon sugar and other refined carbohydrates such as white flour. But most people find that once they shake off the sugar addiction, they feel no strong desire to go back to it. For them, a nutritional approach that allows them to eat a vast variety of meat and fish and salads and vegetables prepared in the most appetizing manner—i.e., with butter and cream and spices and herbs—is anything but austere. Eating Atkins-style is a food lover's dream come true—luxurious, healthy and varied.

3. Atkins is the easiest way to maintain weight loss. The trouble with losing weight on a low-calorie/low-fat diet or on a liquid-protein diet is that the maintenance program is so very different from the weight loss program. So when you go back to your former way of eating, the pounds return with astonishing speed because you are unprepared for maintenance.

There are sound physiological reasons for this. When you restrict the number of calories you eat, your metabolism shifts into a survival mode, meaning it slows down to conserve energy. When you go back to a higher-calorie diet—as you inevitably must—your body is still in its mode of burning calories slowly. So it becomes extremely hard to continue or maintain weight loss.

Success at maintaining weight loss is the great plus while doing Atkins. What most people know about it is that you can usually lose a lot of weight rapidly. And you probably can. But the key point is that the weight doesn't return. One of the reasons is that it doesn't create a big difference in the number of calories you eat during the weight loss and weight maintenance phases.

The Atkins Nutritional Approach is actually a continuum of four phases that transition seamlessly from one to the next. Phase 1, known as Induction, crashes you through most weight loss barriers and will generally introduce even the most metabolically resistant person to weight reduction. Phase 2, Ongoing Weight Loss (OWL), will carry you smoothly toward your goal. Phase 3, Pre-Maintenance, eases you toward adopting permanently a new, healthier way of eating that, with a modest degree of diligence on your part, will allow you to stay slim forever. Phase 4, Lifetime Maintenance, is the game plan that will keep those banished pounds at bay for the rest of your days.

Let me state one crucial fact that you should always keep in mind: For people who comply with all four phases of Atkins, failure to maintain weight loss is very rare.

4. Not only does Atkins not deprive you of the pleasure of eating, it energizes you and makes you feel just plain good. And those two things are definitely factors in keeping the weight off, because few people are willing to go back to feeling lousy once they've experienced the joys of feeling good. As a matter of fact, for about half the patients I see, the most compelling reason they continue to do Atkins is that they feel noticeably worse if they stop the program.

Plus, when you are full of energy, you are more inclined to exercise, enhancing weight loss and replacing fat tissue with muscle, which will also help you cut inches from your measurements. People will see the change in you, enhancing your sense of accomplishment and self-respect.

5. The plan is healthy. Research has repeatedly demonstrated that controlling carbohydrate intake results in improved blood cholesterol and triglyceride levels,

moderation of blood-sugar levels and re
blood pressure. All these indicators result
risk for cardiovascular disease.[15–42] And, i
in my forty years of practice, I've yet to see a single
study that has shown that a high-protein diet causes
kidney problems.

In addition, Atkins can effectively and quickly make
a positive impact on many of the most common annoyances that patients reveal in the privacy of their doctor's office. In all my years of practice, I've heard and
seen it all: fatigue, irritability, depression, trouble con-
centrating, headaches, insomnia, dizziness, joint and
muscle aches, heartburn, colitis, premenstrual syndrome, water retention and bloating. For the lion's
share of patients, Atkins is a specific prescription
against such ills.

6. Atkins works because, as an increasing body of scientific evidence shows, it corrects the basic factor that
controls obesity and influences risk factors for certain
illnesses. That factor is excessive levels of insulin.[43–59]
An essential hormone, insulin governs the basic mechanism by which the body lays on fat. When found in
excessively high levels—we medical folk call that
state *hyperinsulinism*—insulin vigorously promotes
the development of diabetes, atherosclerosis and hypertension. More recently, it has also been linked to increased risk of breast cancer and polycystic ovarian
syndrome.[60–66]

And so the Atkins approach finds itself at the center of
health planning for a long and vigorous life.

What's Wrong With Carbohydrates?

If you mean what's wrong with a spear of broccoli or a
bunch of spinach, the answer is nothing, they're magnificent

,ods. When I speak negatively of carbohydrates, I'm referring to the unhealthy ones—those lurking in the sugar bowl and the bin of white flour, along with milk, white rice and processed and refined foods of all kinds. I also must include concentrates, such as fruit juices.

During the weight loss phase of Atkins, even your intake of potentially healthy carbohydrates such as fruits and whole grains must be controlled. Once you've bid adieu to your extra pounds, you can return to fruits and some starches to the degree that they won't upset your metabolism and reactivate the cravings that result in weight gain. But the refined and processed foods I've just mentioned simply aren't good for you—ever.

Am I advocating a high-fat diet? Not in the long run. As you increase the percentage of carbohydrates, while advancing through the different phases of Atkins, the percentage and actual amount of fat you consume will diminish. However, as long as you are at the lower end of carbohydrate consumption, higher-fat consumption poses no threat to your health.[67]

A Short History Lesson

Let me assure you that eating meat, fish and fowl isn't a health hardship—it's what humans have eaten for millions of years. People ate much the same way in the nineteenth century. They were beef and pork eaters and their use of butter and eggs was unrestricted. In fact, the two most widely consumed fats of all were lard and beef tallow.

In the crucial sixty-year time span between 1910 and 1970, when coronary heart disease escalated from a yet-to-be-recognized problem to the killer of more than half the population, this is what happened to America's diet: The intake of animal fat and butter actually dropped a little, while the intake of cholesterol was not changed. Meanwhile, the intake of refined carbohydrates (mainly sugar, corn syrup and white flour) escalated by sixty percent.[68] (See the graphs on page 27.)

To understand how the human diet in most of the world's developed countries has changed so drastically in the last century, let's take a short historical detour. Even before the onset of agriculture, the human animal was able, for millions of years, to remain strong and healthy in conditions of often savage deprivation by eating the fish and animals that scampered and swam around him, and the fruits and vegetables and berries that grew nearby. Without medicine, without expertise, without insulated housing or reliable heating, our species nonetheless survived. The fact that the dietary side of our primitive lifestyle was enormously healthy undoubtedly helped us.

So what has caused the avalanche of degenerative diseases that now threaten the health of our species? Two hundred years ago the average person ate less than 10 pounds of sugar a year, and white flour was used much less commonly. About a hundred and ten years ago the lid blew off the sugar canister. In the 1890s, the craze for cola beverages swept the nation—which means that when we were thirsty and craved water, we got sugar as well. To make matters worse, the mills that could refine wheat into white, nutritionally barren flour were developed in the same decade.

That was bad enough. But what's worse, once that flour met up with sweetness and saltiness, the junk food industry was off and running.

The Perils of Sugar

The net result was that sugar intake, which had averaged 12 pounds a year per person in 1828, was nearly ten times that in 1928. Remember, too, that if you don't take your sugar straight, you'll find it already sprinkled into a thousand different foods and beverages before they come to your table.

There are marked similarities in the diet eaten in all the

world's developed countries, so, for now, I'll just mention some statistics for the United States. Once you understand what healthy eating can be like, you'll find them as bizarre and shocking as I do.

The latest Department of Agriculture statistics show that the average American consumed 124 pounds of caloric sweeteners (principally refined sugar and high fructose corn syrup) in 1975.[69] By 1999 it had risen to 158 pounds. This translates into an average of nearly 750 calories from sugar a day, which means by conservative reckoning, over one-third of all the calories an adult puts into his or her body each day comes from nutritionally empty and metabolically harmful caloric sweeteners. Those figures represent 190 grams of sugar (and corn syrup) a day. Compare that with the 300 grams of carbohydrate the government expects us to consume each day, and we see that sugar now comprises over sixty percent of the carbohydrate total.

Sugar has no nutritional value and is directly harmful to your health. Despite vociferous attempts to defend it, there are studies that clearly show how harmful (and even deadly in the case of diabetics) its effects can be. I won't go into hyperinsulinism now; it will be covered fully in Chapter 5. For now, simply remember this: Diets high in sugar and other refined carbohydrates radically increase the body's production of insulin, and insulin is the best single index of adiposity. That final word is medical jargon for *fat*.

Sugar, you see, activates certain metabolic processes that are both harmful to your health and folly for your waistline. Sugar is a metabolic poison. You could, of course, ignore this fact and attempt to control your weight by calorie counting and deprivation. That is, you could direct yourself to the quantity instead of the quality of your diet. That's pretty much what conventional diets advise. However, the likelihood that you'll *permanently* lose weight by controlling your caloric intake is almost nil.

The whole problem of sugar was compounded by the low-fat messages we were wrongly bombarded with during the 1980s and 1990s. To make a low-fat product taste good, manufacturers add lots of sugar. Now, in the United States, the aisles in the supermarket are crammed with low-fat or diet cookies and crackers, ice cream, frozen cakes and pies, soft drinks and white bread *filled* with sugar. The United States has "low-fatted" and "dieted" itself to a raging epidemic of obesity and diabetes.

This is not real food; it's invented, fake food. It's filled with sugar and highly refined carbohydrates and with chemically altered trans fats (they are listed as hydrogenated or partially hydrogenated oil on food labels), not to mention plenty of other chemical additives. For thousands of years,

Vive la Difference!

A look at another Western culture is instructive. Only a few decades ago, the Frenchman with his butter-, cheese- and goose-liver-pâté-laden diet had a heart disease rate sixty percent lower than his American peers.[70] (The Frenchwoman did even better—she had the lowest heart disease rate in the western world.) The French also have far lower rates of obesity than Americans do, despite the fact that their diet is higher in fat. They eat comparable amounts of meat and fish, four times the butter and twice as much cheese as Americans. What does it all mean? Could it by any chance have anything to do with the fact that the per capita consumption of sugar in the United States was five times that of France?

By the way, the reason it's more helpful to compare American and French diets of a few decades ago is that the French have now discovered fast food. As their diets become closer to American ones, they are losing some of their health advantage.

human beings were in luck—none of this food existed. Now we're stuck with it. Because it's incredibly profitable, it's also widely distributed. But there isn't a person on this planet who should be eating it.

What Are We to Do?

If you want to be slim and vigorous, you can't eat as I've described. But you can eat the natural, healthy unrefined animal and vegetable foods that people ate and grew robust on in centuries past. Nor do you have to eat like a rabbit; you can eat like a human being. You can enjoy fish, lamb, steak and lobster, nuts and berries, cheese, eggs and butter along with a wonderful variety of salad greens and other vegetables.

In fact, in the ten years since the first edition of this book was published, one of my personal wishes has been granted. Today, a person choosing to follow a controlled carbohydrate nutritional approach has almost as many packaged and prepared food options as people who are, unwittingly, following a low-fat diet. Visit your local natural food store, drug store, supermarket or even mass market store and you will see the wide variety of food products available to someone who understands the benefits of controlled carbohydrate nutrition. Advances in scientific understanding have paved the way for alternatives to foods that are high in carbohydrates, foods such as pasta, bread, muffins, cakes, candy and

---

Changes in How We Eat

Look at the correlation between the decline in fat consumption and the increase in carbohydrate consumption. The pendulum began to swing toward fat restriction in 1975, and for the next twenty years, Americans began to gain weight at an alarming rate (see the following graphs).

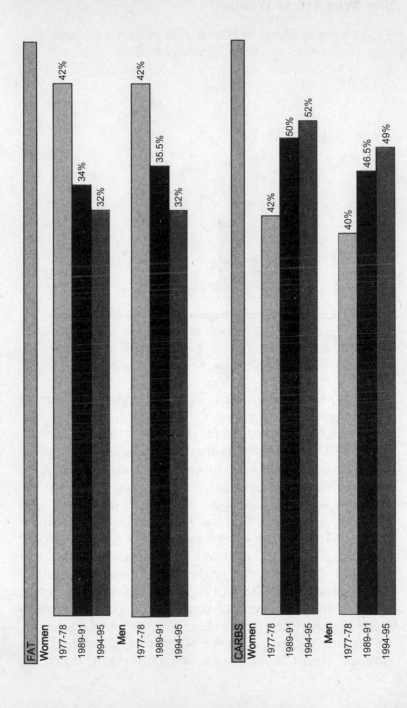

FAT

Women
- 1977-78: 42%
- 1989-91: 34%
- 1994-95: 32%

Men
- 1977-78: 42%
- 1989-91: 35.5%
- 1994-95: 32%

CARBS

Women
- 1977-78: 42%
- 1989-91: 50%
- 1994-95: 52%

Men
- 1977-78: 40%
- 1989-91: 46.5%
- 1994-95: 49%

Number of States in Which 35% or More of Adults Are Overweight

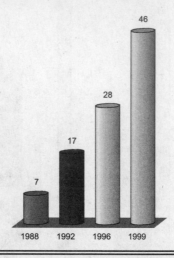

Source: Enns, C.W., et al. Trends in Food and Nutrient Intakes by Adults: NFCS 1977–78, CSFII 1989–91, and CSFII 1994–95, Family Economics and Nutrition Review 10(4) 1997.

even ice cream, not to mention the wide variety of energy bars and ready-to-drink shakes.

On all four phases of Atkins, you select from an increasingly liberal array of foods that are sources of the healthy carbohydrates. Your overall intake of them also gradually increases. Once you've reached your goal weight, you can eat larger helpings of healthy carbohydrate foods, as long as you stay below the Critical Carbohydrate Level for Maintenance (CCLM), which will be explained in Chapters 16 and 17. In simple terms, this means knowing and adhering to a threshold of carbohydrate intake that allows you to neither gain nor lose weight. It's worth mentioning that each person has an individual threshold depending upon age, level of physical activity and other factors.

Common sense dictates that when a lot of people try the same answer to the same problem and most of them fail, there's something wrong with their solution. You may have tried a low-fat diet. I'm sure you've seen other people try one. After a promising start, they often end up as failures. Only people with remarkable self-discipline or those who really don't get pleasure from eating are likely to succeed on low-fat diets. Atkins represents a completely different way.

When you do Atkins, you eliminate virtually all refined sugar and flour and processed foods. Instead, you're in an alliance with Mother Nature, who really did provide for us very well. You bought this book to lose weight, and I'm going to have to make you healthier, too. When doing Atkins, you couldn't separate those results, even if you wanted to.

KEY POINTS!

- It is *not* true that the only way to lose weight is to limit your intake of calories.
- When you control carbohydrate consumption sufficiently, your body will switch from burning glucose, derived from carbohydrate, to burning primarily fat as its energy source.
- You burn more calories when your body is operating on a fat metabolism.
- Atkins has repeatedly been proven to take off more fat than other weight loss programs when an equal number of calories is consumed.
- By drastically increasing the intake of carbohydrate, the American diet has changed dramatically in the past sixty years.
- In the past twenty years the incidence of lifestyle-related diseases such as obesity, diabetes and heart disease has increased by leaps and bounds.

A FREQUENTLY ASKED QUESTION:

Is it true that the Atkins Nutritional Approach is really just another low-calorie diet?
Some people think this, but it's not true. Atkins isn't about counting calories. Those who are doing Atkins may be eating fewer calories as a result of being less hungry and less obsessed with food.

This occurs for two reasons:

1. Stable blood sugar throughout the day ensures that you will have fewer food cravings or false hunger pains.
2. The food eaten by a person doing Atkins (meat, fish, cheese, nuts, eggs, low-sugar/low-starch vegetables and fruit) is less processed and more nutritious than the typical pre-Atkins menu. Give a body fewer empty calories, provide it with more nutrient-dense alternatives, and the body will logically be satisfied sooner and require less food.

TIPS:

- Eliminate from your kitchen sugar and all products that contain sugar.
- When grocery shopping, stick to the aisles on the perimeters of the store. The center aisles are where the junk food and processed food lurk.
- Look for—and purchase—the ever-increasing selection of controlled carbohydrate food alternatives to low-fat, high-sugar foods.
- Use a carbohydrate gram counter—such as the one at the end of this book—to count carbs.
- Even if you are not trying to lose weight, avoid the typical high-carb breakfast choices such as toast, muffins, bagels and cereal.

3

How You'll Succeed

Whether you are an old hand at the weight loss game, or have, at the very least, been on a diet before, the following scenario may sound all too familiar.

Determined to succeed, you vowed to go about slimming down the "right" way. You stopped eating red meat, cooked egg-white-only omelettes with no shortening in a Teflon pan, removed the skin from chicken, ate your baked potato without butter or sour cream and consumed lots of pasta. Frozen yogurt, fruit and sherbet served as dessert. Your breakfast consisted of oatmeal and skim milk or else granola and a banana. A typical lunch was white-meat turkey on a roll and a generous salad, hold the dressing.

And you stuck with your low-fat regimen. You knew it was the right diet because your friends and family congratulated you on your healthy habits. Yet somehow it never felt quite right for you. Nor did it ever work the way you thought it would. You found that you weren't quite satisfied eating this way: You were often hungry and low in energy and—worst of all—permanent, significant weight loss proved elusive. *You never actually achieved the goals that motivated you to go on a diet in the first place.*

Here's the good news: Most of you will now find that your

frustrations are about to end. I have helped tens of thousands of people who have come to me needing to lose weight and improve their health. And I promise I will help you, too.

Diets come and go, but what people hope to get from them remains fairly constant. What would you like from a weight loss program? Let your fancy run free. Would you like to:

- be freed from hunger much of the day?
- eat until you are pleasantly satisfied and full?
- enjoy foods so rich that you've never seen them on any other diet?
- reduce your appetite via a perfectly natural metabolic function of the body?
- never have to count calories again?
- eliminate addictive food patterns?
- experience steady weight loss, even if you have had dramatic failures or weight regain in the past?
- learn a way of eating that will keep any lost weight from coming back?
- enjoy enhanced energy?
- feel better than you have in years?
- be more attractive?
- bolster your self-confidence?
- improve health problems that have accompanied your excess weight?
- minimize your risk factors for certain diseases?
- slow the aging process?

What happens to real people with real problems when they follow the Atkins Nutritional Approach? Well, let me give you a far from atypical example.

Traci Laurens, a 44-year-old restaurant manager and mother of two, had always considered herself a "big-boned girl." Over the years she'd tried many a diet, but her weight continued to oscillate between 190 and 230 on her five-foot four-inch frame. Fortunately, Traci was not experiencing any health problems, and, in spite of her weight, she walked every day.

"I had occasional headaches but no real problems other than the fact that I hated to look in the mirror," she recalls. "I did what all overweight people do: I focused on my face and never stood back and took a long look. My problem was that I couldn't get away from carbs; I craved them. I had been raised on starches and sweets. I am from a family of twelve and that's how my mother stretched meals. I didn't know any other way of eating.

"In 1998, I met my fiancé, Jack. He fell in love with the size-16 me, but I had really gotten tired of being fat. A friend told me about *Dr. Atkins' New Diet Revolution*. I read it cover to cover, and on New Year's Day 2000 I began Induction. I broke through my carb addiction sometime in the first week, and from that point on, doing Atkins was easy. Thirty days later I moved from Induction to OWL [Ongoing Weight Loss], having dropped to a size 13."

Traci and her fiancé had planned two romantic back-to-back cruises in February 2000, a slow time at both their jobs. Even though cruises are floating smorgasbords, Traci stuck to protein and fat and passed up most of the carbs. After the first one-week cruise, she was wearing size 9 or 10 and had to buy some new clothes. At the end of the second cruise, she weighed 146. Newly invigorated, she increased her walking routine to one and a half hours a day. And, like most people, she found that exercise kept her head clear, relieved her anxiety and restored her energy.

Traci has stuck to about 30 grams of carbohydrate daily because she feels good on that level. That way, when she wants to indulge herself a bit, she has some "wiggle room" in case she gains a few pounds. She says she doesn't miss starches at all and hasn't had a piece of bread since December 31, 1999.

"I love to eat sautéed portobello mushrooms in garlic and butter sauce or beef shish kabobs with multicolored peppers and summer squash. If I'm eating breakfast out, I enjoy scrambled eggs and bacon. I am no longer bloated and never tired; I haven't taken a nap in a year and a half. I go to bed at 10:30, sleep through the night and awaken at 5:15, raring to go. When I run into people I haven't seen in a while they say, 'I can hear you, but I don't see you—what happened?' "

Traci plans to continue with Atkins because she now understands it is a whole life change. "With Atkins, I easily keep my weight between 133 and 139 pounds," she says. "I know how quickly 70 pounds can go on. But now I also know the secret to how quickly they can come off."

Change the Way You Look at Your Body

Now we are going to get to the bottom of a mystery and one of the great inequities of life. I bet you know people who eat more than you do, exercise less and yet never seem to put on a pound. They're not lying about the amount they eat any more than you are. They *do* eat a *lot*. Maddening, but true.

Instead of envying them, realize that these slim friends are actually cause for celebration. The fact that they are not fat is living, breathing proof that being overweight needn't mean you're greedy, weak-willed, lazy or self-indulgent. Instead, in all probability, it may mean you are only metabolically less fortunate than they are. Doesn't that make a lot more sense? Most people eat when they're hungry and stop when they're full. And if that's the case, how could they be *over*eating? They're doing what their bodies tell them to do.

Which is why the critical factor is not *how much* you eat, but *what* you eat. And if you're overweight, the *what* is likely an excess of carbohydrates.

It's What You Eat

Do you believe that a man can go from gaining 0.5 pound a week to losing 3.9 pounds a week without significantly altering the number of calories he consumes? Let me introduce you to Harry Kronberg. I want you to pay close attention to his story and try not to give way to disbelief, because these results are real. Harry Kronberg, the 39-year-old manager of a lumberyard, came to me with a heart arrhythmia and a desperate weight problem. He had been chubby even as a child, but now things were out of hand. A few years before, he had gone to a low-fat diet center and had managed to drop from 245 to 185 pounds. Sounds good. But before long, Harry had gained it all back with an added dividend of another 35 pounds.

That's right, when Harry came to see me, he tipped the scales at 280 on a five-foot six-and-a-half-inch frame. In the previous thirty-five months, eating a relatively starchy, low-fat diet of approximately 2,100 calories a day, he had gained 70 pounds, exactly 2 pounds a month.

Harry started Atkins, radically restricting his intake of carbohydrates while eating freely of meat, fish, fowl and eggs. Harry was told he could eat as much as he needed to feel satisfied. The calorie count was strikingly similar to what he had been eating on his previous diet. Three months into his new regimen, he had lost 50.5 pounds (almost 4 pounds a week), and then continued to lose at a steady 3 pounds weekly. His heart symptoms vanished, his total cholesterol level dropped from a mid-range 207 to a dramatically lower 134 and his triglycerides went from 134 to 31.

OK, It's What I Eat, But Will I Still Enjoy Eating?

It will really surprise me if you can't. Let's take a look at Patricia Finley's menu. She's been doing Atkins for three and a half months, and she's lost 31 pounds. Patricia, who used to eat quite a lot of starches and who would sometimes go on massive dessert binges when she was under pressure, has converted to tasty, controlled carbohydrate eating.

For breakfast, she eats a cheese omelette, or some vegetables with blue cheese, or bacon and eggs. Lunch can be tuna fish or chicken with a sumptuous salad. But sometimes she'll have chopped sirloin sautéed with onions, chili powder and peppers. Patricia enjoys having olives or asparagus spears for snacks, but she puts the greatest amount of energy and attention into dinner. She finds that it isn't possible to feel deprived when you're enjoying a meal consisting of guacamole (mashed avocado mixed with tomatoes, onion and seasoning) and strips of chicken and steak. Add to that her passion for grated zucchini in olive oil with butter and nutmeg, her taste for broccoli with lemon butter sauce and her homemade recipe for chicken soup, and what do you get? Starvation? *Not.* Patricia also enjoys lamb shanks with chopped onions cooked with olive oil, herbs and "Crazy Mixed Up Salt." And she assures me this is only a small sample of the food she finds it possible and delightful to eat—doing Atkins.

Yes, that's a weight loss eating plan I've been describing, though it may be hard to believe. I think there's food for thought in such a food story. The Atkins Nutritional Approach allows you to adapt your meal planning to your own individual tastes as long as you eat "acceptable foods" (see Chapter 11). To help you along the path, the "Food and Recipes" section starting on page 367 is full of delicious meals to satisfy your controlled carb taste buds.

Now, let me mention some of the other things this book will teach you:

YOU WILL LEARN HOW TO OVERCOME CHALLENGES SO YOU CAN:

- get right back on track if you occasionally "fall off" Atkins.
- stop binge eating in a matter of days.
- manage cravings for sweets and starches.
- ensure that what you lose is fat and not lean body tissue.
- modify your food choices according to your own metabolism.
- supplement your meals with vitanutrients to help overcome metabolic resistance.
- with your doctor's supervision, eliminate certain medications that helped keep you fat.

I WILL SHOW YOU HOW TO GET HEALTHY SO YOU CAN:

- overcome diet-related conditions such as unstable blood sugar, yeast infections and food intolerances.
- avoid the health catastrophe of hyperinsulinism.
- improve your energy level, which will make exercise easier.
- find the right vitanutrients to complement the foods you eat for complete nutrition.
- lower your cholesterol and triglyceride levels and improve your other blood chemistry values.
- address the medical conditions—especially diabetes, heart disease and high blood pressure—so often associated with obesity.

I'LL HELP YOU DEAL WITH THE DAY-TO-DAY ISSUES SO YOU CAN:

- navigate supermarket aisles to find controlled carb, low-sugar foods.
- dine out with ease in elegant restaurants or even fast food chains.
- attend dinner parties without compromising your weight loss program or offending your hosts.
- explain your new way of eating to family and friends.
- go on vacation or attend special functions without cheating.
- eat comfortably with those whose style of eating remains different from yours.

This Just Might Be the Plan for You

That's an ambitious program I've just outlined: I am happy I don't have to warn you that it's going to be difficult. The truth is that as long as you are committed, it's going to be surprisingly easy. And it's going to literally change your life—and your perception of yourself.

4

Is This You?
Three Types Who Need
to Control Their Carbohydrates

All this is fascinating, you are probably saying, but is it really relevant to my own particular, very individual situation? If you have a weight problem, it is extremely likely that the information contained in this book can help you solve it. My confidence is based on the fact that a long time ago, in 1964 to be exact, I first tried a controlled clinical trial by placing sixty-five subjects on a controlled carbohydrate regimen and sixty-four of them were able to reach their goal weight. The one who did not was still able to lose 90 pounds. In the years since, I have continued to use this program to treat obesity, and I continue to have outstandingly successful results.

So in order to help you understand your individual situation and where you do or don't fit in, I'll profile three typical obese patients. Several characteristic overweight patterns result from carbohydrate metabolism disorders that are instantly recognizable. Do any of the following sound achingly familiar?

Group A: "I Really Don't Eat That Much!"

- Are you overweight despite the fact that you don't eat that much?

- Do you follow standard weight loss diets to the letter, yet make no headway losing weight, or get stuck far short of your goal?
- Have you noticed that many slim people definitely consume more food and more calories than you do?
- Are you just plain unpleasantly hungry on low-calorie/low-fat diets?
- Do you find the amount of food you eat is really the least you can take in without feeling physically unsatisfied?
- Do you feel unfulfilled when you finish a so-called "balanced" meal?
- Do you find that when you eat the amount of food that feels just right, you don't lose—or you even gain?
- Do you find yourself losing and regaining the same 10 to 15 pounds?
- Do you gain weight even though you eat natural, low-fat foods?
- Have you often said, "I'm really very disciplined; it must be my metabolism"?
- Do you ever wonder if your weight problem could be hereditary?
- Do you eat to make yourself feel better?

Group B: "I Crave Food Always!"

- Do you have an inexplicable obsession with food?
- Do you have a habit of eating late at night after dinner?
- Do you have a tendency to binge?
- Do you constantly crave sweets, pasta, bread and other high-carbohydrate foods?
- Do you nibble all day long when food is available?
- Do you have a strong desire to eat again within two hours of eating a filling meal?
- Do you consider yourself a compulsive eater?
- Have you ever said, "I only wish I could control my eating behavior"?

- Do you wish you had more control over how much food you eat?
- Do you have specific symptoms of ill health, such as the ones I'm about to list, that diminish or vanish as soon as you eat? Do you suffer from:
    - irritability?
    - inexplicable drops in your energy level throughout the day?
    - often overwhelming bouts of fatigue, especially in the afternoon?
    - mood swings?
    - difficulty concentrating?
    - sleep difficulties—whether the need for lots of sleep or a habit of waking from a sound sleep?
    - anxiety, sadness and depression for which there's no obvious explanation?
    - dizziness, trembling or palpitations?
    - brain fog and loss of mental acuity?

Group C: "I Can't Live Without This One Food!"

- Do you have a single food or beverage you feel you could not do without?
- Would you pass up an elegant meal to have your most favorite food instead?
- Is there a specific food or beverage that makes you feel better as soon as you consume it?
- Do you ever think, "I wonder if I could be addicted to that food/beverage"?
- Do you feel this way about a category of foods (sweets, soft drinks, dairy products, grains, for example)?

What Your Answers Reveal

First of all, I would find it hard to believe there could be a significantly overweight person who had no "yes" responses.

If your affirmative responses form a pattern, I almost undoubtedly have a solution for your problem.

So let's delve a little deeper. Do most of your "yes" responses place you in Group A? Then you have a metabolic problem, manifested either by an inability to lose weight or keep it off, or by hunger or the inability to achieve and maintain satiety (a feeling of being full or satisfied).

If most of your "yes" responses were to Group B questions, you probably have some form of glucose intolerance. You may suffer from hypoglycemia—more accurately called unstable blood sugar, or, in some cases, pre-diabetes.

If most of your affirmative answers were to questions in Group C, you probably have an addiction to the food or beverage you singled out. Another term for the phenomenon is "food allergy" or the more accurate term of "individual food intolerance."

If the food or beverage you've identified as addictive contains carbohydrates, you have a carbohydrate addiction, and this book will provide you with more answers to your problems than you ever thought possible.

Three Facets of the Same Problem

Individuals whose "yes" answers fell primarily in Groups A and B (and most of you C responders, as well) have a condition that is the common denominator among nearly all overweight people. It is called *hyperinsulinism.* Before I explain the significance of hyperinsulinism and the very good news of how easily you can tame it on Atkins, I want you to reflect on the significance of eating. Stop and ask yourself, "What else do I do in the course of a day that constitutes such a dramatic and intense alteration of my body as swallowing the food I do?"

Between the time you rise and the time you go to bed, you put pounds of organic matter into your mouth. Your body runs on it. So don't be surprised that if you make bad choices, you'll pay a price.

Life Out of Control

Food-obsessive behavior is common. But some of the tougher cases fall beyond the scope of Groups A, B or C and can be a challenge to cure even by doing Atkins. Individuals who binge and fantasize and almost live for food are as much between a rock and a hard place as an alcoholic or a heroin addict. For these people, the best hope is still a metabolic approach to their problem.

Gordon Lingard, a real estate executive, was an extreme example. He was 53 years old when he came to see me, and his five-foot ten-inch frame carried 306 pounds. Gordon had progressed from a normal weight in college (when he was a lifeguard) to extreme obesity by his late twenties. His weight had gone as high as 450 pounds. He had no hormonal imbalances, and he had tried everything—stomach stapling, emetics, laxatives and every diet from B to Z.

Gordon was as inexplicable to himself as to the many doctors he had consulted. All he knew was that he had to eat. The cravings were indescribable. He told me he was constantly planning his next binge. Gallons of ice cream disappeared as swiftly as an ordinary carbohydrate addict downs a candy bar. Sugar was Gordon's master obsession. "There was never a moment I didn't desire it," he recalls. "Often I would shake until I could put some sugar in my mouth. The symptoms were totally physical, and they were really frightening. For me there was nothing else but food. I had an hour's drive from my office to my home, and I knew every restaurant, every diner, every candy machine and every soft drink dispenser along the whole route."

I'd wager you'd be willing to bet Gordon Lingard's obsession was almost entirely psychological—but you'd be wrong. His situation was a special one and, for a while,

treating him was no cinch. In his case, some of the vitanutrient aids I describe in Chapter 23 were a crucial part of the
solution. But what I'd like you to realize is that Gordon's
problem was only a more extreme version of the problems
so many overweight people have. His difficulties were basically metabolic difficulties, and they could be solved metabolically. By doing Atkins under my personal care, Gordon
reached his goal weight for the first time in thirty years, and
he no longer feels driven to consume sugar.

Gordon had failed repeatedly on low-fat/low-calorie diets.
And that's not surprising. His problem lay in his metabolic
response to carbohydrates. To solve an out-of-control situation like this by restricting calories without restricting carbohydrates is like marching into the surf planning to turn
back the ocean.

You may have picked up this book with the secret inner
conviction that you're a "compulsive eater." In all probability, you're a carbohydrate addict. How many compulsive
eaters of steaks have you come across? Not too many, huh?
Let me tell you, it's a rare breed.

Many people ate a so-called "balanced" diet as children,
but by the time they reached adulthood their diets had become progressively less balanced. Eating didn't seem all
that important to them once, but now it does. So they look at
their waistlines, they look at their eating and they realize
they have a problem. Usually they notice that their taste in
food has gone off in a specific direction. Carbohydrates now
form the bulk of what they eat: breads and baked goods,
cakes and candies, pasta and popcorn. Surprising and illogi-
cal food cravings are typical. Do you ever have dinner with a
big dessert and almost immediately afterward find that you
want some candy? That's a sign, as is fatigue, that your carbohydrate metabolism is out of whack.

It's not that you eat when you're not hungry, but you seem
to be always hungry. And yet when you eat the high-
carbohydrate food you crave, you feel better only briefly.
Your situation is the exact opposite of the one you'll experi-

ence when you do Atkins. When doing Atkins, you'll find that your appetite has diminished, but your satisfaction from the food you eat has increased.

Are You a Compulsive Eater?

Many carbohydrate addicts could no more walk past a refrigerator without opening it than Venus or Serena Williams could let a short lob drift overhead without smashing it. I've heard many patients say, "It's irresistible, Dr. Atkins. I'm a slave. How can you possibly help me?"

I say, "That's all right. Your compulsions hold no terrors for me, and soon they won't for you. When you pass that refrigerator, open it, have some chicken salad or a slice of pot roast. If you eat the way I'm asking you to eat, you'll find that food is still delicious, but the compulsions will fade."

You see, your food compulsion isn't a character disorder, it's a chemical disorder called hyperinsulinism, and you have it simply because you've eaten the same unhealthy way that most people in our culture do.

Rebecca Chasen liked baking breads and desserts for her friends. She liked eating that way, too. She had been large since childhood. Now, at age 32, she was carrying 264 pounds on her five-foot eleven-and-a-half-inch frame.

One day, she decided to try on an old pair of pants and found she couldn't bring the button within four inches of the hole. That same week someone at work told her he had lost 50 pounds doing Atkins. Rebecca had tried herbal diets, low-fat diets, the cabbage soup diet ("I was starving") and Fen-Phen ("I thought my heart was going to explode and so I stopped") over the previous decade. It was time for something completely different.

"I was a carbohydrate junkie, so adjusting to Atkins was hard. I desperately wanted bread for the first four days. I struggled to ignore the cravings, and after two weeks I had lost 17 pounds. My size 22 jeans, which were tight before, were now loose."

As Rebecca's cravings stopped, her pounds continued to disappear. One or two friends, in the grip of low-fat illusions, warned her of what terrible risks she was taking on an eating plan that allowed her to eat bacon and eggs for breakfast. Four months into Atkins, she decided to see her physician. "He reviewed my highly favorable cholesterol readings and all my other lab work, put me on the scale and finally said, 'Keep doing whatever you're doing, Rebecca. You're as healthy as a horse.'"

After a year doing Atkins, Rebecca regularly takes walks and rides her bike. She finds she has much more energy, and, so far, she has lost 86 pounds. She has a whole new set of recipes to cook for her friends nowadays. And she never goes anywhere without some controlled carb snacks in her pocketbook.

"My dress size is now a 12 or 14. The old me wouldn't have been caught dead in clothing that showed my shape, but I just went shopping at The Gap and bought medium-sized fitted shirts. I don't recall buying such small shirts since I've been old enough to buy my own clothes. I have vowed to myself that I will never be fat again. I don't know why I didn't try Atkins ten years ago."

If all this still seems amazing to you, I can only say "read on." In the next chapter, we'll learn about the specific metabolic role that insulin plays in obesity.

KEY POINTS!

- A significant number of all overweight people suffer from a metabolic problem known as hyperinsulinism.
- Eating large amounts of foods high in sugar, white flour and other refined carbohydrates can promote or aggravate hyperinsulinism.
- Atkins is a corrective metabolic approach to metabolic problems.

- The protein- and fat-rich foods you eat when doing Atkins stabilize your blood sugar, making food cravings disappear.

TIPS:

- Excess weight around your waist is often the first sign that your body is not metabolizing sugar properly.
- Try not eating your favorite food for a week and see if you notice any changes in how you feel.
- Don't ever go more than six hours without having a meal or protein-rich snack.

5

Understanding the Importance of Insulin

I'm going to talk to you about the hormone whose name you've heard many times: insulin. Some of the content of this chapter is fairly complex, but I think you ought to read it carefully. Because for many of you, the answers to your battle with the bulge and concerns about long-term health issues are here.

Almost everyone knows that insulin is given to people with a certain kind of diabetes, to help control their blood-sugar levels when their own supplies become depleted or insufficient. Insulin is one of the most powerful and efficient substances that the body uses to control the use, distribution and storage of energy. At its most basic, insulin is the control hormone for glucose, a basic form of sugar. So listen up.

Your body is an energy machine, never resting, always metabolically active—and it powers its operations mainly through the use of glucose in the blood, which is why glucose is interchangeably called blood sugar. The body must maintain a certain level of glucose in the blood at all times. So when there is no carbohydrate food source to make glucose, the liver will actually convert protein to glucose. Remarkably, even on a prolonged, total fast, a healthy body can maintain its glucose level within a rather narrow normal range. As a general rule, of course, the body obtains its principal supply of fuel from food.

What Happens to a Meal

You sit down at the table and consume a three-course dinner. Somewhere between chewing and excreting, your body absorbs certain substances from your food, mostly across the surface of your small intestine. From the carbohydrate you eat, your body will absorb sugars, all of which are, or quickly and easily become, glucose. From fat, it absorbs glycerol and fatty acids, and from protein, it absorbs amino acids, the building blocks of all cells.

Obviously, if you eat a lot of carbohydrate, you'll end up with a lot of glucose in your blood. Sounds good, doesn't it? All that energy coursing through your system. Eat sugar, starches and fruits and you're going to get those blood-sugar levels up fast, aren't you? If you love candy bars, perhaps you're saying, "That's great—the more I eat, the more energy I'll have."

Alas, a bad mistake. You see, the human body evolved and primitive humans thrived as hunter-gatherers who subsisted primarily on meat, fish, vegetables, fruit, whole grains and seeds and nuts. Candy bars were few and far between. The human body is used to dealing with unrefined foods as they occur in Nature. Consequently, your body's capacity to deal with an excess of processed foods is pretty poor, which is why our twenty-first-century way of eating so often gets us into trouble.

If you don't understand this yet, let's look at what insulin and the other energy-controlling hormones do when you eat.

As Your Blood Sugar Rises

Consuming carbohydrates impacts your blood-sugar levels. The amount of carbs—and the type—will determine how your blood sugar responds. For example, a food full of refined sugar and white flour, such as a jelly doughnut, will raise blood sugar much more dramatically than does a salad.

To be useful to your body, blood sugar has to be transported to your cells. Think of insulin as the barge that transports glucose from your blood to your cells. Once it reaches the cells, three things can happen to that glucose: It can be mobilized for immediate energy; it can be converted into glycogen for later use as a source of energy; or it can be stored as fat.

Let's delve in a little deeper. Insulin is manufactured in a part of your pancreas called the Islets of Langerhans. As the sugar level in your blood goes up, the pancreas releases insulin to move the sugar out of the blood. It then transports the blood sugar to your body's cells for their energy needs. But as we previously mentioned, when these needs are met the liver converts excess glucose into glycogen, which is stored in the liver and muscles, where it is readily available for energy use. Once all the glycogen storage areas are filled, the body has to do something with excess glucose. And here is the big revelation: The liver converts the remaining glucose to fat, which becomes the "storage tanks" of fat on your belly, thighs, buttocks and elsewhere. That's why insulin is called "the fat-producing hormone."

Since fat is much more efficient—and has more capacity to store energy—than glucose, we can store a lot more fat in our bodies than glucose. That, my friends, results in obesity. And by the way, the main chemical constituent of all this fat (the fat you're reading this book to get rid of) is triglyceride, the very same triglyceride that, in your blood, can be a risk factor for heart disease and stroke.

Insulin is a pretty efficient worker. If it were not, your cells could not get enough glucose, their basic fuel, and blood-glucose levels would rise while the cells searched for other fuels—first for protein in your muscles and organs, and then for fat in your fat stores. That's why people with poorly controlled, insulin-deficient diabetes can lose weight when no insulin is present. And that's why a person on a low-calorie diet may lose lean body mass. (This shouldn't happen on Atkins, where sufficient calories and protein are consumed to meet the body's energy needs.)

On the other hand, excessive carbohydrate intake results in high amounts of blood sugar and may, in turn, overstimulate insulin production. When this happens, it causes a drop in blood sugar, robbing the body of energy for the cells. The result of the process is destabilized blood-sugar levels, quite possibly causing fatigue, brain fog, shakiness and headaches.

The body attempts to adjust by liberating counter-regulatory hormones—such as adrenaline—to raise the glucose level, but another stiff dose of insulin can overpower the effect of those hormones. Fortunately for most of us, this glucose balancing act takes place automatically and our blood sugar stays in a fairly narrow, normal range.

But for some, the bodily insult of massive insulin release to deal with massive blood-glucose levels has been going on for years, causing the glucose-regulating mechanism in the body to break down, initiating unstable blood sugar and eventually diabetes. For more on diabetes, see Chapter 24.

What Is Hyperinsulinism?

Simply put, hyperinsulinism is the condition that results from too much insulin being produced by your body.

It's easy to see how this might happen when you realize that there's a relationship between the kinds of foods you eat and the amount of insulin in your bloodstream. Foods rich in carbohydrates—especially sugar, honey, milk and fruit, which contain simple sugars, and refined carbohydrates such as flour, white rice and potato starch—are readily absorbed through the stomach, so they speedily convert to glucose. When these foods are eaten in excess, they require a lot of insulin for transport. Foods made of protein and fat, on the other hand, require little or no insulin. (Protein in excess converts to glucose in the liver and requires some insulin to transport it to the cells; fat requires essentially none.)

And what happens when there is too much insulin? As an overweight person becomes heavier, insulin's effectiveness may decline. The cells become desensitized to the action of insulin so it can no longer effectively transport glucose to them. This is known in medical circles as insulin resistance, which quickly leads to hyperinsulinism. Numerous studies have shown that insulin resistance is more prevalent among the obese, although even some individuals who appear slim and healthy may actually be insulin resistant.

What appears to happen is that the insulin receptors on the surfaces of the body's cells are blocked, which in turn prevents glucose from reaching the cells for energy use. That's one reason overweight individuals may be tired much of the time. When insulin is ineffective in taking glucose into the cells, the liver converts more and more glucose to stored fat. Your body is, in fact, becoming a fat-producing machine instead of an efficient energy-producing machine.

Your body's hormonal system is now in desperate straits. At this point, insulin is being secreted more and more frequently to deal with high blood-sugar levels, and it is doing its job less and less effectively. Which makes you crave sweets and carbs, which compounds the problem in a vicious cycle. In time, even the insulin receptors that convert glucose to fat start getting worn out, forecasting diabetes.

A Host of Other Health Issues

Here are some further reasons why high insulin levels can lead to big problems:

- Insulin increases salt and water retention, a recipe for high blood pressure.

- Insulin is directly involved in creating atherosclerotic plaques, which, if not controlled, can lead to heart disease.[1-18]
- High insulin levels have been shown to correlate with high levels of triglycerides and low levels of "good" HDL cholesterol.[19-20]
- High insulin levels correlate with increased risk of breast cancer and polycystic ovarian syndrome. (Conversely, the lower the levels of insulin, the better the survival rates for breast cancer.)[21-27]

Obesity increases insulin resistance. This means that you can sharply reduce your risk of blood-sugar disorders—and by extension, heart disease and other ailments—by simply keeping your weight down and controlling carbohydrate intake. Even if you have a hereditary predisposition to diabetes, you may be able to stall or completely avoid its onset.

A Subject of Intensive Study

Don't think the mainstream medical profession hasn't noticed the correlation between insulin resistance and disease. In the past fifteen years—and this is a trend that only keeps building—medical journals have published studies of the powerful association between obesity—usually accompanied by hyperinsulinism—and the probability of heart disease or stroke. All around the world the studies pour in. For example, using data from several epidemiological studies, Dr. B. Balkau found links between high glucose levels and mortality in thousands of men whose medical histories had been followed for two decades.[28] Uniformly, high blood-glucose levels and insulin resistance signified markedly higher risk of death from cardiovascular causes.

American research points in the same direction. The Bogalusa Heart Study followed four thousand children and young adults.[29] Even in childhood, a high insulin level corresponded to higher triglyceride levels and higher VLDL cholesterol—a particularly damaging form of "bad" LDL cholesterol. Not surprisingly, these associations were even more marked in the overweight. We'll go over this ground in greater detail in Chapter 27 when I discuss heart health. For now, just remember a bad diet produces results that are not merely cosmetically unattractive; it flies the black flag of some of the very worst health catastrophes.

Ah, but you came to this book for weight loss. All right, let's make crystal clear the connection between high insulin levels and excess weight.

This Is Why You Can't Lose Weight

I am about to recount a horror story that might be headlined: **Innocent Human Is Turned Upon By Own Hormones!** But we did it to ourselves, you know. Remember, no culture in world history has ever consumed even a fraction of the sugar we twenty-first-century Westerners do.

Perhaps you've been overweight for a long time. Once there was a stage in the progress of your metabolic disease when you could lose weight pretty easily, if you sharply cut your caloric intake. You'd gain the pounds back, but at least at the price of hunger, you could shed them again. Then, although your weight continued to yo-yo up and down, you began to notice that the yo-yo went up easily, but getting it to fall down again was harder and harder.

Now maybe you're past even that stage, and you simply cannot drop pounds. If you are, insulin has really closed the trap. The pancreas, faced with your abuse of simple and refined carbohydrates, has become so efficient at secreting insulin that just a touch of blood sugar will release a flood. In response to high insulin levels, your body has become intent on storing fat by the process I've explained. Group A responders (see pages 38–39) will recognize the role that excess insulin plays in preventing weight loss by giving you an ongoing sensation of hunger that can be satisfied only by constant overeating.

Now that you've reached this understanding of the metabolic basis of being overweight, imagine going into your doctor's office after diligently eating a low-fat diet that was quite possibly high in sugar and carbs. And imagine being told, "Well, if you just had a little more willpower . . ." Sad, isn't it? Willpower is not the issue. To lose weight, you're going to need the controlled carbohydrate nutritional approach offered by this book. You will also need the two other legs of the Atkins triad: regular exercise and nutritional supplementation.

I know I've produced a really heart-sinking analysis of how and why fat accumulates on your body. So, what do you do now? You adjust the insulin spigot. And so far as weight loss goes, the answer lies in two entwined concepts: burning fat and controlling carbohydrates, which we will explore in the upcoming chapters.

KEY POINTS!

- Insulin is the hormone that transports glucose from your blood to your cells, where it can be converted to energy. The liver will convert excess glucose to glycogen, which is stored in the liver and muscles for additional, accessible energy.
- Remaining glucose will be converted to fat and stored throughout the body.
- Excessive carbohydrate intake results in an oversupply of glucose, and thus insulin, in the body.
- An ongoing cycle of excess blood glucose overproduction and insulin overproduction eventually results in hyperinsulinism and ultimately diabetes.
- Hyperinsulinism is what makes it hard for many people to lose weight.
- Atkins can stabilize insulin production to make it easier to lose weight.

- High levels of triglycerides in the blood are a proven risk factor for heart disease and stroke.
- Atkins can sharply reduce your risk of blood-sugar disorders—and by extension, heart disease and other serious ailments.

A FREQUENTLY ASKED QUESTION:

Can I manage my insulin and blood sugar without eating much fat?
No, because when you cut out fat, what is left is protein and carbohydrate, both of which can produce a blood-sugar response. Fat is the only substance that won't have an impact on your blood sugar. It also provides essential fatty acids you can't get from protein or carbohydrates. Contrary to much of what you may have heard, fat can be good for you!

TIPS:

- If you don't stabilize your blood sugar you will have difficulty losing weight.
- If you lower your carbohydrate intake you will lower your insulin levels as well as your triglycerides.
- If you are taking oral diabetes medicine or insulin, consult your physician before starting Atkins. You will need to reduce and then monitor your dosage as you lower your blood-sugar level.

6

The Great Fat Meltdown

Once you've been heavy for some time, you're in a metabolic trap, a sort of high-walled box created in large part by high insulin levels. You may already have noticed that you're trapped. Certainly, trying diet after diet and failing on all of them is depressing. I know from personal experience and from the comments of thousands of my patients just how tightly the lid of metabolic obesity seems to press down. Fortunately, there is a key to unlatch this box. A perfectly natural bodily process called *lipolysis* can lift up the lid and let hope shine in.

The definition of lipolysis sounds like Nirvana to a person longing to lose weight. It means "the process of dissolving fat." Isn't that exactly why we're all gathered here today? Now I will tell you the "secret" to unlocking the latent power of lipolysis.

When you burn fat, it breaks down into glycerol and other fatty acids. How does the process actually work? Are there any drawbacks? There are plenty of laypeople and even physicians who think there must be.

And burning one's fat off sounds like a faddish trick. These folks give a skeptical shrug and say, "I'm sure people lose some weight with your approach, Dr. Atkins, but don't they gain it right back again?"

The interesting thing is that, if they adhere to the four phases of my program, which includes finding their Critical Carbohydrate Level for Maintenance (CCLM), meaning the amount of carbohydrates they can consume and neither gain nor lose weight, not many do. The phase known as Lifetime Maintenance, though more indulgent, evolves naturally from the three weight loss phases, thereby gradually teaching Atkins followers a permanent way of eating that still moderates carbohydrate intake to the degree that is necessary for each individual.

As for the weight loss phases of Atkins, they are simple and overwhelmingly effective. I don't see any reason why I should understate the facts. Lipolysis is one of life's charmed gifts. It's as delightful as sex and sunshine, and it has fewer drawbacks than either of them!

In the earlier editions of this book I used the word *ketosis* to describe this wonderful process. In fact, here is exactly what I said: "The term 'ketosis,' when it applies to the benign, diet-induced type we're talking about, is really a shortening of the term ketosis/lipolysis, which is enough of a tongue twister that you can see why it is commonly referred to only by the name ketosis." Well, experience is a great teacher, and over the years I have learned that in my attempt to simplify things I created confusion.

Let me explain. The Atkins Nutritional Approach stimulates the process of lipolysis, a state I hope you are always in: burning your fat for energy. A secondary process of lipolysis is ketosis. Ketosis occurs when you are taking in a low level of carbohydrates from the food you eat, as you will during the Induction phase of Atkins. Lipolysis results in the creation of ketones (that's ketosis), a perfectly normal and natural function of the body.

In the minds of laypeople (and even some ill-informed doctors) ketosis is often confused with diabetic ketoacidosis.

The latter is the consequence of insulin-deficient subjects having out-of-control blood-sugar levels, a condition that can occur as well in alcoholics and people in a state of extreme starvation. Ketosis and ketoacidosis may sound vaguely alike, but the two conditions are virtually polar opposites. They can always be distinguished from each other by the fact that the diabetic in ketoacidosis has been consuming excessive carbohydrates and has high blood sugar, in sharp contrast to the fortunate person doing Atkins.

To avoid any further confusion, I will use the term lipolysis throughout this chapter to describe the process of burning fat for energy.

Many controlled carbohydrate regimens have been proposed over the years. They work with some degree of effectiveness for some people. However, many of them do not bring carbohydrate intake down to a level that will permit lipolysis. For people who are metabolically obese and have great difficulty losing, that is a grave weakness.

Atkins, on the other hand, starts off at 20 grams of carbohydrates. Each individual then proceeds at his or her own rate, gradually adding back both the amount and the variety of carbohydrate foods. We'll get into the specifics of how you calculate grams of carbohydrate and which carbs you will and will not be eating in Chapter 8. For now, let me assure you that my state-of-the-art weight loss program is the safest, healthiest, most luxurious way to become and stay slim for the remainder of your life.

Going for It

How does lipolysis work? Lipolysis simply means that you're burning your fat stores and using them as the source of fuel they were meant to be.

The by-products of burning fat are ketones. When your body releases ketones—which it will do in your breath and your urine—it is chemical proof that you're consuming your own stored fat. Once more, for emphasis: When a person on a safe, controlled carbohydrate plan such as mine is releasing ketones, he or she is in the fat-dissolving state of lipolysis. This process is simply the most efficient path ever devised for getting you slim. And the more ketones you release, the more fat you have dissolved.

Lipolysis is the biochemical method of weight loss—the alternative to using glucose for fuel, the very process that has made you heavy. Lipolysis can be your life raft, giving you both slimness and health, and distancing you from the obese person's perils of diabetes, heart disease and stroke. Most of all, of course, it is the key to achieving your goal—to use up the fat stored on your body.

The phenomenon of lipolysis or fat burning being the major alternative fuel system has been so well researched that it is simply not disputed in academic circles. It is scientific fact.

Lipolysis vs. Glucosis

Many scientists are of the opinion that you need glucose for fuel. That statement is only partially true. Ketones provide the exception. They are derived from fat when lipolysis is occurring, and are the other source of fuel that energizes our cells and powers our brain and other vital organs. Ketones fuel the body in lipolysis just as glucose fuels the body in glucosis—my term for a carbohydrate metabolism. Glucose and ketones are the only two fuels that come from food. (Alcohol is a third fuel.)

I find that people understand the concept better when I tell them, "If you're not in lipolysis, you're in glucosis." The two fuel sources are your body's alternative, completely parallel options for energy metabolism.

This terminology has helped many of my patients convince their doctors or dieticians that Atkins was the right path. If you have a doctor who tells you lipolysis (and ketosis) is bad, counter with this question, "If I'm not in lipolysis then I will be in glucosis, right? So, why is it so bad for an overweight person like me, with hyperinsulinism, to be living off my own stored fat?"

If you think about it for a moment, you'll understand why such a dual system exists. Before the invention of agriculture, in the first few hundred thousand years of human life, periods of severe food shortage must have been uncomfortably common. Human beings had to be able to burn their own body fat for fuel on those recurrent occasions when the larder was bare. Naturally, our bodies devised a highly efficient system for doing just that.

Have you ever wondered what sustained bears and other hibernating animals during their long winter sleep? It was the utilization of their fat stores. When you dial down the volume of insulin production, as you do in lipolysis, your body is equipped to burn your own body fat in a similar way. It takes place smoothly and is self-sustaining. For you, this is a sort of biologic utopia. The process of losing weight becomes as painless as eating naturally was when you were piling on pounds.

Why Does Lipolysis Work?

You'll remember that insulin's job is to convert all your excess carbohydrate into stores of body fat. In a normally functioning body, fatty acids and ketones are readily converted from fat tissue to fuel. But in overweight people, high insulin levels prevent this from happening.

Most obese people become so adept at releasing insulin that their blood is never really free of it and they're never able to use up their fat stores. By primarily burning fat instead of carbohydrates, lipolysis breaks the cycle of excess insulin and resultant stored fat. So by following a fat-containing, controlled carbohydrate regimen, you bypass the process of converting large amounts of carbohydrate into glucose. When your carbohydrate intake drops low enough to induce fat burning, abnormal insulin levels return to normal—perhaps for the first time in years or decades.[1–3]

Hunger Is Reduced

One of the most attractive features of Atkins is that lipolysis, and the resulting production of ketones if you have triggered the secondary process of ketosis, helps suppress your appetite. Frankly, it first attracted me because back in the 1960s, when I was a young doctor with an ever-increasing paunch, I wanted to slim down. But I knew very well that I couldn't stand being hungry for very long. I had too big an appetite and too little willpower, two facts that haven't changed much.

When I realized that the body could satisfy its hunger by burning its own fat as fuel, I thought I saw an escape hatch. After the first forty-eight hours, the body suppresses hunger and appetite diminishes. Another benefit of lipolysis—and the resulting state of ketosis if your carbohydrate level is low enough—is that it has certain metabolic similarities to fasting.

But there is a significant difference from fasting. A prolonged fast can be dangerous and has one severe metabolic disadvantage: The body burns not only fat for energy, it also burns protein. This means that it burns off some of the body's lean muscle tissue, which is clearly not desirable. Investigation has shown that on an eating plan where you are in lipolysis, and the carbohydrate intake is low enough to result in ketosis, virtually no lean tissue is lost, only fatty tissue.[4–9] And that's why, for extremely overweight individuals, it is possible to be in lipolysis, and at the carbohydrate level that creates ketosis, for six months to a year, and confidently know that they will suffer no ill effects of any kind.[10] These enlightened (and soon to be lightened) people are able to consume their own fat for energy and feel good while they're doing it.

The Message of Smooth and Happy Weight Loss

The beauty of lipolysis is that it bypasses the agony of low-calorie dieting. People who've been burdened with excess pounds for a long time or who've tried weight loss programs often find it very nearly impossible to drop many pounds unless they're in lipolysis. I've treated people who, even on 700 or 800 balanced calories a day, couldn't lose weight. That's less than half the normal caloric intake of an average woman. And yet these pounds finally peeled off when these folks began to do Atkins, even though their meal plans comprised of foods totaling even more calories.

When I make this claim, that you can lose more weight on a higher number of calories, I seem to be breaking the law— one of the hallowed laws: A calorie is a calorie is a calorie, and anyone who claims otherwise is a heretic. If you've counted calories for so long that you could do it in your sleep, you'll be overjoyed to know that lipolysis allows you to take in more calories and still lose more weight as compared with low-fat, calorie-restricted diets.[11] You'll see exactly what I mean in the next chapter.

KEY POINTS!

- Lipolysis is the biochemical process of dissolving fat.
- When you dissolve fat, it breaks down into glycerol and other fatty acids, which in turn break down into by-products called ketones. When this happens you are enjoying a state called *ketosis.*

- Atkins initiates ketosis by restricting carbohydrate intake to 20 grams per day, a level that is then gradually increased as you move on through the phases of Atkins.

A FREQUENTLY ASKED QUESTION:

Are lipolysis and the secondary process of ketosis safe?
Yes. Lipolysis results in the creation of ketones (that's ketosis), a perfectly normal and natural function of the body. Unfortunately, ketosis is often confused with *ketoacidosis*, a condition found in a Type I diabetic person whose blood sugar is out of control and who cannot produce insulin.

Some individuals may experience side effects from ketosis such as bad breath, but the vast majority of individuals do not develop medical problems. Research shows that chronic ketosis without caloric restriction poses no danger to your heart, kidneys, blood[12] or bone health.[13-20]

Is There a Metabolic Advantage?
You Be the Judge.

I can't wait to get you started doing Atkins. But before I do, I want to increase your enthusiasm to a fever pitch. Are you ready to lose more weight and more fat—and keep it off, permanently—than you've succeeded in doing on any other weight loss and weight maintenance plan you've ever tried?

If so, let me introduce you to your ally, mentioned briefly in Chapter 2 and expanded upon here: the *metabolic advantage*.

You'll recall that I said the metabolic advantage would enable you to lose weight on Atkins eating more calories than on its low-fat counterpart. Burning fat takes more energy so you expend more calories when you follow a controlled carbohydrate nutritional approach.

But let me tell you that this enormous dietary bonus is, today, years after it was first studied and a decade after the first edition of this book, still an area of some controversy. In this case it seems appropriate to let you be the judge. The published scientific evidence of the metabolic advantage is so impressive and my own decades of clinical observations so confirming of the conclusions those researchers reached that I'm confident of the outcome. After you read this overview of the actual scientific evidence that underlies the metabolic advantage, you'll have the power of knowledge.

I know many of you are not of a scientific bent and are put off by doctors talking "medicalese" to you. But if you pay close attention to what follows, I promise you'll be privy to some of the most exciting scientific studies ever done on weight loss. And, before the chapter is over, I'll give you a small reward by demonstrating, through one of my patients, just how the metabolic advantage works in the case of a flesh-and-blood person.

I must acknowledge that I owe a debt to two brilliant British researchers, Professor Alan Kekwick and Dr. Gaston L. S. Pawan. In the 1950s and 1960s, the two were in the top echelon of British obesity research, both serving as chairmen of many international conferences. Professor Kekwick was Director of the Institute of Clinical Research and Experimental Medicine at London's prestigious Middlesex Hospital, and Dr. Pawan was the Senior Research Biochemist of that hospital's medical unit. Their seminal experiments (first on mice and then on obese humans) provided the breakthrough concept—including the mechanism, rationale and evidence—that a low-carbohydrate/high-fat diet has a metabolic advantage over so-called "balanced" or "conventional" low-fat diets.

In the early 1950s, the two researchers were struck by the many studies that suggested diets of different compositions of fat, protein and carbohydrate provided differing rates of weight loss. Their subsequent study on obese subjects found that those on a 1,000-calorie diet, comprised of ninety percent protein—and especially those on a diet comprised of ninety percent fat—lost weight (0.6 pound and 0.9 pound per day, respectively). However, when the same subjects were given a diet with the same number of calories, but comprised of ninety percent carbohydrate, they did not lose any weight, but in fact gained a little.[1]

Kekwick and Pawan then replicated a study they had previously done on animals and found the same phenomenon with humans: A diet of 1,000 calories worked well for weight loss so long as carbohydrate intake was low, while a high-carbohydrate 1,000-calorie regimen took off very little weight.[2] They then showed that their subjects did not lose at all on a so-called "balanced" diet of 2,000 calories. But, when their diet contained primarily fat and very little carbohydrate, these same obese subjects could lose, even when they ate as many as 2,600 calories a day. The difference in weight loss between the two programs comes close to being one-half pound per day. Despite the Middlesex doctors' impeccable reputations, the majority of their colleagues remained skeptical, given their "calorie-is-a-calorie" mind set. They set out to disprove this intellectual bomb that Kekwick and Pawan had dropped on them.

Among other things, critics claimed that the impressive results of a low-carbohydrate diet were merely water loss. However, Kekwick and Pawan did water-balance studies that showed water loss to be only a small part of the total weight lost. Kekwick and Pawan then embarked on a two-year study of mice in a metabolic chamber. By measuring the loss of carbon in the feces and urine, they were able to show that the mice on the high-fat diet excreted considerable unused calories in the form of ketone bodies, as well as citric, lactic and pyruvic acids. At the end of the study period, they analyzed the fat content of the animals' bodies and found significantly less fat on the mice that had been fed a high-fat, low-carbohydrate diet.

Perhaps the most provocative aspect of Kekwick and Pawan's work is that during the time they were proving the metabolic advantage of a low-carbohydrate diet, they detected and extracted a substance from the urine of people on the regimen. When that substance was injected into mice, it caused the same metabolic results they had observed in the mice on low-carbohydrate diets, indicating that fat was "melting" off their bodies. The carcass fat decreased dramatically, the ketone and free fatty-acid levels rose and, most significantly, the excretion of unused calories via urine and feces rose from a normal ten percent to thirty-six percent. They named this substance fat-mobilizing substance (FMS).

Kekwick and Pawan attributed hormonal properties to FMS. Unfortunately, their findings on FMS have never been investigated by scientists. But I am hopeful that research will be underwritten that will seek to duplicate and investigate further this phenomenon. I intend to do my part, through the newly formed Dr. Robert C. Atkins Foundation, which will sponsor further research on the metabolic advantage and other aspects of controlled carbohydrate nutrition.

Now let's look at some other research that supports the fat-burning theory, this time from the Oakland Naval Hospital.[3] Impressed with the Kekwick and Pawan success, Frederick Benoit and his associates decided to compare a 1,000-calorie, 10-grams-of-carbohydrate, high-fat diet with fasting (the same principle that Kekwick and Pawan found most effective), using seven men weighing between 230 and 290 pounds. They used state-of-the-art body composition technology. After ten days, the fasting subjects lost 21 pounds on average, but most of that was lean body weight; only 7.5 pounds was body fat. However, on the controlled carbohydrate regimen over the same period of time, 14 of the 14.5 pounds lost was body fat. Think of it. By eating foods low in carbohydrate and high in dietary fat, subjects burned their fat stores almost twice as fast as when they ate nothing at all!

Benoit's other exciting discovery was that on a fat-burning regimen, subjects maintained their potassium levels, while subjects who fasted experienced major potassium losses. (Potassium depletion can cause heart arrhythmia, which, in severe cases, can be fatal.)

Still not convinced? Try this one. Charlotte Young, professor of clinical nutrition at Cornell University, compared the results of overweight young men placed on three diets, all providing 1,800 calories, but with varying degrees of carbohydrate restriction.[4] The regimens contained 30, 60, and 104 grams of carbohydrate, and subjects followed them for nine weeks. Young and her colleagues calculated body fat through a widely accepted technique involving immersion underwater. Those on 104 grams of carbs lost slightly better than 2 pounds of fat per week, out of 2.73 pounds of total weight loss—not bad for 1,800 calories. Those on 60 grams of carbs lost nearly 2.5 pounds of fat per week, out of 3 pounds of actual weight loss—better.

But those on 30 grams of carbs, the only situation that produced lipolysis and the secondary process of ketosis, lost 3.73 pounds of fat per week—approximately one hundred percent of their total weight loss. These results are a perfect example of the benefits the metabolic advantage provides. That's what has enabled most of my patients to succeed. And it will make you a success, too.

Before we leave Charlotte Young, I've got good news for those of you who have been trying to lose weight on low-fat plans, most of which typically comprise sixty percent or more carbohydrate. Dr. Young's most liberal regimen contained only thirty-five percent carbohydrate. She discovered that the more carbs consumed, the less body fat was lost. In treating many thousands of weight loss patients, I have observed the same thing. And virtually every other scientist who has actually studied controlled carbohydrate nutrition has confirmed that the more carbohydrate consumed, the less the amount of body fat lost. And that may be one of the major reasons you are struggling with your weight and getting nowhere.

Several other studies have shown that you can consume more calories and lose more weight than on low-fat programs. For example, Ulrich Rabast and associates at the University of Wurzburg studied forty-five hospitalized patients for five weeks.[5] Once again the controlled carbohydrate approach to weight loss demonstrated a significant metabolic advantage: This time an extra 9.24 pounds were lost on the low-carbohydrate version of a 1,000-calorie-a-day diet in contrast to the 1,000-calorie-a-day, low-fat diet. Moreover, careful water-balance studies demonstrated that the proportion of those extra pounds that could be attributed to water loss was insignificant. This trend continued in other trials, even when calories consumed were greater than 1,000.

The Beat Goes On

The massive revival of interest in controlled carbohydrate approaches to weight management that flowered in the 1990s has provoked exciting new research. And the results have only fueled the fire. The metabolic advantage is very real.

Five studies are worth noting. The relevance of the first four of these is limited by the fact that the carbohydrate content of the "low" carbohydrate diet being studied was still a good deal higher than you would experience during the first weight loss phase of Atkins. Therefore the metabolic advantage was relatively small, though it still existed. One study done in Glasgow described overweight women who after three months had lost 14.5 pounds on a thirty-five-percent carbohydrate diet of 1,200 calories and 12.3 pounds on a fifty-eight-percent carbohydrate diet of 1,200 calories. That's fairly slow weight loss and pretty strict caloric deprivation. The advantage went to the lower-carbohydrate diet as always, but the lesson is that stricter carbohydrate control makes for an even more successful weight loss plan.[6]

Three other recent examples[7-9] also didn't go low enough in carbs and thus had limited metabolic advantage, but two facts should be noted: First, in all cases, the lower-carbohydrate group did lose more weight than the higher-carbohydrate group. Studies that show the opposite are, believe me, more rare than pink elephants in the streets of Boise. Second, in two of the studies cardiovascular risk factors improved significantly—but only in the subjects who were on a lower-carbohydrate intake. The folks who got put on a high-carbohydrate diet showed no significant improvements in these health indicators.

That leaves one last study, which was really a blowout. Published in the *Journal of Adolescent Health* in 2000, it reported on a group of obese adolescents put on a controlled carbohydrate diet with no restriction on calories for three months and meticulously monitored throughout that period. By design, the regimen was based on the Atkins approach. The group was compared with a control group put on a low-fat diet.

The results? Well, naturally, the adolescents lost significantly more weight on the controlled carbohydrate diet than on the low-fat diet. The written records indicated that at the end of the trial, the adolescents in the controlled carbohydrate group had averaged 1,830 calories daily, while the adolescents in the low-fat group had consumed 1,100 calories. The controlled carbohydrate group averaged 21.7 pounds lost, compared to 9.1 pounds for the low-fat group, and a significant improvement in body mass index (BMI), compared with the low-fat dieters.[10]

As studies like this become increasingly common, opposition to a controlled carbohydrate nutritional approach should fall away even more quickly than has already been the case in recent years.

The Metabolic Advantage in Action

Perhaps you will now understand how Harry Kronberg, the patient I mentioned in Chapter 3, was able to lose fifty pounds in three months on an eating plan containing an abundance of nutrient-dense, high-calorie foods. And he did so, even though in the previous three years on a moderately low-fat balanced diet he had gained 70. This does not contradict reason; instead, it is an outstanding example of metabolic advantage.

When you study both of Harry's menus, you'll see that when doing Atkins, he ate an average of only 200 calories less than he ate on his low-fat diet, but he has gone from gaining an average of 0.5 pound a week to shedding almost 4 pounds.

The metabolic advantage is there. It can't be disguised, evaded, put down to water weight or wished away.

Harry Kronberg's Before and After Menus

A Typical Pre-Atkins Day

Breakfast	Calories
Cheese Danish	308
Coffee (decaf with half 'n' half)	2

Lunch	
French Fries (3½ oz)	175
Pastrami/Corned Beef (4 oz cooked)	410
Rye Bread (2 slices)	140
Pretzels (3 oz)	220

Snacks	
Nestle Crunch Bar (1 oz)	138
Orange	71

Dinner	
Kippered Herring (4 oz)	217
Vegetables (1 cup cabbage)	24
Small Green & Tomato Salad	80
Crackers (4 rye thins)	52
Diet Soda	0
Vanilla Ice Cream (1 cup)	290

Total	2,127

A Typical Atkins Day

Breakfast	Calories
Tuna Salad (1 cup)	240
½ Grapefruit	41
Decaf Coffee (with half 'n' half)	2

Lunch

Grilled Chicken (light meat, 6 oz)	280
Small Green & Tomato Salad	80
Salad Dressing (1 oz)	170

Dinner

Rib Steak (6 oz)	490
Summer Squash (½ cup)	19
Small Green & Tomato Salad	80
Salad Dressing (1 oz)	170
Seltzer	0

Snacks

Almonds (1 oz)	176
Sugar-free Coleslaw	174
Cucumber (½ medium)	8

Total	1,930

Now it's your turn. Do you want an edge, a bonus and the odds on your side? You could bet the ranch on it. May the Edge be with you.

KEY POINTS!

- Only by doing Atkins can you lose weight eating the same number of calories on which you used to gain weight.
- Burning body fat has a metabolic advantage over so-called "balanced" or "low-fat" diets.
- The breakthrough concept of fat-mobilization was first discovered over forty years ago.
- Numerous studies have reinforced the metabolic advantage of burning fat for energy.

A FREQUENTLY ASKED QUESTION:

Why have you never published your findings on the various benefits of the Atkins Nutritional Approach in a scientific journal?

I am a full-time practitioner and not a researcher. As a physician I am responsible for the health of my patients and would never use some of them as a control group in the interest of research.

But I have taken a series of important steps to share the benefits of the Atkins Nutritional Approach with the medical community throughout the world. Working with a number of leading academic and research institutions, I have developed a series of Continuing Medical Education courses for health professionals. These courses explore the available research and clinical relevance of controlled carbohydrate nutrition.

Additionally, the Dr. Robert C. Atkins Foundation sponsors further research in all aspects of controlled carbohydrate nutrition. The Foundation is funded through Atkins Nutritionals Inc., our food products and nutritional supplements company. ANI, as I call it, has the added benefit of helping to supply the demand we now see of people seeking controlled carbohydrate foods. All of our products are developed to support the Atkins Nutritional Principles. Interestingly, our products have encouraged other food companies to develop additional new products.

TIPS:

- Count carbs, not calories.
- Spread your carbohydrate intake throughout the day to avoid blood-sugar spikes.

8

The Complexities of Carbohydrates

Carbohydrate is a major category of food, including all the fruits, vegetables, grains and starches. If you choose—as I hope you will—to do Atkins for a lifetime, you must bring some exacting standards to the process of deciding what carbohydrate foods you intend to eat. And make no mistake, I'm determined to teach you how to fashion a great way to eat—long term—not simply a weight loss regimen.

When doing Atkins, you will control the number of grams of carbohydrates you eat and will focus on certain food groups rather than others. One reason you will need to do this is because not all carbohydrate found in food is created equal. Most carbohydrate is digested by your body and turned into glucose—and most nutritionists refer to this as *digestible carbohydrate*. However, some carbohydrate can be digested by your body but not turned into glucose (glycerin is one example), and some carbohydrate is not digestible at all, such as fiber (see "Fiber: A Form of Carbohydrate," opposite) and is therefore eventually excreted by your body. These last two types of carbohydrate don't have an impact on your blood-sugar levels. Understanding the different behavior of carbohydrate in your

Fiber: A Form of Carbohydrate

Perhaps your grandmother called it roughage; physicians call it bulk. No matter what it's called, dietary fiber is traditionally used for relieving constipation, an important consideration when changing the way you eat as you do when you start Atkins.

What exactly is fiber? Simply put, dietary fiber is the indigestible parts of plant cells. Although it is a carbohydrate, fiber does not convert to glucose and thus does not raise your blood-sugar level the way carbohydrates typically do.

In fact, fiber actually slows the entry of glucose into the bloodstream. This in turn reduces the blood-sugar spikes that cause insulin production and encourage the body to produce and store body fat.[1] And by slowing down food's transit time in the digestive tract, fiber helps you feel full longer, resulting in fewer food cravings.

But that's just the beginning. Fiber also:
- binds to cholesterol in the intestine, helping rid the body of it.
- absorbs and then eliminates bacterial toxins in the intestine.
- reduces the likelihood of getting diverticulitis.
- speeds the excretion of gallstone-promoting bile.
- supports the immune system by crowding out harmful bacteria in the colon.
- bulks up the stool and make it easier to pass.

Supplementing With Fiber

Fiber-rich foods include vegetables, nuts and seeds, fruits, beans and whole unrefined grains. During Induction, your primary source of fiber will be vegetables. (In later phases you will be introducing the other sources of fiber in the order aforementioned.)

How can you get the benefits of fiber without the carbs contained in these foods? The answer is supplementation. I recommend that you take one tablespoon of psyllium husks daily. Be sure to select a sugar-free product. You can also take one tablespoon of coarse wheat bran or flaxseed meal. Although it's derived from grain, coarse bran is pure fiber and therefore it too contributes zero to your carb count. Psyllium husks should be mixed with water. You can sprinkle bran over your vegetables or blend flaxseed meal into a shake.

Drinking the recommended eight glasses or more of water daily is also essential to avoid constipation. You need to accompany any increase in fiber intake with plenty of water.

Be aware that fiber is one place where less is more. Consuming too much can block mineral absorption because food simply doesn't stay in the digestive tract long enough for your body to extract valuable nutrients. Gas, flatulence or constipation can also result. If you haven't been eating significant amounts of fiber, increase your intake gradually to allow the intestinal tract to adjust.

---

body can help you make smart food choices.

But you cannot necessarily rely on food labels. Recently (in 2001) the Food and Drug Administration (FDA) rejected a request by numerous health food manufacturers to allow non-digestible and non-metabolized carbohydrates to be listed separately on packaging, so that diabetics and other people with glucose/insulin disorders would be able to have the information upon which to make health-promoting decisions. I can't tell you I agree with this decision, and I certainly don't agree with the apparent notion that all carbohydrates are the same and affect your body the same way.

The Carbs That Count

The fact that fiber is not converted to blood sugar makes for an interesting benefit for people doing Atkins, allowing you to sneak in a few extra carbs in the form of high-fiber foods. Let me explain what I mean by "sneaking," because it is most definitely not the same thing as cheating.

Let's compare a cookie made of white flour and sugar with a couple of fiber-rich crackers. Both contain 10 grams of carbs. But there the similarity ends. Eat the cookie and you'll send all 10 grams of carbs coursing into your blood stream. But when you chomp into the crackers (which have, say, 4 grams of fiber) only 6 of those 10 grams impact on your blood sugar. Basically, you can deduct the grams of fiber from the food's total carb count. I call the net number of grams, "The carbs that count when you do Atkins." In the case of those crackers, you got a 4-gram free ride.

Consider the possibilities! By merely choosing fiber-rich foods over their flab-inducing, refined counterparts, you can benefit your health and get more bang for your carbohydrate buck. And determining which carbs count is simple: Check the total fiber grams listed on the food label and subtract that number from the total grams of carbohydrate listed. (For more on how to read a food label, turn to Chapter 19, pages 241–245.)

To know how many grams of carbohydrate a portion of a certain food contains, you will likely need a carbohydrate gram counter. And so one has been provided for you in this book. An even more extensive version, continually updated, is available on our website at *www.atkinscenter.com.*

In a moment I'm going to show you how to choose foods that supply the maximum nutritional bang, while they cost you only the very smallest metabolic price. When you combine your own personal preferences with the information in this chapter, you will be ideally situated not only to start doing Atkins (as you will learn in detail in Part Two) but also to continue doing Atkins for life.

But first, two points:

1. A controlled carbohydrate way of eating provides you with a powerhouse of nutrients to support your newly stabilized blood-sugar levels and your freshly unburdened body (yup, the one that soon won't be carrying so much weight around!). For many years, misinformed individuals have been claiming that you just couldn't get enough nutrients doing Atkins. After they've read this chapter, I'm going to let them puzzle out how they could possibly have said that.

2. As it relates to foods containing carbohydrates, you will need to make certain tradeoffs as you do Atkins. Once you've read this chapter, you'll have a much better understanding, both logically and intuitively, of how I came up with the lists of acceptable and unacceptable foods that you will find in Chapter 11 and the food decisions I'll be asking you to make. You'll know, for example, why a green salad is a good choice during the Induction phase and a carrot isn't.

So, let's take a quick look at the science of food.

The Glycemic Index—A Beautiful Tool

It is, too. The glycemic index is a numerical scale that tells you how fast glucose enters your bloodstream after a specific food is eaten. Most versions of the index, including the one I'll use (see pages 80–82), assign pure glucose the number of 100 and measure the effects of other foods in descending order from there. It's a highly effective system. Note, however, that the glycemic index doesn't tell you how much carbohydrate is in a serving of a particular food—that is why the glycemic index works hand-in-hand with a carb gram counter. Since there is no single standard glycemic index yet, the numbers may vary in different versions, but the relative order of foods on the various indexes is pretty consistent.

For someone controlling his or her intake of carbohydrates, the implication of such an index is obvious. By using it, you get to know—in advance of eating it—how a given food will affect both your blood-sugar levels and your insulin response. By choosing low-glycemic foods you can insure yourself a stable, smoothly running metabolic engine. That translates into plenty of energy and lays the foundation for both long-term health and disease prevention. The controlled carbohydrate foods you'll eat during the weight loss phases of Atkins have a good deal of overlap with the low-glycemic foods you'll see listed on the glycemic index table on the following pages.

As you can see, this is a tool for measuring only *carbohydrate* foods. That's because fat causes virtually no blood-sugar elevation and protein very little elevation.

It's interesting to browse through the list. Notice that a baked potato ranks exceptionally high. Starch converts to glucose in the bloodstream with great rapidity. That explains the high-glycemic index of another vegetable, the carrot. White rice, white bread and many cereals are well up there. Bananas and pasta are in the high-mid range.

(Pasta lovers who intend to try to squeeze in a little once they reach the Lifetime Maintenance phase, I have a tip for you: Note that cooking your pasta *al dente* significantly lowers its glycemic effects. Here's why: The shorter cooking time leaves the long chains of starch that are in pasta more closely packed together than longer cooking time; as a result, it is harder for your body's enzymes to break down this starch so there is less of an effect on your blood-sugar levels. Of course, the best idea is to purchase one of the great-tasting controlled carbohydrate pastas now available to you.)

Glycemic Index

Food	Glycemic Index (glucose = 100)
Bakery products	
Muffins	
Apple made without sugar	48
Blueberry	59
Bran	60
Corn	49
Breads and pastry	
Bagel, plain, frozen	72
Croissant	67
Hamburger bun	61
Melba toast	70
Pita bread	57
Pumpernickel	41
Waffles	76
White bread	70
Breakfast cereals	
All-Bran	42
Corn Flakes	84
Grape-Nuts	67
Muesli	66
Puffed Wheat	74
Shredded Wheat	69
Grains	
Barley	25
Couscous	65
Rice, brown	55
Rice, instant	91
Rice, white, low-amylose	88

Food	Glycemic Index (glucose = 100)

Fruits

Apple	36
Banana, ripe	52
Cherries	22
Grapefruit	25
Grapes	43
Orange	43
Peach	28
Pear	33
Pineapple	66
Plum	24
Watermelon	72

Legumes

Baked beans	48
Chickpeas	33
Kidney beans	27
Lentils	29

Pasta

Linguine	46
Macaroni and cheese, boxed	64
Spaghetti	41
Spaghetti, boiled 5 minutes (al dente)	37

Snack foods and candy

Corn chips	73
Jelly beans	80
Peanuts	14
Popcorn	55

Cookies

Oatmeal	55
Shortbread	64
Vanilla wafer	77

Food	Glycemic Index (glucose = 100)
Vegetables	
Carrots	71
Peas, green	48
Potato, baked	85
Sweet corn	55
Sweet potato	54

Source: Women's Health Watch—Harvard Health Online.

One of the latest installments of the famed Harvard Nurses Study—conducted for almost two decades (it started in 1984) by Simin Liu and Walter Willett and their associates—confirms the importance of the glycemic index. Researchers tracked the dietary habits and the health of 75,521 nurses for ten years. The research team discovered that the consumption of carbohydrates with a high-glycemic index was strongly associated with an increased risk of heart disease. They also discovered, although the data was not as strong, that "total carbohydrate intake, representing the replacement of fat with carbohydrate, appeared to be positively related to CHD [coronary heart disease] risk."

The Harvard researchers concluded, in my view quite correctly, that eating foods high on the glycemic index leads to elevated blood-sugar and insulin levels, which in turn leads to hypertension, undesirable cholesterol and triglyceride levels and other risk factors for heart disease. Since this is the largest long-term epidemiological study being conducted in America, these conclusions will not go unnoted in the scientific community.[2]

This is a good time for me to disabuse you of the long-held notion that there was some enormous difference between so-called "simple" and "complex" carbohydrates. That theory held that simple carbs such as sugar and white flour sent glucose rushing into your blood stream faster than complex carbs such as fruits, potatoes and whole grains. But, Liu and Willett and the other researchers found that two foods that contribute most to elevating blood sugar to an excessive level (called the "glycemic load") are baked potatoes and cold breakfast cereals. These foods were traditionally classified as complex, as opposed to simple, carbohydrates. However, they behaved just as simple carbohydrates do. So the glycemic index appears to be a better gauge of the impact of various carbohydrates on your blood sugar. As research continues to associate high-glucose load with increased risk of heart disease, we need to pay closer attention not only to the amount of carbohydrates consumed, but also to their position on the glycemic index.

Choosing your carbohydrate foods from the lower end of the glycemic index is fundamental common sense, and, for a person doing Atkins, an important building block for permanent weight loss.

In addition to being helpful for weight loss, the glycemic index has enormous potential as a tool for minimizing the risk factors associated with certain diseases. As the message spreads that hyperinsulinism is a factor in certain illnesses and disease—and it has spread like wildfire in the medical establishment over the last five or six years—the glycemic index becomes an ever more important tool for selecting foods. In my practice most of my patients have symptoms of unstable blood sugar (you may know it as *hypoglycemia).* Time and time again I have found this condition dramatically clears up when a diet inducing a lower glycemic response is followed. Also, doctors who specialize in diabetes are learning not only how important it is to control their patients' intake of carbohydrates, but how the glycemic index can help their patients do that intelligently.

Interestingly, it has also been shown that reducing your glycemic load appears to diminish your risk of developing colo-rectal cancer.[3] One likely reason is that cancer cells feed off sugar. Another possibility is that sugar may compromise the integrity of the intestinal tract. Moreover, hyperinsulinism, in response to a high-glycemic load, may increase the risk of cancer. Furthermore, recent studies on women who have had breast cancer have shown that women with lower insulin production have a better survival rate and a decreased incidence of recurrence than women with higher insulin levels.[4-5]

Two other recent studies have shown that hyperinsulinism has also been associated with higher risk for polycystic ovarian syndrome.[6-7] It all goes back to lesson one in eating for health: Avoid glycemic load. Don't cause your metabolism to struggle incessantly with high insulin levels, weight gain and looming cardiovascular and other health tragedies.

Now let's look at another, equally exciting way to rate carbohydrate foods.

The Promise of the Positive

Let us sing a song of veggies. Such beautiful, health-enhancing, varied foods. Adaptable to every cuisine world-wide, nothing in the world of cooking has more variety of taste and texture. I am waxing rhapsodic about vegetables, but their virtues are firmly grounded in scientific research.

Vegetables, if you choose the right ones, are very high-powered nutrient packages. These advantages come—once again if you choose your vegetables carefully—at a relatively low metabolic cost. That means that you are getting high fiber and phytochemicals with relatively low numbers of calories and carbohydrates.

So if some misguided individual tells you that you won't eat vegetables when you do Atkins, wave this chapter (with a stalk of celery, for good measure) at him or her. You will. And, it's just possible, if you are a typical American, that you will eat more vegetables than you ever ate before. Because despite what Mom, and countless other mothers before her, advised, most people do not eat nearly the amount of vegetables they should.

But let's look at the other side of the coin. In encouraging you to eat your vegetables, I certainly have no intention of compromising the basic weight loss principles of Atkins. Yes, I want you to consume plenty of nutrients, but you must do so without eating so many carbohydrates that you sabotage your weight loss efforts.

Each person has a Critical Carbohydrate Level for Losing (CCLL), and if you stay below that highly individual number you will lose weight. However, if you exceed that level—even with all healthy foods—your body will not switch to burning fat as the primary source of fuel. We need a way to focus on health-promoting vitanutrients that also provide blood-sugar stability and weight loss.

Fortunately, we're in luck. Nature dovetails with the Atkins plan beautifully, and the vegetables densest in nutrients happen to be those lowest in carbs. Salad greens and other leafy greens—escarole, spinach, parsley, watercress, arugula, Boston and romaine lettuce—are nutrient powerhouses that are low on the glycemic index.

Some other excellent health choices include asparagus, bamboo shoots, broccoli, cabbage, cauliflower, collard greens, eggplant, kale, kohlrabi, leeks, okra, onions, pumpkin, scallions, snow peas, spaghetti squash, string or wax beans, Swiss chard, tomato, turnips, water chestnuts and zucchini.

Even during Induction, the first phase of Atkins, and the one which is most restrictive of carbohydrates, most of you will be able to eat one cup of those vegetables daily, as well as two cups of salad vegetables (or just three cups of salad vegetables). As your metabolism permits, most of you will add more vegetables during the increasingly liberal phases that follow. By the time you are in the Lifetime Maintenance phase, you may well be able to eat most every vegetable, although some in moderation or only rarely. Still, it is always a good idea to make the high-nutrient/lower-carbohydrate ones your primary choices.

Nuts and Seeds:
The Original Functional Foods

Nuts and seeds have been an important component of the human diet since the days when mankind survived as hunter-gatherers. I suspect that nuts and seeds were the original dessert in caveman days. The two combine protein, fat and carbohydrate in one tidy package. The protein content of nuts ranges from ten percent in walnuts to seventeen percent in almonds; the fat content ranges from about thirty-five percent in coconuts to over seventy percent in macadamia nuts; the remainder is carbohydrate, including a significant amount of fiber. Obviously, the higher the fat content, the lower the carb count, which is one reason my personal favorite is the macadamia nut.

These little powerhouses are also densely packed with nutrients. Almonds are a rich source of calcium. Almonds, sunflower kernels and hazelnuts are particularly good sources of vitamin E. Nuts also provide a long list of other nutrients, including niacin, vitamin B_6, folic acid, magnesium, zinc, copper and potassium, plus a number of phytochemicals, including many antioxidants.

After the first two weeks of Induction, when you can introduce nuts and seeds into your menus, you will find they make excellent snacks and often an unexpected and tasty ingredient in an entrée or vegetable dish. You can also use ground nuts and seeds in lieu of breading before baking or sautéing chicken breasts, veal scallops or fish fillets. Like all good things, nuts and seeds should be eaten in moderation. An ounce of most nuts or seeds contains roughly 5 grams of carbs.

Tasty and nutritious as they are, nuts and seeds should be a component of any healthy nutritional regimen. Numerous studies have shown that regular consumption of nuts and seeds minimizes your risks of coronary heart disease. A number of epidemiological studies (studies of populations over time) have shown that people who eat nuts regularly are less likely to have a heart attack than people who do not consume nuts and oil-containing seeds.[8–10] Moreover, the greater the frequency of consumption, the lower the incidence of heart attack. Lignans in seeds and nuts lower LDL (bad) cholesterol, as do the heart-protective vitamin E, betaine and arginine.

People on low-fat diets often eliminate nuts and with them a powerful source of omega-6 fatty acids and other nutrients. When you do Atkins, one of the many culinary pleasures is being able to enjoy the multiplicity of fat-rich and nutrient-dense nuts and seeds.

Giving It a Number

One way to look at nutrient value is to measure the concentration of antioxidants in food. Antioxidants are a special group of vitamins and phytochemicals that protect your cells from the ravages of environmental pollution, stress, disease and aging. Researchers at Tufts University School of Medicine in Boston studied the antioxidant capacity of common vegetables and assigned each vegetable an antioxidant score.[11] I've taken that score and divided it by the number of grams of carbohydrate in the same-size serving of each vegetable or fruit and thus computed what I now call the Atkins Ratio.

The higher the number, the more antioxidant protection you get per gram of carbohydrate. Talk about bang for your buck. If you used this tool to maximize your nutrient intake and simultaneously exercised regularly and controlled your carbohydrates by following Atkins, I would defy you not to be an outstanding physical specimen.

Look at the numbers in the Atkins Ratio below. As you can see, garlic is in a class by itself. The cruciferous vegetables—broccoli, cauliflower, kale, Brussels sprouts and cabbage—which extensive research has shown to be a group of potent cancer fighters, are well up there. Onions also play a starring role. From this already rich list, let's identify some vegetable all-stars.

Atkins Ratio

Garlic (1 clove)	23.2
Leaf Lettuce (1 leaf)	8.2
Kale (½ cup raw)	6.5
Onion (1 tablespoon)	6.2
Spinach (½ cup raw)	5.0
Broccoli (½ cup raw)	3.2
Red Bell Pepper (½ cup raw)	2.5

The world of vegetables is filled with natural chemicals that help protect you from illness. Scientists now call these defenders phytonutrients—*phyto* being Greek for plant. Here, for instance, are three phytonutrients that have been shown to lower the risk of cancer. Bear in mind that a complete list would be long enough to fill an entire book.

1. **Beta carotene**: You'll find a rich supply in green vegetables such as spinach, kale, broccoli, Brussels sprouts and beans, as well as in squash, peppers and yams.
2. **Lycopene**: The king of this nutrient hill is the tomato, and there is very good reason to think it will help protect you from prostate cancer. Note, however, that fresh tomatoes contain less lycopene than tomato purée or tomato juice.
3. **Lutein**: This carotenoid has been identified with reduced breast cancer risk, and it can be found in kale, collard greens, spinach and yellow squash.

How (and When) to Eat Your Veggies

Choose a good lineup of vegetables, then follow these five tips:

1. *Consume vegetables little by little throughout the day.* If you save up your carb allowance for a giant veggie splurge, it might produce a surge in your blood sugar.
2. *When you eat higher-carb vegetables, such as yams or winter squash, do so along with proteins and fats.* They will slow the passage of carbs through your digestive system and minimize their impact on your blood sugar.
3. *Look for recipes in which a variety of vegetables are included* with meat, fish or fowl as part of a complete entrée, such as stews and dishes based on Asian cuisine.
4. *Don't drink your vegetables.* Juicing removes the fiber, which has the double merit of helping you feel full and maintaining a healthy digestive system. Juices also concentrate the sugars from vegetables, increasing the risk that they'll spike your blood sugar.
5. *Cook carefully.* Vegetables are usually most nutritious when crisp—not overcooked. An exception to this recommendation and to #4, above, is the tomato; its cancer-fighting chemical lycopene becomes more bioavailable when heat breaks down the tomato's cell walls or even when it is served as juice.

A Message to My Friends, the Die-Hard Carnivores

Of course, there are lots of people who start Atkins more than a little pleased with the fact that I certainly won't discourage them from eating meat, fish and fowl. I'm a carnivore, too. But I'm also an omnivore—meaning I eat anything that's healthy.

I know there are some people who simply don't like vegetables. Or, at least, they don't like the ones they've eaten so far. The funny thing is that a lot of folks who do Atkins eventually find vegetables they can love. Perhaps it's because many people who follow the program end up trying many recipes and dishes they have never eaten before. They are

---

Berries Are Best!

One important lesson learned from the Tufts study previously mentioned is that, as evaluated by the Atkins Ratio, the lumping together of fruits and vegetables as being essentially equal in benefits is not true. Relatively speaking, vegetables have considerably more antioxidant value per carbohydrate gram than fruits and thus represent a much more valuable dietary choice.

Even so, after the Induction phase of Atkins, you may use some of your daily carb ration to add the more valuable fruits to your menu. Berries, including blueberries, raspberries, blackberries and strawberries, are the fruits highest in antioxidant value.[12–13] Berries are also lower in carbs than other fruit and are relatively low on the glycemic index scale. Moreover, the phytonutrients in certain fruits can slow pre-cancerous growths.[14]

---

making all sorts of healthy changes in their eating habits, and, in that context, sampling new foods doesn't seem particularly revolutionary. If you've always been a grudging consumer of vegetables, I hope you'll become a vegetable-eating convert.

Look at the recipe section in the back of this book. Pick out a few vegetable concoctions that sound at least tolerable to your carnivorous personality. How surprised you will be if you like some of them. Then try a few more. Vegetables don't have to become your favorite food, but if you can lure yourself into dietary habits that put more of them on your plate than most Americans eat, you will be doing your noble, hard-working body an immense favor.

Think of all the things your body does for you. I'm sure you'll agree that it's payback time.

KEY POINTS!

- All fruits, vegetables, grains and starches contain carbohydrates.
- The more carbohydrate an individual consumes, the less body fat he or she will lose. That's why low-fat diets usually don't work.
- All carbohydrates are not created equal.
- The glycemic index measures the relative rate at which glucose enters the blood stream after a specific carbohydrate food is eaten.
- Low-glycemic vegetables contain relatively less sugar.
- Choosing foods that are low in carb grams, have a low-glycemic index value and are high in antioxidants is your passport to weight loss, increased energy and improved overall health.

A FREQUENTLY ASKED QUESTION:

What is the difference between a carbohydrate gram counter and a glycemic index?
A carbohydrate gram counter typically lists the total carbohydrate value of a food item. (The carbohydrate gram counter starting on page 492 also lists the level of digestible carbohydrates you should count when doing Atkins.) The glycemic index is a measure of a given carbohydrate's effect on your blood-sugar levels. You can use the glycemic index to choose carbohydrate foods that will have a relatively low impact on your blood sugar. But remember, when doing Atkins your total carbohydrate intake is of ultimate importance.

TIPS:

- Keep a carbohydrate gram counter and a glycemic index on your refrigerator (and use the electronic versions at *www.atkinscenter.com*).
- Eat whole vegetables instead of drinking juices.
- Overcooking vegetables destroys nutrients.
- Adding some fat and/or protein to a salad minimizes the impact of the carbs on your blood-sugar level.
- Vegetables most dense in nutrients are lowest in sugar and should be your primary choices.
- When you think fruit, think berries.

9

~m~

Facts and Fallacies About the Atkins Nutritional Approach

I'm almost certain that you are reading this book because you know of someone who has lost weight—and likely overcome other health problems—by following the individualized nutritional approach you've been reading about here. And you've decided you want to feel good, look good and be revitalized, too.

But you may be wondering why not everyone acknowledges the fact (and it is a fact) that controlling carbohydrates the Atkins way is the ideal eating strategy for losing weight and promoting good health. One reason the Atkins Nutritional Approach has not been a part of mainstream teaching (although the tide is beginning to change, as well it should) has been misinformation.

If you've encountered these critical articles suggesting that Atkins is dangerous, not to mention ineffective, you may have mixed feelings about starting a lifetime of controlled carbohydrate eating. Let me ease your misgivings: It is clear to me—and to every doctor I've met who has had adequate experience with Atkins—that this program should be the "treatment of choice" not only for obesity but for diabetes and several other diet-related disorders. The misinformation saddens me, because it has prevented so many people in need from using and benefiting from the best treatment available. In effect, these ill-informed reviews are propagating epidemic, life-threatening conditions.

That is why I am taking the time here, before we start "Part Two: How to Do Atkins—Today and for Life," to address these criticisms. I don't want you to have any lingering questions or doubts as you read through the remaining sections of the book. Too much is at stake: namely, your health and well-being.

Modern medical history contains few examples of such vast discrepancies between what is said in print and the truth. You may find that the explanations in this chapter sound a bit scientific. This was done on purpose. I want you to have the full complement of information at your disposal to counter any challenge you get. Armed with information gleaned from my forty years of clinical experience, and with the support of specific scientific studies, you will be able to hold your own—and likely to sway opinion—in any debate that comes your way.

Fact vs. Fallacy

Fallacy #1: Ketosis is dangerous and causes a variety of medical problems.

Fact: Our bodies have only two fuel delivery systems to provide us with energy. Our primary fuel is based on carbohydrate and is delivered as glucose. People who eat three so-called "balanced" meals every day get virtually all their energy from glucose. But the alternate, back-up fuel is stored fat, and this fuel system delivers energy by way of ketones whenever our small supply of glucose is used up (in a maximum of two days).

When a person doing Atkins releases ketones, he or she is in ketosis. Ketosis occurs when you are taking in a very low level of carbohydrate from the food you eat, as you will during much of the weight loss phases of Atkins. Ketones are secreted in the urine (and at times in one's breath), a perfectly normal and natural function of the body. The more ketones you release, the more fat you have dissolved.

Part of this fallacy is the claim that ketones can build up to dangerous levels in the body. Studies show that ketone bodies are very tightly regulated in the body and will not increase beyond the normal range in healthy individuals. (Uncontrolled diabetics, alcoholics, and people who have been on prolonged fasts might see an increase in ketones beyond the normal range.) The body regulates ketone levels the same way it regulates blood-glucose or pH levels.[1–4] And in the clinical setting of my practice, it has been repeatedly demonstrated that overweight patients produce just enough ketones to meet their immediate needs for fuel—and no more. A person will have no more ketones after three months of controlling carbohydrates than they do after three days. It is highly unlikely that people, other than insulin-dependent diabetics, will build up ketones.

Confusion about ketosis often comes from people mistaking it for ketoacidosis, a condition found in Type 1 diabetics; this occurs when a person's blood sugar is out of control and he or she cannot produce insulin. No doctor should have trouble differentiating physiologic ketosis, which you will experience doing Atkins, from ketoacidosis. Further, since people are often overweight specifically because of an overabundance of insulin, it is essentially impossible for them to be in ketoacidosis.

Some individuals at the ketogenic level of controlled carbohydrate eating may experience mild symptoms such as unusual breath odor and constipation (see Fallacies #12 and #14). However, the vast majority of individuals do not develop problems. One study of a severely ketogenic diet showed that ketosis was benign, with no complications or side effects when studied in metabolic ward conditions. The month-long study documented heart, kidney, liver and blood-cell functions in the patients and found no adverse effects.[5]

In other studies, it has been shown that bone health was not compromised[6-12] and that renal (kidney) function was found to be stable[13-16] on controlled carbohydrate diets. Supporting what we know from years of clinical practice, there is even scientific literature on hyperlipidemia (elevated blood fats—i.e., cholesterol and triglycerides), showing improved values on controlled carbohydrate diets.[17-28]

So the next time you read that the ketosis produced by the Atkins Nutritional Approach is dangerous, challenge the writer (in a letter to the editor, if necessary) and ask: "What is so dangerous about using up your stored fat?"

Fallacy #2: *The Atkins Nutritional Approach is only effective for weight loss because calories are restricted.*

Fact: While some people who follow the Atkins Nutritional Approach may eat fewer calories than before, it certainly is not because the program limits calorie intake. People doing Atkins may end up eating fewer calories because they are generally less hungry and no longer obsessed with food. This occurs for two reasons:

1. Stable blood sugar throughout the day ensures that you will have fewer food cravings and false hunger pains.
2. The food eaten by a person doing Atkins (meat, fish, cheese, nuts, eggs, and low-sugar/low-starch vegetables and fruit) is less processed and more nutritious than that on the typical pre-Atkins menu. Give a body fewer empty calories, provide it with more nutrient-dense alternatives and it will logically be satisfied sooner and require less food.

   Let's look at the results of the study mentioned in Chapter 7 that supports these conclusions. Researchers at New York's Schneider Children's Hospital studied forty obese patients, ages 12 to 18, who were split into two groups. We already mentioned that the low-fat group lost half as much weight on 1,100 calories per day as did the controlled carbohydrate group, which was allowed unlimited calories and, on average, ate 1,830 calories per day.

What's even more exciting is that the controlled carbohydrate group enjoyed further health benefits—far from suffering the dangers some warn of with the controlled carbohydrate nutritional approach. Lipid profiles (cholesterol and triglycerides) improved more than those on the low-fat program.

Also, those on the controlled carbohydrate diet showed better long-term compliance than those on the low-fat diet. A year later, seven out of eight of those following the controlled carbohydrate approach were still involved with the program as opposed to none on the low-fat diet.[29]

Fallacy #3: *The weight lost on the Atkins Nutritional Approach is mostly water, not fat.*

Fact: It is typical of any weight loss plan, including the Induction phase of Atkins, that during the first few days, or even the first week, some of the weight loss will be water loss. However, when you follow a controlled carbohydrate eating plan, your body switches from burning carbohydrate to burning stored fat for energy, resulting in the loss of stored fat. In fact, research shows that even when water is lost during the first few days on a controlled carbohydrate nutritional approach, the water balance soon returns to normal, and the weight loss comes from burning body fat for energy.[30] The most dramatic sign of this loss is seeing the inches drop off your measurements.

Fallacy #4: *The Atkins Nutritional Approach is unbalanced and deficient in basic nutrition.*

Fact: The Atkins Nutritional Approach actually provides more nutrients than the typical American diet. It deliberately rebalances your way of eating. It is probable that the eating pattern that led to your weight gain was improperly balanced in the first place. The evidence showing that overproduction of insulin is responsible for most weight gain is quite impressive, and the best way to correct an insulin disorder is to avoid foods that stimulate insulin activity—that is, foods high in carbohydrates.

However, the Atkins Nutritional Approach does not exclude these foods (fruits, vegetables and grains). The Induction phase of Atkins, which people often mistake for the entire program, is the most strict, permitting only 20 grams of carbohydrates each day. Those 20 grams come in the form of green, leafy vegetables and also can include nutrient-dense, high-fiber, low-carbohydrate vegetables such as broccoli, asparagus, eggplant and spinach. Hardly foods lacking in nutrients!

A sample Induction menu containing 2,000 calories and 20 grams of carbohydrate was analyzed using the highly regarded "Nutritionist V" program (the computer program used by nutritionists worldwide). Results of the analysis found the menu to meet or exceed Recommended Daily Intake (RDI) requirements of nineteen of the twenty-four vitamins, minerals and trace elements, and the remaining few (panthothenic acid, sodium, magnesium, copper, chromium and molybdenum) can easily be replaced with a supplement (see page 134).

Once they complete Induction and begin the next phase of the program, individuals can raise their carbohydrate gram count. This phase prescribes even more nutrient-dense, green, leafy vegetables and fruits such as strawberries. With these additions, the plan far exceeds requirements for fiber.

The second part of this criticism is more thought-provoking. I, for one, am deeply committed to finding a vitanutrient solution for most health problems. This means that I believe no eating pattern contains optimal nutrition, and that all of us can improve our health by taking vitanutrients that are targeted to our individual health problems, disease risks and nutrient deficiencies.

That said, let's look at the essential-nutrient contributions made by the foods people eat on low-fat diets. These foods are low in the fat-soluble vitamins A, D, E and K and the essential fatty acids, our number-one deficiency in this country. They also may be low in nutrients we get from meat, such as vitamin B_{12} and carnitine. And if people overeat foods made from white flour—which is often the case on low-fat diets—they will be low in half the B complex nutrients (the half that isn't included in the mandatory enrichment) and most of the essential minerals. People on a low-fat diet need supplementation desperately.

Fallacy #5: *People doing Atkins may feel tired, weak and lacking in energy.*

Fact: Fatigue may occur during the first few days of doing Atkins, while the body adapts to the switch in metabolic pathways. It typically takes about three to four days for the body to convert from a sugar metabolism to a primarily fat metabolism. Your body can store carbohydrates for only up to forty-eight hours, so you can be confident that your metabolic switch will occur, as long as you are doing Atkins properly.

After the transition, those people who were tired at first usually report high energy and clear thinking throughout the day. The explanation is simple: They have rebalanced their nutrition so that their blood sugar is stabilized. They avoid blood-sugar peaks and valleys throughout the day, putting an end to mood swings and periods of lethargy. And those people who consume a full vitanutrient program are much less likely to feel weak or tired even at the start of Atkins.

Fallacy #6: *You eat too much protein when doing Atkins, which is bad for the kidneys.*

Fact: Too many people believe this untruth simply because it has been repeated so often that even intelligent health professionals assume it must have been reported somewhere.

But the fact is that it has never been reported anywhere. I have yet to see someone produce a study for me to review, or even cite a specific case in which a protein-containing diet causes any form of kidney disorder.

The only remotely related phenomenon is the fact that when someone is *already suffering* from far-advanced kidney disease, it is difficult for that person's body to handle protein. But protein has nothing to do with the *cause* of the kidney problem.

Fallacy #7: Atkins is high in fat, and we all know that fats cause gallbladder disease.

Fact: There is now overwhelming scientific evidence that gallstones (responsible for over ninety percent of gallbladder disease) are formed when fat intake is *low*. In a study that examined the effects of a diet that provided 27 grams of fat per day, gallstones developed in thirteen percent of the participants.[31] The reason is that the gallbladder will not contract unless fat is taken in, and if it doesn't contract, a condition called *biliary stasis* develops and the bile salts crystallize into stones. Our gallbladders need to be kept active to prevent stone formation.

It is not uncommon to find gallstones in people who are obese, although the gallstones may not be causing discomfort. People with existing stones may, however, have trouble with high-fat meals. If you are one of these people you may have to slowly increase the level of fat you eat according to your own tolerance—meaning, how you feel. Remember, gallstones are not formed overnight. So anyone who tells you they started doing Atkins and two weeks later developed gallstones doesn't fully understand the medical situation.

Fallacy #8: The Atkins Nutritional Approach is deficient in bone-building calcium and has a negative impact on calcium absorption.

Fact: While you're doing Atkins you will get one hundred percent of the RDI of calcium from foods such as cheese, broccoli and kale. (Milk is only one source of calcium, so even if you're not drinking it, you can still meet your needs.) In addition, in a study published in the *American Journal of Nutrition,* researchers followed four male adults and studied the short-term and long-term effects of a high-meat diet on calcium metabolism. The study found no significant changes in calcium balance, nor was there any significant change in the intestinal absorption of calcium during the high-meat diet.[32]

Fallacy #9: A nutritional approach that promotes a liberal intake of high-fat meats and dairy products will raise cholesterol levels, ultimately leading to heart disease.

Fact: I certainly do not deny that every major health organization, as well as the United States government, endorses a low-fat diet in the unquestioned belief that fat causes heart disease. But are they right? A good deal of compelling evidence points in the opposite direction.

A growing body of scientific literature demonstrates that a controlled carbohydrate eating plan, if followed correctly, promotes heart health and improves clinical health markers. One study, conducted by Jeff S. Volek, MS, RD, PhD, while at Ball State University, showed the positive effects of a controlled carbohydrate nutritional approach on triglyceride levels. The study consisted of twelve healthy men, ages 20 to 55, who followed a controlled carbohydrate program adhering to the Atkins protocols for eight weeks. Upon completion of the study, each participant lowered his triglyceride levels by an average of fifty-five percent.[33]

Furthermore, this study showed that a higher-carbohydrate diet results in increased levels of triglycerides and decreased levels of HDL cholesterol (the good kind). These factors have been associated with higher risks of myocardial infarction, ischemic heart disease and coronary heart disease events.[34] In addition, various researchers have demonstrated that high triglycerides and low HDL alone—as opposed to the total cholesterol number most of us focus on—may be the most important factors in heart disease and stroke.[35]

We also can look at the research that's come out of Framingham, Massachusetts—the community studied for fifty years by Harvard researchers—to glean meaningful information about the cause of heart disease. This research showed that the risk of heart disease increased both with high cholesterol levels and obesity, but their data showed that weight gain and cholesterol levels were inversely correlated with dietary fat and cholesterol intake! In other words, consuming less fat and cholesterol resulted in more weight gain and higher blood cholesterol.

More recently, the Framingham researchers reported on a study in which the young, healthy, male population of the community was followed for several decades to see which dietary patterns might lead to having a stroke. To their amazement, they found that those with the highest intake of saturated fats had the fewest ischemic strokes (the most common kinds), a whopping seventy-six percent less than those with the lowest intake of saturated fat.[36]

Fallacy #10: The Atkins Nutritional Approach is the "most severe" of the controlled carbohydrate plans and is most likely to have immediate adverse effects.

Fact: Since there's nothing harmful about a controlled carbohydrate nutritional approach, the concept of severity isn't especially meaningful. The idea of severity surely comes from the low level of carbohydrate consumed during the Induction phase. Induction's purpose is to jump-start the body chemistry into fat mobilization. Throughout the other phases of Atkins, each individual seeks the most permissive level of carbohydrate intake that still results in weight loss or weight maintenance.

Fallacy #11: *The bad thing about Atkins is that it makes you crave sweets!*

Fact: Craving is a symptom of addiction, and the surefire cure for addiction is abstinence. Atkins, with the help of chromium and glutamine supplements, allows you to get on with the project of dealing with your addiction. For almost everyone with sugar addiction, Atkins is the most effective treatment.

I have treated thousands of patients whose cravings come back as a result of a few unfortunate deviations from the plan. These cravings can be reined in simply by adhering to Atkins. Incidentally, in my experience, the controlled carbohydrate approach can be an extremely effective adjunct to the processes of breaking other addictions, including alcohol and cigarette dependencies.

Fallacy #12: *Atkins causes bad breath.*

Fact: Well, actually, it causes ketone breath. Ketones, which impart a sweetish smell, do not cause what I would call bad breath. It's a different breath smell to be sure, but not an offensive one. I have not noticed it among my patients for years; perhaps I simply consider it normal. In any case, this condition, if it exists at all, is likely to last only as long as you are doing the Induction phase of Atkins. Try drinking more water, or every now and then chew a little fresh parsley. And, on the positive side, it is proof that your body has switched to the alternative metabolic pathway of burning fat for fuel.

Fallacy #13: *People on Atkins learn to eat fatty foods like bacon and eggs, so if they stop doing the program they are worse off than before.*

Fact: For an overweight person, Atkins provides the single best opportunity to find a nutritional approach he or she can live with, without developing the desire to abandon it. The fact that it includes some high-fat, rich foods is exactly what enables people to follow this nutritional plan, eat things that feel satisfying and enjoy the good overall health the plan promotes.

Fallacy #14: The Atkins Nutritional Approach causes constipation because it lacks fiber.

Fact: The Atkins Nutritional Approach includes fiber-rich foods such as spinach, eggplant, broccoli, asparagus and leafy greens. It also includes fruits such as berries. In addition, if more fiber is needed during the Induction phase, I recommend a fiber supplement. This is unnecessary in the Ongoing Weight Loss phase and beyond because more fruits and vegetables are introduced into the eating plan.

Fallacy #15: It is impossible to keep off the weight lost on the Atkins Nutritional Approach for the long term.

Fact: That statement applies better to low-fat or low-calorie diets. After all, nothing is more difficult to endure for a lifetime than being constantly hungry. Atkins, from the start, allows you to eat until you feel satisfied. Furthermore, the variety of foods allowed on Atkins provides a diverse menu that is neither complicated nor boring and helps people stay motivated to change their eating patterns forever.

Don't just take my word for it—turn to the "Food and Recipes" section beginning on page 367 and see for yourself. Additionally, in the time since the last edition of this book was published, numerous companies have introduced controlled carbohydrate versions of bars, shakes, syrups, candy, chips, desserts, bread, ice cream and more, including my own company. It has never been easier to stay with an eating plan that offers you the full spectrum of delicious foods in quantities that leave you satisfied.

PART TWO

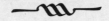

How to Do Atkins —
Today and for Life

10

Before You Begin

You are probably raring to start Atkins and begin losing weight. But there are two medically important steps and several practical preparations that will lay the groundwork for your success. First, a crucial warning: People with severe kidney disease (creatinine over 2.4) should not do any phase of Atkins unless ordered to do so by their physician. Also, pregnant women and nursing mothers may do the Lifetime Maintenance phase but should not do any of the weight loss phases of Atkins.

The first thing you must do is review any medications you take and make a doctor's appointment to get a complete physical, including some blood work and other tests. I'd like you to understand why having a medical workup before beginning Atkins is so important, both from a health perspective and to help motivate you to follow the program faithfully.

A patient of mine named David French—a 52-year-old stockbroker—had tried countless diets and failed on all of them. He came to me somewhat reluctantly—nagged, I suspect, by his wife and children. During our first conversation, he quickly expressed his skepticism, groaned at the thought of taking vitamins and seemed to me like someone who would not stick with the program. Although he weighed 206 pounds at only five feet eight inches tall, he had no obvious health problems other than generalized fatigue and difficulty with even very mild physical exertion.

"Let's at least check your blood lipid levels, Mr. French," I said, "and then we'll have some idea of whether you have anything to worry about." (The word *lipids* is medicalese for cholesterol and triglycerides, traditionally regarded as the main blood indicators for heart disease risk.) The blood tests were enlightening. His total cholesterol was a whopping 284 and his triglycerides level was an incredible 1,200. At our next meeting, I let him have it with both barrels: "If you don't do something soon, I'd say you're probably going to die in the next year or two, Mr. French."

That caught his attention. In all probability, I told him, a heart attack or a stroke would be his undoing. He also showed signs of being a borderline diabetic. His condition was completely reversible, but when he left my office that day I didn't think he'd make the effort to reverse it.

I was wrong. Dave started doing Atkins, and six months later, he weighed 162 pounds, his total cholesterol was 155 and his triglycerides were 90. He had been a carbohydrate eater his whole life—he'd hit the coffee cart for bagels and rolls, stop on the way home from work for a calzone and drank soda pop every day—but Dave thrived on my program, reassured by the fact he could eat until he was completely satisfied. "If you're hungry, eat," I said.

I also persuaded Dave to do a half hour of exercise four times a week. He soon found that he slept better and felt far less tired during the day. Also, physical exertion was no longer beyond him.

Dave is a slim and healthy man now and he won't let himself slip into his old ways. "I have a picture that I keep on the desk in my office that shows the maximum me," he says. "I look like I'm going to have a baby. I keep the photo right there where I can see it, to remind me of what I'll never be again. Nowadays, I don't even look like the same person."

Even more important, Dave French probably wouldn't be alive today if the results of his blood work hadn't shocked him into changing his ways.

Review Your Medications

With that sobering thought in mind, let's look at those medical steps you should take before you begin to change your eating habits. You will need to stop taking any unnecessary over-the-counter medications, such as cough syrup or cough drops, antacids, sleep aids, antihistamines or laxatives. Many prescription medications also inhibit weight loss. For a list of these medications, please turn to Chapter 20, page 262. If you take one or more of the drugs listed, you may be disappointed in your weight loss results. Talk to your doctor to see if an alternative can be found. You can also refer to *Dr. Atkins' Vita-Nutrient Solution* for more natural approaches to deal with your symptoms.

There are also several categories of drugs that can cause adverse effects when taken while on a controlled carbohydrate eating plan. First are the diuretics, because reducing your carbohydrate intake alone can have a dramatic diuretic effect. Second, since Atkins is so effective at lowering high blood sugar, people who take insulin or oral diabetes medications that stimulate insulin can end up with dangerously low blood-sugar levels. Third, Atkins has a strong blood pressure lowering effect and can easily convert blood pressure medications into an overdose. If you are currently taking any of these medications, you will need your doctor's help to adjust your dosages.

Checkup and Blood Work

When you go to your doctor, I recommend that you get your blood chemistries and lipid levels measured—and quite possibly the glucose-tolerance test (with insulin levels drawn at fasting and at one- and two-hour intervals)—before you start the program. Lipid levels will reveal your total cholesterol, HDL (good) and LDL (bad) cholesterol and triglycerides. These indicators often change with drastic dietary intervention. The blood chemistries will measure baseline glucose, kidney and liver function. Be sure your doctor also measures your uric acid levels. Since many people wrongly believe that these indicators are negatively affected by doing Atkins, you may later regret not having a "before" baseline to compare with your "after" results.

If you choose to keep track of those hidden physical changes that are measured in your blood, you'll find that, after you start Atkins, they should begin improving steadily (see "Before and After Tests," opposite). I don't want you to wait to have your initial lab work done until *after* you start Atkins, because then you may think any abnormalities are the result of your new way of eating. You may well have had even higher cholesterol and triglycerides before you began.

Your doctor will also check your blood pressure. High blood pressure—known as "the silent killer"—and being overweight often go together. Having high blood pressure (also called *hypertension*) puts you at clear risk for stroke and heart disease and may indicate elevated insulin levels. What happens to high blood pressure on Atkins? It goes down. Nothing is more consistently or more rapidly observed than normalization of blood pressure.

Lou Stazzio was a good illustration of that. This 40-year-old New York policeman had gained 50 pounds over the previous twenty years and had, in the process, acquired a roof beam-raising blood pressure of 180/110. He was on medication and was constantly fatigued. Doing Weight Watchers only introduced him to the pleasure of starvation.

One day, he read an article about how overweight teenage children lost weight more easily on a controlled carbohydrate plan than on a low-fat diet. Well, why not him? He

Before and After Tests

After you have been doing Atkins for six weeks or so, have your blood work redone; you may be surprised at the dramatic improvements. A whole body of published literature suggests that you ought to be terrified of eating liberal amounts of eggs, fat and meat. In fact, the most common question I'm asked when I tell a patient what I expect him to eat is "But won't my cholesterol go up?" I have no hesitation in answering, "It will probably go down." And in cases where your total cholesterol goes up, what you will almost invariably find is that your HDL (good) cholesterol goes up more than your LDL (bad) cholesterol does, thus improving the all-important HDL/LDL ratio.[1–3]

Typically, triglycerides plummet within the first month on Atkins, then HDL begins to rise. In some cases, LDL will rise. If it does, ask your doctor to test for the subtypes of LDL to determine whether it is the low-risk type of LDL or the high-risk type that has risen. Low-risk LDL, large fluffy lipo-protein A, is so designated because it doesn't cause plaque to form in the arteries. Research has shown that high-fat diets will raise the beneficial low-risk LDL.[4]

Your kidney and liver functions should also be excellent.[5–6] In fact, in my clinical experience, some individuals who have previously had elevated liver levels due to fatty deposits in the liver have shown improvement after doing Atkins. Your uric acid levels should test normal. If you have elevated uric acid prior to going on the program, you must be sure to keep your water intake up and monitor your uric acid level. An elevated uric acid level can lead to gout; if you suffer from gout I recommend you consult *Dr. Atkins' Vita-Nutrient Solution*, since certain vitanutri-

ents can help you control your uric acid levels. You
can also ask your physician about the drug allopuri-
nol, which consistently lowers uric acid levels.[7]

---

decided to give Atkins a try. In eight months on the plan, Lou
lost 60 pounds, was taken off his blood pressure medication
and now has an unmedicated blood pressure of 118/74—a
first-class advertisement for cardiovascular health.

You should also ask your doctor about your thyroid function. A sluggish thyroid is often responsible for obesity. If
you have an underactive thyroid, getting the correct treatment may help solve your weight problem. For a detailed
discussion of thyroid problems, turn to Chapter 20.

The Blood-Sugar Test

Let's talk about the laboratory test most relevant to people starting Atkins—the five-hour glucose-tolerance test
(GTT). If, after reading the last few chapters, you suspect
you may have a blood-sugar or insulin imbalance that is
contributing to your weight problems, discuss it with your
doctor and request a five-hour GTT with insulin levels.
Since the onset of diabetes is insidious and damage to the
body can occur even before full-blown diabetes is first discovered, it is vitally important to be aware of the possibility
you have pre-diabetes and of the degree of risk you may already suffer (see Chapter 24).

If you are hesitating, consider this: We are not talking
about headaches, acid indigestion or ingrown toenails here.
Need I remind you that the conditions the GTT with insulin
levels can detect can be precursors to diabetes? Sixteen million people have diabetes.[8] One in three doesn't know he or
she has it.

If you don't want to be drafted into the diabetic army, it

pays to find out right now if you are a potential recruit. I. your blood tests show you that you're well along the road, you will suddenly have a reason for doing Atkins that is far stronger than your desire to shed excess poundage. (If you became overweight early in life, this may have serious implications for your children, too. Check your blood-sugar and insulin levels so that you can know what condition they may have inherited from you. Taking early action to address the same issues in their diets can make a big difference.)

The GTT measures your blood sugar after twelve hours of fasting and then over the course of five to six hours after you drink a sugary liquid with no other food or beverage. Any variation from the normal range may be viewed with suspicion. If the highest reading is over 160 mg/cc, it may suggest pre-diabetes; if the lowest reading is thirty percent below your baseline, or below 60 mg/cc, you may have reactive hypoglycemia (more accurately called *unstable blood sugar*), an early stage of diabetes. If the difference between the highest and lowest readings is over 90 mg/cc, it may indicate a problem, as does a drop in sugar level of 60 points or more within an hour. Many other criteria exist to show deviations from normal—all of which take on more importance if other symptoms exist, such as dizziness, trembling, palpitations, brain fog, craving sweets, bingeing or other compulsive eating behaviors. If you have a family history of diabetes, it is essential that you be properly tested.

Insulin levels should be measured along with your blood-glucose levels, at the fasting and one- and two-hour stages. Your fasting insulin should be below 19 units. One hour after the glucose drink, your insulin should be under 100, and two hours after it should be below 60. I see some people in my practice with readings as high as 600.

Note: The GTT results are not considered accurate unless you are consuming at least 150 grams of carbs a day for at least four days before you take the test. Therefore, doing it after you start Atkins would mean

have to go back temporarily to eating a high-
ydrate diet (and almost certainly regain some
pounds you have just successfully lost).

If your GTT results point to problems in your body's ability to metabolize sugar, this alone should motivate you to change your diet. If your results are normal, you can count yourself fortunate that your new way of eating will forestall any future blood-sugar and insulin problems.

Let me remind you that although the Atkins plan has a positive effect on many conditions, if you have serious health problems, you must see your doctor before starting! You will need his or her help in monitoring your changing metabolism.

Now that you've addressed the medical issues, it's time to ready your kitchen, your loved ones and your own mind set. Don't skip any steps; each one will help make this one of the most rewarding experiences of your life.

TAKE YOUR MEASUREMENTS

Before you begin doing Atkins, use a tape measure to record some vital statistics. Measure your chest, waist, hips, upper arms and thighs, and write down those numbers! When you measure yourself again in a couple of weeks, you'll be happy you did; the more ways you have of gauging your success, the more encouraged you'll be.

FILL OUT THE BLOOD-SUGAR SYMPTOM TEST

This quiz on pages 150–151 is a great way to quantify how much better you'll soon be feeling. Go ahead and fill it out now but make a copy because you'll do it again in a couple of weeks, at which point I'm confident it will help spell out exactly how significantly your new way of eating will have affected your quality of life.

CONSIDER ADOPTING AN EXERCISE PLAN

If you aren't already exercising, I strongly urge you to start doing so now. Even a half hour of brisk walking four times a week will make a big difference, especially if you are almost completely inactive now. Exercise has enormous benefits for your health, and will speed your weight loss! It's a critical element of the healthy new you, and its importance cannot be underestimated.

HAVE THE RIGHT FOOD ON HAND

Stock the refrigerator and the cupboards with the food you're going to eat, including plenty of your favorite protein goodies. The next chapter will give you complete lists of acceptable and unacceptable foods specified for the Induction phase of Atkins.

When you go to the supermarket or health food store, avoid the aisles where the high-carbohydrate temptations are found. Whenever I give this advice, I think of John Connor. He was a 19-year-old, six-foot four-inch patient who dropped his weight from 290 pounds to 209 in six months by doing Atkins. He told me he'd often go to the supermarket to buy legitimate food, get sucked into one of the sugar-saturated aisles and end up walking out of the store with a package of candy bars. During his drive home, self-control would reassert itself, and he'd lower the car window and throw the package into the street!

What acceptable foods are your favorites? Do you love deviled eggs, turkey, chicken, shrimp salad, cheese? Have all these foods and more readily accessible in your refrigerator, along with plenty of low-carbohydrate vegetables and salad makings. I can't stress that enough. Better that a little food should be wasted than you should find yourself running out of the right foods and tempted by the wrong foods when hunger strikes.

Next, get rid of all the foods and beverages you won't be consuming. This is easiest if you live alone and don't need to worry about what anyone else wants in the refrigerator. Invite friends over to finish off the ice cream. Have a "carb blowout" party! Give away all your forbidden foods, perhaps to a shelter for the homeless or a food bank. As a last resort, just toss them. Alter your mental picture—for you, these foods no longer exist.

In addition to stocking up on the right foods, you'll want to purchase a good supply of the nutritional supplements I recommend and lipolysis testing strips, all of which you will learn about in Chapter 11. You'll also want to stock up on the wide variety of controlled carbohydrate foods available in your local health food store, drugstore or in most supermarkets.

GET YOUR LOVED ONES ON YOUR TEAM

If you don't live alone, prepare the people who live with you for the "shock" of your new eating style. Actually, unless your nearest and dearest are vegetarians, it shouldn't be too shocking. You will be eating things you've always eaten, but passing up the dishes and items full of carbohydrates.

If you are the chief cook and bottle washer, unless you can convince the other members of your household to share the Atkins experience with you, you'll simply have to cook for yourself and prepare a few additions for them. If they want bread, potatoes and dessert, you may have to suffer a little temptation, but if you really want to lose weight you'll bite the bullet and not the breadstick.

Keep this comforting thought in mind: Human beings are remarkably adaptable, and, in as little as a week, your tastes will start to change. Soon you'll find that sugar and refined carbohydrates don't tempt you as much as they used to. Your other great ally will be the appetite suppression that I've told you is a natural consequence of this nutritional plan.

If, for the first few days, you find it a downer watching other folks eating foods that you're fond of and can't touch, remind yourself that right now weight loss is your destiny. These moments of temptation are fleeting. Tell family mem-

That's What Friends Are For

Some people are lucky—they don't do Atkins alone. Ernesto and Donna Santiago had the perfect buddy system: The two both wanted to lose weight. Ernesto is a construction worker, and, at five feet eleven inches and 258 pounds, this 42-year-old was definitely hefty. At five feet nine inches tall Donna weighed 210. One day this 36-year-old saw pictures of herself on videotape and broke down in tears.

The two of them decided to come to the Atkins Center for Complementary Medicine and soon began doing Atkins.

Ernesto says: "When I was tempted to cheat, Donna helped me stay strong. And when she was tempted, I'd help her." As they were slimming down, they started taking martial arts classes together, and this brought them even closer. After two months doing Atkins, they had each dropped 30 pounds. It took about eight months for Donna to reach 147 and Ernesto to get down to 182. I've seen pictures of them training in ju-jitsu, and they look like a pretty trim couple to me. Incidentally, Donna lowered her LDL cholesterol from 189 to 137 and raised her HDL from 58 to 74. And Ernesto lowered his LDL from 159 to 126 and raised his HDL from 42 to 62. No cardiologist could ask for anything more.

It is often easier to try something new if you have a partner to share your experience with. If you don't have one, come to our website at *www.atkinscenter.com*. We'll serve as your surrogate partner and help reinforce that your efforts will provide you with a healthier life. Or find a friend or co-worker to support each other's efforts.

bers that you need a strong show of support and understanding. You certainly don't want them tempting you with illicit food and saying such inappropriate things as "Don't worry, this tiny piece of cake won't hurt you." It will!

Tell people in advance that you take Atkins seriously and that you'd appreciate their doing the same. We all know what a tricky, emotion-laden business food is. It's not uncommon for families to have issues surrounding food. I understand that the other people in your house may not be entranced with your new eating regimen. In the nicest possible way, tell them it's your lifestyle, not theirs. All they need to do is show respect for the major decision you've made. You're about to lose a lot of weight and gain a lot of health. After you've done Atkins, you won't need to request respect for it; the results will speak for themselves.

A Matter of Morale

Psychologically, have you made a firm commitment? Don't start something this important with the shallow notion of "Oh well, I'll give it a whirl." At the least, you should have decided that you're going to commit two weeks of your life—without deviation or compromise—to doing Atkins.

If you can commit yourself to that, I expect great things for you. By the end of two weeks, you'll be walking with new energy, getting out of bed in the morning with new zest and joyously anticipating your encounters with the bathroom scale. You'll be so impressed with how you look and feel, continuing with the program for life will be a foregone conclusion!

A note about that new energy and zest: Are you ready to increase your current level of physical activity? Another important step in getting ready is to read Chapter 22 and have your exercise plan in place. (You may not want to implement this plan, however, until after the first two days on Atkins. In that forty-eight-hour period, you may feel tired and a bit off-kilter as your body makes its conversion from burning glucose to burning fat as its primary fuel.)

KEY POINTS!

- Over-the-counter and certain prescription drugs can interfere with weight loss.
- Get a medical checkup to determine your overall physical health and have blood and other tests done that will serve as a baseline for comparison later.
- A five-hour glucose-tolerance test with insulin levels will evaluate the degree of stress on your glucose-insulin-regulating mechanism before you begin Atkins.
- Typically, after six weeks doing Atkins, you can expect to see improvement in virtually all health indicators.
- Practical and psychological preparation is also key to success on Atkins.

A FREQUENTLY ASKED QUESTION:

My cholesterol has gone up since I started doing Atkins. What can I do about it?

Examine the foods you've been eating. Have you been doing Atkins correctly? If you are just starting, be sure you follow the Rules of Induction (see Chapter 11). You may also want to consider a couple of other things that could be happening. First, the increase might be temporary. When a person loses weight, cholesterol usually rises because the body must break down stored fat for energy. Your total cholesterol should drop within two months.

Also, remember to look at your HDL (good cholesterol) levels. A rise in total cholesterol levels could even be a good thing, if it's all attributed to HDL cholesterol. Total cholesterol may temporarily go up due to the rise in HDL.

If you've been following the Atkins Nutritional Approach for some time and your cholesterol levels have not come down, something else is going on. Exercise is an important component, as is cutting back on processed meats, such as bacon, sausage and cold cuts, and limiting your intake of hard cheese. You may also need to look at a third component of your blood tests: triglycerides. Cholesterol rises in some people when triglycerides drop significantly. If that drop is greater than the LDL increase, your lipid profile may, again, be improved overall.

High cholesterol that has a genetic component usually responds to changes in diet, but may be difficult to address with diet alone. You may still need to take supplements such as pantethine, essential oils, garlic and fiber. For a detailed discussion of cholesterol-lowering nutrients, see *Dr. Atkins' Vita-Nutrient Solution*.

TIPS:

- Give your high-carb foods to a soup kitchen or homeless shelter.
- Stock the pantry and refrigerator with your favorite protein goodies.
- Your children may have inherited your blood-sugar imbalances. Eliminating sugar- and white-flour-laden junk food from their diets too may be the greatest gift you ever give them.
- Ask your family and friends for their support.
- Find an Atkins buddy to share your weight loss journey.

CAUTIONS:

- People with severe kidney disease should not do Atkins.
- The weight loss phases of the Atkins Nutritional Approach are not appropriate for pregnant women and nursing mothers.
- If you are currently taking diuretics, insulin or oral diabetes medications, you must undertake Atkins only under the guidance of a physician. Your decreasing reliance on these medications must be monitored and carefully adjusted.

11

And Away You Go: The Induction Phase

First of all, let me welcome those of you who are starting the book at this point. While I admire your sense of efficiency, I think you are cheating yourself of the information that will provide long-term success. Only by reading the first ten chapters will you have a full understanding of *why* Atkins *works* and of the preparations that will increase your chances for permanent lifetime control of your weight, long-term health and well-being.

Induction is only the first phase—the way you get the weight loss ball rolling—not the whole Atkins Nutritional Approach. I call it Induction because its purpose is to *induce* weight loss by changing your body's chemistry so that you will achieve, perhaps for the first time in your life, lipolysis and the companion process of ketosis, as explained in Chapter 6. Induction is designed to do all of the following for you:

- Efficiently switch your body from a carbohydrate-burning metabolism to a primarily fat-burning (your fat!) metabolism.
- Stabilize your blood sugar and abruptly halt a myriad of symptoms indicative of unstable blood sugar, such as

fatigue, mood swings, brain fog and an inability to function at your best.

- Curb your cravings by stabilizing your blood sugar.
- Break addictions to foods such as sugar, wheat or corn derivatives, alcohol, caffeine, grain or any other food. For people addicted to sugary, high-carb or high-glycemic foods—just as for alcoholics—moderation simply does not work.
- Let you experience firsthand the metabolic advantage discussed in Chapter 7.
- Knock your socks off by demonstrating how much body fat you can burn, while eating liberally, even luxuriously, off the fat of the land.

The Induction phase is not going to be your lifelong way of eating. It will last a minimum of fourteen days, after which you should see a significant result.

In a later phase, I will teach you a series of steps that will enable you to craft your own personalized eating plan. This plan will be geared to create the best possible balance between your metabolic responses, your tastes and lifestyle and your total health profile.

Rules of Induction

Another purpose of the Induction phase is to demonstrate to you that *even you* can lose weight while eating luxuriously. But it must be followed precisely for success! If you do it at all incorrectly you may prevent weight loss and end up saying, "Here is another weight loss plan that didn't work." So I want you to memorize the following twelve rules as though your life depends upon it. It does.

1. Eat either three regular-size meals a day or four or five smaller meals. Do not skip meals or go more than six waking hours without eating.

2. Eat liberally of combinations of fat and protein in the form of poultry, fish, shellfish, eggs and red meat, as well as of pure, natural fat in the form of butter, mayonnaise, olive oil, safflower, sunflower and other vegetable oils (preferably expeller-pressed or cold-pressed).

3. Eat no more than 20 grams a day of carbohydrate, most of which must come in the form of salad greens and other vegetables. You can eat approximately three cups—loosely packed—of salad, or two cups of salad plus one cup of other vegetables (see the list of acceptable vegetables on pages 125–126).

4. Eat absolutely no fruit, bread, pasta, grains, starchy vegetables or dairy products other than cheese, cream or butter. Do not eat nuts or seeds in the first two weeks. Foods that combine protein and carbohydrates, such as chickpeas, kidney beans and other legumes, are not permitted at this time.

5. Eat nothing that is not on the acceptable foods list. And that means absolutely nothing! Your "just this one taste won't hurt" rationalization is the kiss of failure during this phase of Atkins.

6. Adjust the quantity you eat to suit your appetite, especially as it decreases. When hungry, eat the amount that makes you feel satisfied but not stuffed. When not hungry, eat a small controlled carbohydrate snack to accompany your nutritional supplements.

7. Don't assume any food is low in carbohydrate—instead read labels! Check the carb count (it's on every package) or use the carbohydrate gram counter in this book.

8. Eat out as often as you wish but be on guard for hidden carbs in gravies, sauces and dressings. Gravy is often made with flour or cornstarch, and sugar is sometimes an ingredient in salad dressing.

9. Avoid foods or drinks sweetened with aspartame. Instead, use sucralose or saccharin. Be sure to count each packet of any of these as 1 gram of carbs.
10. Avoid coffee, tea and soft drinks that contain caffeine. Excessive caffeine has been shown to cause low blood sugar, which can make you crave sugar.
11. Drink at least eight 8-ounce glasses of water each day to hydrate your body, avoid constipation and flush out the by-products of burning fat.
12. If you are constipated, mix a tablespoon or more of psyllium husks in a cup or more of water and drink daily. Or mix ground flaxseed into a shake or sprinkle wheat bran on a salad or vegetables.

ACCEPTABLE FOODS

Foods you may eat liberally:

All fish including:	All fowl including:	All shellfish including:	All meat including:	All eggs including:
tuna	chicken	oysters*	beef	scrambled
salmon	turkey	mussels*	pork	fried
sole	duck	lobster	lamb	poached
trout	goose	clams	bacon**	soft-boiled
flounder	cornish hen	squid	veal	hard-boiled
sardines	quail	shrimp	ham**	deviled
herring	pheasant	crabmeat	venison	omelettes

---

*Oysters and mussels are higher in carbs than other shellfish so limit them to four ounces per day.
**Processed meats such as ham, bacon, pepperoni, salami, hot dogs and other luncheon meats—and some fish—may be cured with added sugar and will contribute carbs. Try to avoid meat and fish products cured with nitrates, which are known carcinogens. Also beware of products that are not exclusively meat, fish or fowl, such as imitation fish, meatloaf and breaded foods. Finally, do not consume more than four ounces of organ meats a day.

OTHER FOODS ACCEPTABLE DURING INDUCTION

Cheese
You can consume three to four ounces daily of the following full-fat, firm, soft, and semi-soft aged cheeses*, including:

cheddar
cow, sheep and goat cheese
cream cheese
Gouda
mozzarella
Roquefort and other blue cheeses
Swiss

Salad Vegetables
You can have two to three cups per day:

alfalfa sprouts	daikon	mushrooms
arugula	endive	parsley
bok choy	escarole	peppers
celery	fennel	radicchio
chicory	jicama	radishes
chives	lettuce	romaine
cucumber	mâche	sorrel

These salad vegetables are high in phytonutrients and provide a good source of fiber.

---

*All cheeses have some carbohydrate content. The quantity you eat should be governed by that knowledge. The rule of thumb is to count one ounce of cheese as equivalent to one gram of carbohydrate. Note that cottage cheese, farmer's cheese and other fresh cheeses are not permitted during Induction. No "diet" cheese, cheese spreads or whey cheeses are permitted. Individuals with known yeast symptoms, dairy allergy or cheese intolerance must avoid cheese. Imitation cheese products are not allowed, except for soy or rice cheese—but check the carbohydrate content.

Other Vegetables

You can have one cup per day if salad does not exceed two cups—these vegetables are slightly higher in carbohydrate content than the salad vegetables:

artichoke	celery root	pumpkin
hearts	(celeriac)	rhubarb
asparagus	chard	sauerkraut
bamboo	collard greens	scallions
shoots	dandelion	snow peas
bean sprouts	greens	spaghetti squash
beet greens	eggplant	spinach
broccoli	hearts of palm	string or wax beans
broccoli rabe	kale	summer squash
brussels	kohlrabi	tomato
sprouts	leeks	turnips
cabbage	okra	water chestnuts
cauliflower	onion	zucchini

If a vegetable, such as spinach or tomato, cooks down significantly, it must be measured raw so as not to underestimate its carb count.

Salad Garnishes

crumbled crisp bacon
grated cheese
minced hard-boiled egg
sautéed mushrooms
sour cream

Spices

All spices to taste, but make sure none contain added sugar

Herbs

basil	garlic	rosemary
cayenne	ginger	sage
cilantro	oregano	tarragon
dill	pepper	thyme

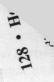

For salad dressing use oil and vinegar (but ~~~ vinegar, which contains sugar) or lemon juice a~~~ spices. Prepared salad dressings without added s~~~ more than two carbs per tablespoon serving are a~~~

Fats and Oils

Many fats, especially certain oils, are essential to good nutrition. Olive oil is particularly valuable. All other vegetable oils are allowed, the best being canola, walnut, soybean, grapeseed, sesame, sunflower and safflower oils, especially if they are labeled "cold-pressed" or "expeller-pressed." Do not cook polyunsaturated oils, such as corn, soybean and sunflower oil, at high temperatures or allow to brown or smoke.

Butter is allowed. Margarine should be avoided, not because of its carbohydrate content, but because it is usually made of trans fats (hydrogenated oils), which are a serious health hazard. (Some non-hydrogenated margarines are available in health food stores.)

You need not remove the skin and fat from meat or fowl. Salmon and other cold-water fish are an excellent source of omega-3 fatty acids.

I cannot stress strongly enough that trying to do a low-fat version of Atkins will interfere with fat burning and derail your weight loss.

Beverages

clear broth/bouillon (not all brands; read the label)
club soda
cream (heavy or light); limit to two to three tablespoons
    a day; note carbohydrate content
decaffeinated coffee or tea*

Excessive caffeine may cause unstable blood sugar and should be avoided by those who suspect they are caffeine dependent. Everyone should try to avoid caffeine. Grain beverages (coffee substitutes) are not allowed. Alcoholic beverages are also not permitted during Induction; those low in carbohydrates are an option, in moderation, in later phases.

et soda made with sucralose (Splenda®)
essence-flavored seltzer (must say "no calories" and must
   not contain aspartame)
herb tea (without barley or any fruit sugar added)
lemon juice or lime juice (note that each contains 2.8
   grams carbohydrate per ounce); limit to two to three
   tablespoons
mineral water
spring water
water

Artificial Sweeteners

You must determine which artificial sweeteners agree
with you, but the following are allowed: sucralose (marketed
at Splenda®), saccharin, cyclamate, acesulfame-K. Natural
sweeteners ending in the suffix "-ose," such as maltose, fructose, etc., should be avoided. However, certain sugar alcohols such as maltitol do not affect blood sugar and are
acceptable.

Saccharin has been extensively studied, and harmful effects were produced in the lab when fed to rats only in extremely high doses. The Food and Drug Administration
(FDA) has removed saccharin from its list of carcinogens,
basing its decision upon a thorough review of the medical
literature and the National Institute of Science's statement
that there is "no clear association between saccharin and
human cancer." It can be safely consumed in moderation,
meaning no more than three packets a day. Saccharin is
marketed as Sweet 'N Low®. We discourage the use of aspartame (marketed as NutraSweet® and Equal®). The FDA
has approved the herb stevia for use only as a supplement,
not as a sweetener.

My preference, however, is sucralose (Splenda®), the
only sweetener made from sugar. Sucralose is safe, non-
caloric and does *not* raise blood sugar. It has been used in
Canada for years, and the FDA recently approved it after re-

viewing more than one hundred studies conducted over the past twenty years.

Note that each packet of sugar substitute contains about 1 gram of carbohydrate, so don't forget to include the amount in your daily totals.

Special Category Foods

To add variety, each day you can also eat ten to twenty olives, half a small avocado, one ounce of sour cream or three ounces of unsweetened heavy cream, as well as two to three tablespoons of lemon juice or lime juice. But be aware that these foods occasionally slow down weight loss in some people, and may need to be avoided in the first two weeks. If you seem to be losing slowly, moderate your intake of these foods.

Convenience Foods

Although it is important that you eat primarily unprocessed foods, some controlled carb food products can come in handy when you are unable to find appropriate food, can't take time for a meal or need a quick snack. As I mentioned earlier, more and more companies are creating healthy food products that can be eaten during the Induction phase of Atkins. Just remember two things:

1. Not all convenience food products are the same, so check labels and carbohydrate content. I can vouch for any product carrying the Atkins brand name! (See Chapter 19 for more on these convenient options.)
2. While any of these foods can make doing Atkins easier, don't overdo it. Remember, you must always follow the Rules of Induction.

Avoid Pitfalls!

Here are five common pitfalls to avoid:

1. During Induction you must not eat *any* fruit, bread, grains, starchy vegetables or dairy products other than cheese, cream or butter.
2. Stay away from diet products unless they specifically state "no carbohydrates." Most such foods are for low-fat diets, not controlled carbohydrate plans.
3. The words *sugarless, sugar free* or *no sugar added* are not sufficient. The label must state the carbohydrate content; that's what you must go by.
4. Many products you do not normally think of as foods, such as chewing gum, breath mints, cough syrups and cough drops, are filled with sugar or other caloric sweeteners. They must be avoided.
5. Be wary of prepared salads at salad bars or deli counters. For example, cole slaw or even tuna fish salad may have been prepared with sugar.

How to Fashion a Food Plan from the Acceptable Foods List

During Induction and the other weight loss phases of Atkins, you will be consuming the types of foods and beverages aforementioned. Quality counts! Always aim for unprocessed natural foods and select the freshest produce you can find. If possible, purchase organic meats and dairy products.

Now that you know what foods you can eat, a meal plan should leap out at you. You should instantly see that for breakfast a ham, cheese and mushroom omelette, or nitrate-free bacon and scrambled eggs, or slices of smoked salmon wrapped around cream cheese would start off the day on the right note.

For lunch, the typical chef's salad with chicken, nitrate-free ham, cheese and hard-boiled egg on a bed of greens, covered with a creamy garlic dressing, will qualify, as will a cheeseburger without the bun. (Avoid ketchup, which contains sugar.) Or maybe a chicken Caesar salad (skip the croutons) or a scoop of homemade tuna or chicken salad.

Base your dinners around your favorite protein main courses—lamb chops, poached salmon, roast chicken, filet mignon, buttered lobster tails, seafood mixed grill or whatever you fancy—plus a salad. You might even have an appetizer such as shrimp cocktail with a mustard and mayonnaise sauce (cocktail sauce has carbohydrates), paté or steamed clams in garlic butter. And for dessert, have assorted cheeses or flavored gelatin made with sucralose and topped with whipped heavy cream.

You are more likely to enjoy gourmet meals doing Atkins than on the low-fat diets that still wearily make the rounds. But, for the moment, I merely want to introduce you to the notion that gourmet dining will be yours once you master all the possibilities offered by a nutritional plan that allows an intelligent and reasonable use of high-fat ingredients, including butter. Here and now, your attention should be totally focused on whether you feel you are in control of your eating and whether you feel healthy. Remember, during Induction my intention is to make you realize it is possible to be liberated from constant food cravings aggravated by unstable blood sugar. When you experience this liberation—and most significantly overweight people do—try to savor it. Notice how different it makes you feel. And remember it's something you can enjoy only on a controlled carbohydrate eating plan.

Nutritional Supplements

The foods you will be eating are tasty and nutrient-rich. But in starting people on my program, I have found that their vitamin and mineral reserves are often so depleted from the way they were eating before that it frequently takes a week or two of supplementation with vitanutrients to build them up again. This is one of the many reasons that, after a few days on Induction, you're likely to experience a burst of energy.

Some critics of controlled carbohydrate weight reduction have made the suggestion that Atkins is so restrictive of certain foods that I have no choice but to advise everyone who goes on it to take vitamin and mineral supplements. There's only a smidgen of truth in this; when you go down to a low level of vegetable consumption during Induction—the strictest phase of the program—you may be getting inadequate portions of certain nutrients. I stress *may*, because if you choose nutrient-dense foods, it is easy to consume adequate amounts of most vitanutrients.

On the facing page is a sample daily menu to be followed by a person in the Induction phase. The two graphs on page 134 show that the menu, as analyzed using the most widely accepted nutritional software program, "Nutritionist V," provides the recommended daily intake of almost all vitamins and minerals.

Sample Daily Menu of 20 Grams of Carbohydrate

Breakfast
Three-egg omelette with avocado
Mozzarella cheese and tomato
Decaffeinated coffee with cream

Lunch
Beef round steak (8 oz)
Spinach and mixed leaf salad with mushrooms, onions, celery and parmesan cheese

Dinner
Broiled salmon (9 oz)
Kale topped with garlic, lemon and sesame seeds

But the real reason you'll need vitanutrients is because of the way you've likely been eating for years, or because of the low-fat diet that you may be following even as you read this. If you have been on a low-fat diet, your need for supplementation may be profound. You will have to play catch-up to make up for possible deficiencies of essential fatty acids, vitamin B_{12} and the fat-soluble vitamins A, D and E. Several minerals are also in short supply on virtually all low-fat diets.

If you've been bingeing on junk food full of sugar and bleached flour, then you've been consuming anti-nutrients, and your nutritional needs are even greater. When you eat such foods you're doing more than just depriving yourself of sufficient supplies of important vitamins and minerals. Metabolizing those empty refined foods uses up what little stores of nutrients remain. I am always surprised when I encounter anyone over 35 years of age who eats the typical American diet of refined carbohydrates and isn't chronically tired. Chromium, zinc, manganese, magnesium, vitamin B_6

In this nutrient analysis of the sample Induction menu on page 133 with 20 grams of carbohydrates, even the strictest phase of the Atkins Nutritional Approach meets or exceeds the recommended daily allowance of almost all VITAMINS.

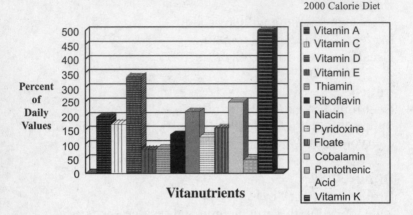

In this nutrient analysis of the sample Induction menu on page 133 with 20 grams of carbohydrates, even the strictest phase of the Atkins Nutritional Approach meets or exceeds the recommended daily allowance of almost all MINERALS.

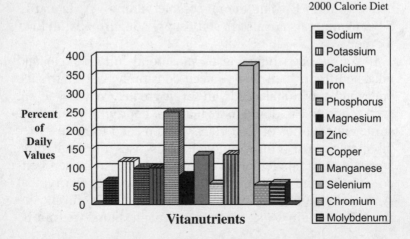

and folic acid are among the nutrients that are used up faster than they can be replenished on such a diet. In fact, many Americans are deficient in chromium, a mineral needed to metabolize carbohydrate.

Another reason you need vitanutrients is to maximize your body's ability to function optimally as a fat-burning unit.

Supplements for Everyone

The more I learn about nutritional supplements, the more I discover nutritional components that can help nearly everyone. With the increasing depletion of nutrients in our soil, there is simply no way we can ensure that we get all we require from food. In fact, I consider individualized prescription of vitanutrients programs to be one of the two pillars of nutritional medicine. For the overweight, this program, of course, is the other pillar. (Actually, controlling carbohydrate intake is the key to good health in general, even if you do not have a weight problem.) The operative word is *individualized*, for each person requires a different roster of vitanutrients, depending upon his or her individual health profile.

I won't spend a lot of space in this book describing all the many ways vitanutrients can help you overcome health problems. If you ever need information on how nutrients can solve health problems better than drugs do, you'll find it in *Dr. Atkins' Vita-Nutrient Solution.*

In this chapter, however, all I want to do is provide adequate nutritional support for Induction. When you opt to become a lifetime Atkins follower (notice, I didn't say "if"), you will have to familiarize yourself with the content of Chapter 23. But for now, these are the nutritional supplements you should be taking during Induction:

- A broad multiple vitamin and mineral supplement that contains considerably more than the recommended daily intake (RDI) of B complex factors and vitamin C, and that also contains at least thirty other different nutrients (and no iron). Ideally, chromium picolinate or polynicotinate (between 200 and 600 mcg) should be included.

- Essential fatty acids (EFA). EFA-deficiency may be the most prevalent dietary shortage in our culture, thanks to the misguided obsession with avoiding dietary fat and the overconsumption of trans fats instead of healthy natural fats. An EFA supplement should include gamma-linolenic acid (GLA)—primarily found in primrose or borage oil—and omega-3 fatty acids from fish oil or flaxseed oil. (You can, of course, also eat salmon and other cold-water fish.)
- If you have sugar cravings, you should also take 500 mg of L-glutamine (one or two tablets) prior to each meal. L-glutamine has been shown to curb alcohol addiction as well. If you previously ate lots of carbohydrates, this will help to ease the transition to controlled carbohydrate eating.

As mentioned in the Rules of Induction, you should also be supplementing with one or another form of fiber, usually wheat bran or psyllium husks, to prevent constipation. For more on the benefits of fiber, see "Fiber: A Form of Carbohydrate" on pages 75–76.

Blast Off! You've Begun—Munch Away.

So, here we go. You're doing Atkins, and naturally you begin by eating—something you've previously done with some degree of guilt. Say good-bye to all that. It's time to plow into those prime ribs and that cheese omelette. You must have faith. As you savor high-calorie food you always thought would make you fat, you can now relax. When carbohydrates are sufficiently reduced, the body has no choice

Lipolysis Testing Strips: Proof Positive

Lipolysis testing strips (LTS) measure the ketones—the markers that confirm your body is in lipolysis and the secondary process of ketosis—in your urine. The strips will change to pink or purple, depending upon how many ketones are present. The more ketones you excrete, and therefore the greater degree of ketosis you are in, the darker the color. (Lipolysis testing strips are available under the brand names of Lipostix, which are designed for people following a controlled carb weight loss program, or Ketostix, which are designed to warn of ketoacidosis in diabetics. However, both are quite serviceable as lipolysis testing strips. LTS are relatively inexpensive.)

You don't have to use LTS, but doing so can be an extremely convenient aid to doing Atkins. My patients often tell me that they find the strips psychologically supporting. To see them go from beige to pink or purple is to receive in chemical code the message "you're burning fat." On the other hand, if you're not getting the results you expect, they will surely help clear up the mystery of what is standing in your way.

After all, the clear premise for Induction is to switch you into a primarily fat-burning metabolism by sharply controlling carb intake. Your LTS will help measure the extent to which you've done so. Later, as you move through the other phases and increase your carbohydrate intake, the strips are no longer needed. As long as you continue to lose weight gradually, lose inches, have your appetite under control and experience none of your old symptoms, you are clearly burning fat. Moreover, in most cases the LTS will no longer turn pink or purple once you are taking in 50 or more grams of carbs a day, so they are of no use as people get above that level of carb intake.

What If They Don't Turn?

First, make sure that none of your foods—except your salad and other vegetables—contain carbohydrate, meaning no hidden sugars, no breading, etc. Then strictly follow Induction for five days. If the LTS still haven't changed to at least pink, measure your salads to make sure you are not eating too many veggies. Still no change? Try cutting out tomatoes and onions, which are both relatively high on the glycemic index. Finally, make sure you are not consuming excess quantities of protein. When eaten to excess, protein converts to glucose.

However, should your LTS not turn pink or purple, despite the fact that you are doing everything correctly, you may still show a decrease in appetite, an improvement in well-being, a loosening of your clothes and a slow but steady weight loss and reduction in inches. This simply means that you are not producing enough ketones to register on the LTS but enough to burn fat. Remember, the strips are tools; making them change color is not the sole object of the game.

---

but to burn its own fat. Moreover, at this stage, eating rich, fatty foods can only be advantageous.

I encourage you to eat until you're satisfied. Just don't confuse being satisfied with being stuffed. If you have been overweight for a long time, it may take you a while to distinguish between the two sensations. If you are not sure, stop eating before you feel full and see if you are still hungry a few minutes later. If you are, have a few more bites and stop again. Repeat until you are satisfied. Soon you will discover you are pleasantly full sooner and can avoid that feeling of getting up from the table feeling as stuffed as a Thanksgiving turkey.

For the first few weeks, I want you to be unafraid of natural fat (butter, cream, cheese, olive oil and the fat in meats, poultry and fish), but remember to stay away from those evil trans fats, which are labeled as hydrogenated and partially hydrogenated fats. The ease of getting into deep lipolysis is based on the ratio of fat (not protein) to carbohydrate. Thus, you should strive for an adequate amount of fat during this initial period, and, in doing so, you will almost certainly find yourself experiencing the most appetite-suppressing aspects of Atkins.

What's the First Thing You'll Notice?

After a couple of days you will find you are in control of your appetite. That's because once your body's two-day supply of glycogen (stored glucose) diminishes and you make the switch to primarily burning fat, lipolysis suppresses your appetite. Suddenly, you find yourself eating moderate portions without constant hunger pangs and no longer obsessing about food. You know you're in lipolysis when you find yourself saying, "You mean lunchtime was an hour ago?"

When you consume a so-called "balanced" diet high in carbohydrates, the first fuel your body burns for energy comes from those carbohydrates. Now that you've lowered your carbohydrate consumption to a level that can't finance your energy expenditures, you must burn your stored fat. Your body draws upon those stores of fat—easily, if you're metabolically average; reluctantly, if you're metabolically resistant.

You may be a person for whom incessant, almost hourly food cravings have been a way of life. Remember Gordon Lingard, the patient who came to see me weighing 306 pounds? He used to say, "I'd always be planning the next binge. I'd be in a business meeting, very serious, a lot of money at stake, and one-half of my brain would be figuring out what I would eat, how much I would eat, when and where I would eat. Food had seized my brain."

Now that's enslavement to food. Gordon ultimately succeeded, and if he could do it, you can, too. Superhuman willpower is not required to do Atkins, only the wisdom to put yourself into a position where you won't need it.

Welcome Back: Your Old Friend Energy

The next thing that will strike most of you is a sense that you've latched onto some misplaced, long-lost energy level. Typically, this feeling arrives around about the third or fourth day. Some people experience a slight euphoria. Most simply find they no longer have to suffer those dreary, weary periods that used to hit them a couple of times a day.

That said, there are a few people who experience fatigue or light-headedness during their first week doing Atkins. Most often this means that the process is going too fast for their particular metabolism—they're losing weight too fast, losing water and certain minerals too fast, and their bodies can't keep pace with these quick changes. One sign is ascent weakness: You feel weak walking up stairs. These reactions can be aggravated by hot weather, when you are already losing minerals through sweat, or by taking a diuretic. Obviously, drinking lots of water is essential.

Usually, I advise patients who have these problems to slow down the weight loss. They should add another helping of vegetables to their evening meal or one or two ounces of nuts or seeds. Although their bodies would almost certainly adjust during the second week, there isn't any good reason for feeling washed out and sickly for even one day. After the symptoms abate, go back to the lower level of carb intake.

Another problem people occasionally experience is leg cramps at night due to a rapid excretion of calcium, magnesium or potassium. Be sure you are getting enough of these minerals in your multivitamin or take a separate multimineral supplement. If you are still getting leg cramps, you may need to add more. Bear in mind that the FDA does not allow over-the-counter sales of anywhere near the proper amount of potassium you may need; therefore, you may need a doctor to write you the proper prescription.

Addiction and Withdrawal

Another mechanism that can cause adverse reactions is withdrawal symptoms. Quite a few people have addictions to foods they consume every day without being aware of them. When you suddenly stop eating a food or ingredient you are used to, as you do when you start Atkins, you may experience withdrawal. Common offenders are caffeine, sugar, wheat and other foods capable of quickly changing blood-sugar levels. Withdrawal symptoms vary widely, ranging from fatigue, faintness and palpitations to headache and cold sweats.

Bad as they seem, experiencing withdrawal symptoms is really good news. The withdrawal process is usually completed within three days, and afterward you should feel better than ever, unless, of course, you re-addict yourself. If you cannot stay the course and progress through withdrawal, do it gradually by consuming progressively smaller amounts of an addictive food until you get to zero. (For help on identifying which food is causing the problem, see Chapter 26 on food intolerances.) The more severe your withdrawal symptoms, the more you stand to gain from abandoning the food that is causing them. A food that demands to be eaten daily is often a key to a disordered metabolism. It can run your life, as well as ruin it.

Most people—even people with food addictions once withdrawal symptoms abate—experience a significant energy lift. It tends to send them roaring on through Induction because it's such clear evidence of the positive influence their dietary change is having on their metabolism.

You'll notice that I have not yet mentioned weight. Unless you are extremely metabolically resistant, you will start losing considerable weight during Induction. The amount and rate at which you lose can vary dramatically depending upon your age, level of activity, whether you are taking hormones or other drugs, your degree of metabolic resistance and other factors. The median weight loss from two weeks doing Induction is 10 pounds for overweight males and 6 pounds for overweight females. But do understand this: On any weight loss program, the first weight lost is water weight. Atkins is a particularly effective diuretic, so the water weight tends to come off fast on my program. But be assured that after four to five days, the pounds that come off are primarily fat.

Congratulations! You are really doing Atkins now. I'm very happy for you. With my help, Induction will be just the first step of a natural progression to your permanent way of healthy eating.

KEY POINTS!

- Induction is designed to switch your body from burning carbohydrate for energy to burning primarily fat for energy.
- Fat burning helps control your appetite.
- Withdrawal symptoms, caused by food addictions, may occur, but will subside within a few days.
- By the end of the first week most people find that they have more energy and feel better.
- Lipolysis testing strips (LTS) measure the presence of ketones in your urine, gauging your fat-burning status.

A FREQUENTLY ASKED QUESTION (OR TWO):

I'm used to counting calories. How many am I allowed during Induction?
There is no need to count calories. The Atkins Nutritional Approach counts grams of carbohydrates instead of calories. At the beginning of Induction you are allowed 20 grams of carbohydrates, gradually adding them in 5-gram increments as you progress from Ongoing Weight Loss to Pre-Maintenance, and finally to the Lifetime Maintenance phase of Atkins.

Although there is no need to count calories, they do matter. Gaining weight results from taking in more calories than you expend through exercise, thermogenesis (the body's own heat production) and other metabolic functions. Research has shown that on a controlled carbohydrate program, more calories are burned than in a low-fat/high-carb diet, so there is a certain metabolic advantage to the controlled carb approach. But understand that this does not give you a license to gorge.

No matter what I do, I can't get into ketosis, or the shade of purple on the LTS is very light. What am I doing wrong?
There are many reasons why a person's lipolysis test strip would be varying shades of purple. Each person's metabolism is different and therefore will turn the sticks a varying degree of purple. In addition, the time of the day, whether or not you exercise and what you ate at your last meal will all affect the test strips. Don't worry about the exact level of ketosis indicated by the strip. The important thing is to see how your clothes are fitting and what the scale says. And, remember, you don't necessarily need to use the strips at all.

TIPS:

- Limit sweeteners to three packets a day.
- If you use lipolysis testing strips to measure ketone output, be sure to do so at the same hour each day.
- When looking at food labels, be aware that "low fat" generally means "high carb."
- If you start Induction before or during a menstrual period, it may take longer for weight loss to register.
- Try not to weigh yourself every day, and, if possible, aim for just once a week.
- Don't make the common mistake of eating less fat to get into ketosis; the opposite is actually true.

12

Time to Review Your Results

You did it! After doing Atkins for a mere fourteen days, you're probably so blown away by the changes you've experienced that you have no desire to go back to your old way of eating. That's why the two-week marker is a logical time for evaluation. You will be past any difficulties you faced during the transition and should be feeling slimmer and more energetic already.

You Gotta Hang in There

Of course, some people have difficulties at the very start. At 39, Alan McCarthy was a successful insurance executive, married and with a child on the way. Two months before his son's birth, Alan's father died of a heart attack. A year later, Alan's total cholesterol level hit 264.

"I was practically a clone of my father," recalls Alan. "Same pants size, same shoe size, same sky-high cholesterol." He worried that it would mean a quadruple bypass followed by premature death for him, too. Alan didn't know which way to turn.

Then fate, in the form of a co-worker, took a hand. His office buddy had succeeded on Atkins and believed it was particularly effective at reducing cholesterol. That was good enough for Alan.

But when he started Induction, sugar deprivation made him feel so lousy that, for the first two days, he thought he'd give up. Alan had always been a regular 300-grams-of-carbs-a-day American. Bean burritos, ice cream and every sugary treat that came within reach of his fast-moving hands went down the gullet.

"But then on the third and fourth days, my energy started ratcheting up to the same levels I used to have when I was younger and exercising regularly. I actually felt my metabolism increase; it was as if the furnace had been turned on. I lost 10 pounds in the first two weeks and by week four I'd dropped 15 pounds."

When Alan had his total cholesterol checked, it had dropped to 211. Twelve weeks after starting Atkins, he had lost 25 pounds and reached his goal weight.

His wife did her bit by cooking Atkins recipes. And Alan actually found that his tastes had changed. Sugary desserts, on the rare occasions that he tried them, now tasted too sweet.

"I used to avoid confrontation by telling people I was on a no-sugar diet," Alan says. "Now, I love converting skeptics. I also love being at my high school weight of 165 and having a total cholesterol of 179! Results don't lie!"

Will You Go On?

This is a logical time for you to decide whether you will continue doing Atkins. I hope you will. Most people do so not only because they're losing weight, but also because they feel so good. For many of you, especially if you're over 40, the most significant revelation of controlled carbohydrate eating is the discovery that some nagging physical ills, from headaches to various aches and pains, have completely vanished.

Some Questions to Ask

Before you decide anything, let's review your results to date, and I don't mean just how many pounds you have lost. Ask yourself these questions:

1. Is my appetite under control?
2. Am I experiencing food cravings?
3. Am I constipated?
4. Do I have leg cramps?
5. Have I noticed a difference in my measurements as well as in my weight?
6. Am I enjoying the food I'm eating?
7. Am I sleeping better? Do I have fewer aches and pains? Is my energy level during the day more stable than before? Am I able to concentrate better?

ANSWERS

1. **Hunger**
   Let's consider your answer to the first question. If you were hungry, you weren't following my counsel to eat as much as you needed to feel satisfied. Remember: If you have a tendency to become hungry between meals, pop a few olives, an ounce of cheese, a scoop of tuna salad, a slice of pot roast or a convenient controlled carbohydrate bar or shake.
2. **Cravings**
   If cravings continue, are you eating adequately and not skipping meals? Is there a hidden source of sugar in something you are eating? If none of the above applies, and you are just looking for a taste of something, consider a substitute product such as a controlled carb bar or something made with controlled carb bake mix.
3. **Constipation**
   A certain amount of constipation is common during the first week, but it can be resolved quickly and easily. As

you progress to later phases where you increase your carb consumption and thus your fiber intake, constipation should not be a problem. Meanwhile, follow the instructions in the previous chapter (See "Rules of Induction," #12). If the problem isn't solved, you may try a tablespoon of wheat bran sprinkled on your salad or other vegetables. If you are sensitive to grain products, add ground flaxseed to a shake or psyllium husks to a glass of water instead. (None of these fibers contain the kind of carbohydrates that impact on your blood-sugar levels.) Most important: Be absolutely sure to consume a minimum of eight 8-ounce glasses of water a day.

4. **Leg Cramps**

If you have leg cramps, it probably means you are losing too many electrolytes, which are full of minerals. Starting any weight loss program has a diuretic effect, which is one of the reasons it is so important to stay hydrated. Supplement with potassium, magnesium and calcium in addition to your multivitamin, and the cramps should disappear.

5. **Measurements**

I hope you've followed my suggestion to measure your chest, waist, hips, upper arms and thighs with a tape measure. The loss of inches is an indication of real success and sometimes occurs when weight loss is only marginal. Also, your weight can fluctuate from day to day, even from hour to hour, depending upon fluid balance, hormonal cycles, and the effects of medications, to name a few things. And exercise, if you go at it vigorously—and I hope you are following my advice to get moving—can cause some weight gain because it increases muscle mass, and muscle is denser than the fat it displaces. This is a good thing.

Even if these various factors cause you to lose pounds more slowly than you want, your tape measure will reveal that you are slimming down all over. Your loss of inches is of fundamental importance, for it represents real fat loss—the emptying of your fat cells. And I never underestimate the psychological importance of knowing one has made progress. But as with the scale, do not become obsessed with the tape measure either. You'll know the inches are disappearing because of the way your clothes fit. Pick an outfit that you can barely get into because it is so tight, then try it on every week and see if it doesn't start to feel more comfortable.

6. **Food Preferences**

Fortunately, most people enjoy protein food. If you are a strict vegetarian, you really can't do the Induction phase. (The three later phases could be managed but the food selections on a regimen that restricts carbohydrate and simultaneously excludes animal foods are limited.) In general, I've found that a person who will not eat any animal foods will not do Atkins permanently. They find it too boring. But if you are willing to eat fish and chicken, plus eggs and cheese, you can certainly do Atkins without eating red meat.

The rest of you can enjoy a delicious and satisfying way of eating. That is not to say that many people don't miss pasta and bread, as well as fruit and juice, the first two weeks. Soon enough in the later phases you will be able to add back fruit and even special controlled carb baked goods.

So why are people willing to do without foods that used to be so important to them to continue on Atkins? Simply this: The upside is so much larger than the downside. Weight loss, of course, but feeling physically better and in control of your eating are also paramount issues. I challenge you to tell me honestly that you do not feel better now than you did two weeks ago. And this is just the beginning.

7. **Feeling Good**

Now I want you to retake the test on pages 150–151 that you originally took in Chapter 10. If you have experienced improvements in some of these areas, this exercise will help motivate you to continue to do Atkins.

If you've been overweight for a long time, you will

almost certainly have suffered some of the symptoms in this test. No doubt you thought them a normal part of aging. Isn't it wonderful to see that you can make them go away simply by changing the way you eat?

Doing Atkins, you'll find that you're cleaning out a lot of metabolic garbage from your life, in addition to excess pounds and junk food. Many of my patients have discovered that instead of a weight loss program, this is for them a rejuvenation program. Now take the test, and see if I'm right!

Blood-Sugar Symptom Test

Choose each symptom according to the following:
0 = Never
1 = Mild and/or rare
2 = Moderate and/or up to twice a week
3 = Severe and/or more than twice a week

	0	1	2	3
hunger between meals				
eat candy, cake, soda				
drink alcohol				
drink more than 3 cups coffee/cola				
cravings for sweets or coffee				
irritable before meals				
shakiness inside especially if hungry				
faint if food is delayed				
tired all of the time				
depressed				
can't fall asleep easily				
waking during the night				
fearful				
difficulty making decisions				
difficulty with concentrating				
poor memory				
worried a lot				
feel insecure				

	0	1	2	3
emotional				
moodiness				
feel like crying				
outbursts of anger				
make mountains out of molehills				
feelings of hopelessness				
bored				
bad dreams				
anti-social behavior				
phobias				
can't work under pressure				
headaches				
sleepiness during the day				
sleepy after food				
slow starting in the morning				
poor motivation				
eat when nervous				
fatigue relieved by food				
excessive thirst				
nervous stomach/cramps				
allergies or sinus problems				
can feel heart beat				
gastritis, gastroesophageal reflux disorder, ulcers				
abdominal bloating				
cold hands and feet				
shaking of the hands				
blurring vision				
lightheaded/dizziness				
lack of coordination				
excessive sweating				
frequent urination				

Add each column and multiply by the number at the top of that column.

Add all together (Remember, all in the 0 column = 0).

If score is more than 50 = Positive for blood-sugar stress.

The Pounds Won't Move?

Though I've just emphasized the importance of measuring inches, I'd certainly also like to see you losing some weight. If you don't seem to be losing on the program, turn immediately to Chapter 20. Sometimes, very simple problems can get in the way of positive results. And simple problems usually mean simple solutions. Failure to lose weight doing Atkins is a rare phenomenon, and the odds are good that I can give you the ammunition you need to resolve your body's resistance to weight loss.

Success and Long-Term Satisfaction

The Atkins Nutritional Approach has four phases; moreover, it can be individualized for every person. The high-fat, deep-lipolysis Induction phase you've just experienced is the first and most carbohydrate-restrictive one. The vast majority of the time people spend doing Atkins is not spent in this first phase (after all, there's a phase called Lifetime Maintenance, which speaks for itself). The basic theme of any good nutritional approach is adaptability. With my help, you can easily map out your own, personalized plan within the Atkins approach.

The next chapter addresses the next step: Do you continue Induction or move to the next phase? Either way, what is important is being comfortable, contented and healthy. I want you to feel at ease doing Atkins: physically well, satisfied, pleased with your daily menu, comfortable in your body, confident that this time you will succeed for the long term.

Too Soon for New Tests

If you got your first round of blood-lipid and other tests done before you started Atkins, you may be chomping at the bit to have them redone to confirm your good results—and dispel any lingering concerns you have. I wholeheartedly agree that you should have new tests done, but not yet. Two weeks is too early to show significant changes; instead, wait at least six weeks. By then you'll have chemical confirmation of the wisdom you showed in deciding to do Atkins.

KEY POINTS!

- Induction lasts a minimum of fourteen days but can be safely followed much longer.
- After two weeks doing Induction, most people begin to feel dramatically better.
- Symptoms such as difficulty sleeping, aches and pains and general malaise are often related to excess weight and blood-sugar stress.

TIPS:

- Have a small controlled carbohydrate snack high in fat or protein if you are hungry between meals.
- Don't include decaf coffee or tea or other beverages as part of your daily water intake.
- Potassium, magnesium and calcium supplements will help prevent leg cramps.
- Wait at least six weeks to repeat your blood work.

13

Are You Ready for Phase Two?

By now you've probably seen some pretty dramatic changes in your body and are likely feeling euphoric as it begins to dawn on you that it's within your power to achieve the new you I talked about in Chapter 1. You are probably now catching glimpses of that new person on the horizon—if not in your own mirror. That new you is thinner, happier, healthier and more confident.

Now it's time for you to take a serious look at your body and decide what you want to do with it and how you want it to look. Be realistic. In all probability, you don't expect to be an Olympic athlete or a fashion model. On the other hand, you may be selling yourself short by setting goals that are too modest. Are you willing to accept "pleasingly plump"? Many of my patients come to me thinking that such goals would be quite all right—or even more than they dare hope for.

Frankly, I think you should set your sights higher than that. How about a weight target based on your height, age and bone structure? How about excellent health and vigor that's surprising for someone your age? Trust me, that's not being overly ambitious. That's being truly realistic.

What Is Your Goal Weight?

Ask yourself when in your life did you look and feel your very best? How much did you weigh then? Can you comfortably weigh that again? What size did you wear then? Don't skip over these questions. As I always say, you're the greatest expert on your body. Whatever that wonderful weight—and size—was, you can almost certainly reach it again. Was it 120? 140? 170?

Most people have a pretty good sense of that number. They held that weight for a good part of their lives and found that they gained weight only after specific events, such as getting married, having kids, quitting cigarettes, starting or stopping medication or experiencing certain hormonal changes. Why not go for it?

On the other hand, is that "perfect" weight unrealistic now that you're couple of decades older? Menopausal women particularly often have a hard time staying as slim as they once were. So perhaps a more realistic approach is to ask what is the weight you would be comfortable with today. The trick is to come up with a figure that is attainable without setting yourself up for disappointment.

Ted Asher set himself a goal weight of 170 pounds when he began Atkins. At five feet eight inches tall, this 34-year-old had reached a modestly prodigious 227 pounds. Could it be his bachelor's breakfast of two Pop-Tarts washed down with a can of soda? And perhaps that nutritional approach was causing his occasional bouts of gastrointestinal distress? One weekend Ted read an earlier edition of this book and started doing Atkins.

He stayed on Induction for a couple of months, and then gradually moved through the stages toward Lifetime Maintenance, stopping well short of 100 grams of carbs. He had lost 47 pounds by that time, taken up golfing and shared his doctor's pleasure at his cholesterol and triglyceride improvements. Along the way, he decided he felt pretty good at

180 pounds. He says he'd like to lose 10 more pounds but thinks they'll come off with a bit more exercise. I hope he gets that exercise, but he's right not to obsess over the last 10 pounds; he looks and feels fine, and his blood work shows the inside of him is now as healthy as the outside.

If you don't recall ever being a weight you were happy with, the Body Mass Index (BMI) chart on the opposite page should give you a ballpark figure to aim for. Be aware that the BMI is just a guideline: If you are very muscular, for example, your BMI will often come out too high.

You'll see that the BMI chart gives you numbers at the top. By checking your height and weight below and running your finger up the column to where the BMI figures are, you will find your BMI number. Based on these figures, the federal government has announced guidelines that create a new definition of a healthy weight—a BMI of up to 24.9. A BMI of 25 or above is considered overweight. If your BMI is 26 or 27, you are approximately twenty percent overweight. Individuals who fall within the BMI range of 25 to 34.9 and have a waist size of over forty inches for men and over thirty-five inches for women are considered to be at especially high health risk.

For most people, this chart is helpful as a general guideline—ranges that are considered the norm—but I can't emphasize this too strongly: The best weight for you is the one at which you feel comfortable and attractive and can enjoy your life. It also needs to be a weight you can maintain.

Say your best friend and you are the same height and generally the same build, but she wants to be rail thin, while you are comfortable with 10 pounds more on your frame—if it feels good to you, that's what counts. Remember, too, that if you are physically active and have a low BMI, you can weigh more than your sister, who thinks lifting a pencil is exercise.

This isn't climbing Mount Everest; you can reach your goal weight. I know that if you're metabolically similar to the tens of thousands of overweight patients I've treated over the last forty years, you have an excellent chance of succeeding.

Body Mass Index Chart

	19	20	21	22	23	24	25	26	27	28	29	30	31	32	33	34	35
Height (inches)					Body	Weight	(pounds)										
58	91	96	100	105	110	115	119	124	129	134	138	143	148	153	158	162	167
59	94	99	104	109	114	119	124	128	133	138	143	148	153	158	163	168	173
60	97	102	107	112	118	123	128	133	138	143	148	153	158	163	168	174	179
61	100	106	111	116	122	127	132	137	143	148	153	158	164	169	174	180	185
62	104	109	115	120	126	131	136	142	147	153	158	164	169	175	180	186	191
63	107	113	118	124	130	135	141	146	152	158	163	169	175	180	186	191	197
64	110	116	122	128	134	140	145	151	157	163	169	174	180	186	192	197	204
65	114	120	126	132	138	144	150	156	162	168	174	180	186	192	198	204	210
66	118	124	130	136	142	148	155	161	167	173	179	186	192	198	204	210	216
67	121	127	134	140	146	153	159	166	172	178	185	191	196	204	211	217	223
68	125	131	138	144	151	158	164	171	177	184	190	197	203	210	216	223	230
69	128	135	142	149	155	162	169	176	182	189	196	203	209	216	223	230	236
70	132	139	146	153	160	167	174	181	188	195	202	209	216	222	229	236	243
71	136	143	150	157	165	172	179	186	193	200	208	215	222	229	236	243	250
72	140	147	154	162	169	177	184	191	199	206	213	221	228	235	242	250	258
73	144	151	159	166	174	182	189	197	204	212	219	227	235	242	250	257	265
74	148	155	163	171	179	186	194	202	210	218	225	233	241	249	256	264	272
75	152	160	168	176	184	192	200	208	216	224	232	240	248	256	264	272	279
76	156	164	172	180	189	197	205	213	221	230	238	246	254	263	271	279	287

Source: Clinical Guidelines on the Identification, Evaluation, and Treatment of Overweight and Obesity in Adults, National Instititutes of Health, National Heart, Lung, and Blood Institute, June 1998.

How to Keep It Going

Now, let's talk about sustaining that weight loss, which you've so happily begun. You undoubtedly know exactly how much weight you lost during the first fourteen days of Induction. That number will help give you a general understanding of your personal degree of metabolic resistance. As you can see on the metabolic resistance table on page 158, a woman who has 40 pounds to lose and sheds 3 pounds in two weeks during Induction has a high degree of metabolic resistance as compared to a woman with similar weight loss goals who drops 8 pounds. For a complete discussion of metabolic resistance, please turn to Chapter 20.

Weight Loss During the First Two Weeks on a Fat-Burning Program for Patients at Three Levels of Obesity

Degree of Metabolic Resistance for Men

Pounds Lost in First 14 Days When Metabolic Resistance is high, average or low:

Pounds to Lose	High	Average	Low
Less than 20	4	6	8
20–50	6	9	12
Over 50	8	12	16

Degree of Metabolic Resistance for Women

Pounds Lost in First 14 Days When Metabolic Resistance is high, average or low:

Pounds to Lose	High	Average	Low
Less than 20	2	4	6
20–50	3	6	9
Over 50	4	8	12

As I'm sure you've guessed, the degree of resistance to weight loss that your body shows corresponds to your degree of difficulty in getting well into lipolysis. By definition, resistance to weight loss is resistance to lipolysis.

During Induction you were consuming about 20 grams of carbs per day. The carbohydrate level was extremely low because I wanted to demonstrate that it is possible for virtually everybody to experience lipolysis, or fat burning, from the person who can lose weight quite easily on almost any program to the hardest case—the person who, until doing Atkins, thought that losing weight was almost impossible.

I am sure that almost all of you found that you were losing weight. Those who didn't should look at Chapter 20 and work with the special weight loss plan I've devised for patients with extreme metabolic resistance. Many of you, however, are now looking forward to liberalizing your menu.

More Induction?

Before you even think about stepping up from Induction, consider the possibility of staying with it for a while longer. A lot of people think of Induction as *only* two weeks, but it can be followed for a longer time. If you have a lot of weight to lose or have difficulty losing weight, you might want to do Induction for quite a while. That way you'll see dramatic progress before moving on to the more moderate phases of the program.

Although Induction offers plenty of advantages, there are lots of valid reasons for progressing: boredom with the food choices, modest weight loss goals (say 20 or 30 pounds) and perhaps the chance to avoid becoming dependent on a "crash diet" mentality. When people learn that they can lose weight quickly, as they do during Induction, they sometimes take their ability to lose weight for granted. They don't think in terms of a lifetime commitment to the Atkins lifestyle— just a quick fix for overindulgence. The result of this faulty thinking is yo-yo dieting and metabolic resistance to weight loss. While the next phase—Ongoing Weight Loss or OWL—may likely slow your rate of weight loss, this is not a bad thing. The slower the progress, the more chance you have to permanently change bad habits over the long term.

In order to decide if this is the right time for you to move on, I suggest you answer the following four questions:

1. Are you bored with Induction?
2. How much weight do you have to lose?
3. How metabolically resistant are you to weight loss?
4. Are you willing to slow down the pace of weight loss in exchange for more food choices?

If you are bored, and this boredom could lead to not complying with the Rules of Induction, by all means move on to OWL after two weeks. However, if you are comfortable staying in this phase, and you still have a lot of weight to lose, you can do Induction safely for six months or more. If you do not have much more weight to lose, it is advisable for you to advance to OWL so you can cycle through all the phases of the program.

If you are metabolically resistant to weight loss, which you will know by how much weight you lost in the first two weeks and by comparing your results with the categories in the metabolic resistance tables on page 158, you will lose weight relatively slowly. People with high metabolic resistance can benefit from doing Induction longer because it gives them time to correct metabolic imbalances they may have developed over time. These include insulin resistance, blood-sugar imbalances, carbohydrate addictions and allergies. Once the metabolic imbalances are corrected, weight loss may speed up.

But after all is said and done, to a large degree, your decision to continue Induction or move to OWL will depend on your personality and lifestyle. If you are the type to just go for it and can easily make your life work around the Induction eating program, you may decide to stick with it until you drop some more weight. Another person, who perhaps is under a lot of stress and wants to relax a bit about food choices, might choose to move to the more liberal phase of OWL. This brings us to the last, and ultimately the only, answer that matters. Is a longer period of time until you get to your goal weight the tradeoff you're willing to make to have more food choices? It's up to you.

The Choice Was Theirs

The two people I am about to introduce you to are good examples of how much individualization is possible in the transition process from Induction to OWL. A high school principal, Dan Wilson was up to 323 pounds on a five-foot ten-inch frame, when he stumbled upon his mother-in-law's copy of a previous edition of this book.

In his first two weeks doing Induction—abandoning his usual breakfast of M & M's washed down with Mountain Dew—Dan lost 18 pounds. Pleased with his progress, he went immediately to OWL, and within a few weeks he was consuming between 30 and 40 grams of carbs a day.

A former gym teacher, Dan resumed a high level of physical activity and continued to lose weight so easily that after a month he moved into Pre-Maintenance, where he ascertained his Critical Carbohydrate Level for Losing (CCLL) was 80 grams a day, on which he managed to lose 95 pounds in only four months.

If Dan represented the proverbial hare in the old fable, Carol Kitchener could be the tortoise. She held to the 20 grams of carbs permitted during Induction for almost two years. Carol is a nightclub performer, but as she puts it, feathers and sequins notwithstanding, there is nothing beautiful about a size 24 dress. Standing five feet five inches tall, her weight was 274 pounds before she began, and her blood pressure was edging into the danger zone. By her reckoning, she must have tried Weight Watchers twenty-five times. She had never found a weight loss plan that worked for long.

Atkins did. She skimmed off 129 pounds over twenty-four months—approximately 5 pounds a month. Slow but steady. There were a few tortoiselike patches in there, but Carol noticed that even when the scale wasn't budging, her dress size kept dropping. Besides, once she realized that she enjoyed the food and was no longer plagued with cravings, she was perfectly willing to let success come at its own pace.

It's easy to see how much less metabolic resistance Dan had than Carol, and even easier to understand why they took the paths they did. If Dan had continued Induction, he would have lost his weight so quickly that it would probably have been harder for him to convert to a Lifetime Maintenance plan. If Carol had moved on to OWL, her weight loss would have slowed so radically that she might have given up in despair. It sounds to me like Dan and Carol made the right choices. Certainly they both reached their goal weight and felt enormous satisfaction in doing so.

Proceed With Caution!

If you have decided to move to phase two, I want to remind you not to regard it a time to cut loose and undo all the good work you have just completed. Ongoing Weight Loss has a couple of fundamental differences from Induction, which I will explain in Chapter 14, but it is also very similar to Induction in that you will continue to derive the majority of your carbohydrates from vegetables low in carbs. You will add more portions of vegetables, and most people are later able to add nuts, seeds and even some berries. It's important to understand that you will not be shifting significantly away from protein and fat and to carbs, although you will be gradually changing the ratio of carbs to that of fat and protein.

But the one thing we don't want to do is get you out of lipolysis and halt your forward momentum. If that happened, we would have to resume Induction, or, as I chide so many of my patients, "It's back to square one." On the other hand, know that if you get into trouble, you can always return to Induction for a few days to get your metabolism fired up again.

Look at the Big Picture

In one sense, doing Induction is the easiest part of Atkins. You're following a strict regimen that almost always works. Now, as you learn in the next few chapters how to liberalize that regimen, you will be re-entering the "real" world. That doesn't have to be the bad world of junk food and uncontrollable cravings. But it is a world of greater choice, and certainly one in which you will be closer to the place where weight gain is a possibility.

If being overweight has been a big problem in your life, I don't want you to muff this opportunity. Over the course of the next few months, you can teach yourself a whole new way of life that will keep you healthy for decades. That is what doing Atkins is really all about.

When you begin OWL, you will be at a crucial stage for learning the parameters of your lifetime program. You'll find out what's the most liberal level of carbohydrate consumption your metabolism can handle while continuing to take off excess pounds. Pay close attention: This important number is your Critical Carbohydrate Level for Losing (CCLL).

KEY POINTS!

- Be realistic and determine for yourself the weight you would be comfortable with today.
- Knowing exactly how much weight you lost during the first fourteen days of Induction will help give you a general understanding of your personal degree of metabolic resistance and help you set goals and determine your pace of weight loss.

- The key question in the decision to stay on Induction or move on is "Am I willing to trade slower weight loss for more food choices?"

TIPS:

- Be aware that the Body Mass Index is just a guideline.
- People with high metabolic resistance can benefit from doing Induction longer than two weeks because it gives them time to correct the metabolic imbalances they may have developed over time.

14

Ongoing Weight Loss: The Second Phase of Atkins

If you're starting Ongoing Weight Loss (OWL), I know that you've succeeded doing Induction. Congratulations on reaching the first stage of your goal! OWL is where you'll start tailoring Atkins to fit your special tastes; it's what makes Atkins so unique and such a pleasure.

Although more lenient than Induction, OWL will continue to reveal the wonders of dissolving fat. Expect a gradual decrease in the rate at which the pounds and inches disappear—this is a deliberate part of the plan. I have to repeat one caveat: Allowing a few more carbs in at this phase is not a license to return to your old habits of dining on foods full of sugar, white flour and other "junk" carbs. The quality of the carbohydrate foods you eat continues to be as important as the quantity.

Focus on the positive changes you have already begun to enjoy! Now you—not that nameless, food-obsessed demon—are the one in charge of your appetite. And what delicious things you can have on your plate! In all likelihood, the crispy duck in Chinese restaurants or cheese omelettes garnished with thick slices of avocado were among the luxuries you had to do without when you were watching your fat intake. And you're on a nutritional plan that's healthier than any other you've tried before.

But I know that what initially brought you to this book was probably your concern with being overweight. So let's look at the big weight loss picture, and, as the chapter unfolds, you'll understand how OWL is the key to becoming a *former* fat person.

Make Your Goal Specific

You've set a goal now, and that's great! But make sure your goal is specific. Planning to lose 35 pounds, for example, is far better than planning to lose "some" weight. You will likely lose some weight, but you probably won't lose the full 35 unless you hold it in your mind as the destination of your journey.

The journey metaphor is apt. Imagine getting in the car to go on a family vacation without a clear idea of where you wanted to go. You'd drive around aimlessly, and you would certainly get somewhere, but it probably wouldn't be the same place you'd end up if you'd chosen a destination at the start. It's the same thing with weight loss. Any behavioral psychologist will tell you that you are more likely to achieve change in your life if you have a specific picture in your mind of how you want to change.

Visualize!

In other words, once you've said, "Okay, I will lose 35 pounds and I will weigh 140 pounds again," go even further. Instead, imagine how your body will look, think about the clothes you hid in the back of the closet that you'll be able to wear again and the admiring looks from your friends and family. Imagine actually being comfortable in shorts or a bathing suit or feeling confident on the ski slopes or going for a jog! If you are like many people, over the years that you've gained weight your world got a bit smaller. When you went to a pool party, you came up with some excuse to avoid going in the water. When your kids wanted to play, you just weren't up for it. When your friends hiked up a hill with ease, you had to lag behind, huffing and puffing—or just had to call it quits. At work, you may have had a great idea at a meeting but been too self-conscious about getting up in front of the group to express yourself. Imagine all the things that you will be doing with ease and pleasure with your friends, family and co-workers. Visualize, visualize and visualize. Then go out and make it happen!

Having a specific goal also helps you keep tabs on your progress as week after week you get to see the pounds vanishing. So when you've sent 15 of those 35 pounds reeling into oblivion, you know you're almost halfway there. After so many years as the enemy, the bathroom scale and the measuring tape are about to become some of your best friends. The mirror, too. You know that mirror, the one you could barely look at? And when you did, some overweight person you barely recognized stared back.

I'd like to remind you yet again that there are people who don't ultimately succeed doing Atkins because they can't get past the notion that a diet is something they get on and then get off, as you would a bus. But a true "diet" is not an excursion. Such individuals—who get on and then off Atkins—are often the people who need to lose 40 pounds but lose interest at 28. Then they go back to their old way of eating, and four or five months later they're back where they were to begin with. Typically, each "excursion" and retreat leaves them with a few more pounds than the last time. Don't be that kind of person!

A Second Chance

I'd like to introduce you to someone who did get off the Atkins bus. Fortunately—in the long run anyway—he got back on the bus and has committed to being a permanent passenger. Back in 1979, Gary Rizzio, a computer programmer from Colorado who is now 45, lost 60 pounds doing Atkins. But while recuperating in bed from a broken ankle, he alleviated his boredom with all-out indulgence in the junk foods he used to eat. That broke the spell, and before long his weight was back up to 250, and there it stayed for the next eighteen years, when he had a mild heart attack. His family history in heart disease and diabetes ran deep. His doctor was blunt: "Diet and exercise," he said, "or you'll have a short life."

Gary tried a low-fat diet and lost 1 pound in three weeks. So he came back to me. It took him six months to lose 50 pounds, during which time he became a creative cook. He says he might make an omelette with turkey, avocado, sour cream and cheese, or he'll sauté red onions and add them to scrambled eggs. He also eats a lot of chef's salads and seafood and chicken salads. And he now exercises forty minutes a day, five days a week.

Gary had been on his way to becoming diabetic, but Atkins improved his blood-sugar levels so much that his primary-care physician took him off one medication and decreased another. His total cholesterol has dropped from 212 to 178. With all these changes, it's no surprise that he now feels great. It's just too bad that it took a mild heart attack for Gary to get back on board. I hope you will heed the message before getting such a wake-up call.

What OWL Does for You

Your goal—for a large percentage of you, your destiny—of reaching your desired weight and staying there for life is best met by realistically considering which levels of carbohydrate intake apply to you. In OWL, you will take the physical and emotional well-being promoted by fat burning and combine that with the gustatory pleasure of an increasingly varied diet. Specifically, on OWL you will:

- continue to burn and dissolve fat.
- maintain control of your appetite sufficiently to control cravings.
- learn your threshold level of carbohydrate consumption, which will allow you to continue to lose weight.
- eat a broader range of healthy foods, selecting those that you enjoy most.
- learn to make the most nutrient-rich choices among carbohydrate foods.
- deliberately slow your rate of weight loss in order to lay the groundwork for permanent weight management.

How to Do OWL

There are three key differences between Induction and OWL. The first is obvious: You will consume more carbohydrates. Second, whereas during Induction you ate your protein and fat foods, plus three cups of salad and other veggies (and the special foods such as avocado, olives and sour cream), OWL allows you much more choice. That means now you can craft a weight loss regimen that is uniquely yours. But it also means—and here's the third key—that counting grams of carbohydrate is truly your responsibility.

If you don't count, you could get in trouble. Fortunately, counting is easy with the help of the carbohydrate gram counter in this book, which will familiarize you with the number of grams of carbs in common foods. For a more comprehensive guide, refer to *www.atkinscenter.com* or purchase a copy of *Dr. Atkins' New Carbohydrate Gram Counter*. After you have been doing Atkins for a while, you will begin to have a natural feel for the carb counts of your favorite foods, but it is always a good idea to keep your carb counter handy so you can check out new or unfamiliar foods.

Your Own Private, Personal Number

Life in the twenty-first century means lots of numbers to remember, what with cell phone numbers, bank PIN numbers and the like, but I'm going to give you the tools to find out another number that is just as essential for your lifestyle. Remember these two basic principles:

1. When you do Atkins, your rate of weight loss is generally proportional to the amount of carbohydrate you consume.
2. The level of carbohydrate you consume can be measured. By attaching numerical quantities to the carbohydrate foods you're eating, you know how much you can safely eat.

I refer to your daily threshold of carbohydrate consumption as your Critical Carbohydrate Level for Losing (CCLL). Stay below this number and you will experience ongoing weight loss. Go above it and your weight loss stalls. Here's how you'll determine your CCLL: Each week, you'll incrementally increase the quantity of carbohydrate you eat beyond the salad and one cup serving of vegetables allowed during Induction. These increments should measure roughly five grams of daily carbohydrates, representing what I call one "level."

During the first week on OWL, increase your daily carb intake from the 20 grams a day on Induction to 25 grams a day—going up one level. I recommend you add either another salad, half an avocado, a cup of cauliflower or six to eight stalks of asparagus or another vegetable. Continue to eat this way for the rest of the week. As long as your weight loss continues steadily, you can go up another level—to 30 grams daily—the following week. If you are a veggie lover, you may be happy continuing to add more salad greens and other vegetables. Or you may choose to add a half-cup of cottage cheese, an ounce of sunflower seeds or a dozen macadamia nuts. If you have been feeling fruit deprived, now is the time to add berries, the fruits lowest on the glycemic index. (Thirteen average-size strawberries contain 5 grams of carbs.)

Look at "The Power of Five" on pages 174–175 for other suggestions of foods you can add to your daily menu. Most people find it best to add back foods in a certain order— what I call the Carbohydrate Ladder (see below).

Note that few people will be able to add back *all* these food groups in OWL. Those on the second half of the list tend to rank higher on the glycemic index and are more commonly introduced in Pre-Maintenance. Following this order tends to minimize blood-sugar surges that could reactivate cravings.

CARBOHYDRATE LADDER

1. More salad and other vegetables on the acceptable foods list
2. Fresh cheeses (as well as more aged cheese)
3. Seeds and nuts
4. Berries
5. Wine and other spirits low in carbs
6. Legumes
7. Fruits other than berries and melons
8. Starchy vegetables
9. Whole grains

Each week you'll go up another level, adding another 5-gram increment until eventually you'll reach a number at which you stop losing. That's how you find your CCLL. Above it, you lose no more, or you begin to gain. Below it, you continue to lose. The lower your metabolic resistance to weight loss and the greater your level of physical activity, the higher that number will be.

Once you calculate your CCLL, you'll be able to say to another Atkins follower, "My Critical Carbohydrate Level for Losing is 45 grams. What's yours?" Or it might be higher—say 50, or as low as 25. To get an idea of the range that is possible, see the "Carbohydrate Gram Levels and Metabolic Resistance for Losing" table opposite. As I've mentioned before, metabolic resistance is influenced by age, gender, activity level, hormone issues, level of physical activity, prescription medications and other factors, so the range in CCLLs can be great.

If you eat beyond your CCLL, your scale and measuring tape will herald that you've crossed a line and you'll make adjustments accordingly. Most people simply drop back down to the prior level of carb consumption.

Lipolysis testing strips can also help you ascertain your CCLL in many cases. They generally stop turning color at a point a little bit below your CCLL. When that happens, your CCLL will be only a few carbohydrate grams higher. However, you should be aware that once you are consuming 50 or more grams of carbohydrates a day, the LTS will no longer register a change in color. So long as you continue to lose pounds and inches and experience no recurrence of your pre-Atkins levels of hunger, cravings and other symptoms, rest assured that all is well. You are still functioning on a primarily fat-burning metabolism even though you may not be producing enough ketones to show up in your urine.

You should be aware that everybody hits plateaus—periods during which no weight comes off. We will discuss this occurrence in depth in the next chapter.

Carbohydrate Gram Levels and
Metabolic Resistance for Losing

Metabolic Resistance	Approximate CCLL Range
High	<15 grams of carbs per day
Average	15–40 grams of carbs per day
Low	40–60 grams of carbs per day
Regular exerciser*	60–90 grams of carbs per day

In this context, a regular exerciser is someone who does vigorous exercise five days a week for at least forty-five minutes.

Your CCLL is an even more precise way to determine your level of metabolic resistance than the amount of weight you lost during Induction. As you continue to do Atkins, you will, by glancing at this table, have a more accurate idea of your degree of metabolic resistance.

The Wise OWL Mind Set

The OWL phase is all about choice. The choices you make should focus on healthy and pleasurable additions, with a strong emphasis on foods that contribute both. As you add foods in roughly 5 gram carb increments, you can probably move beyond vegetables to other foods, such as nuts, berries and possibly grains. Although you will be eating primarily natural, unprocessed foods, you will find an increasing number of convenience foods created for people seeking to follow a controlled carbohydrate nutritional approach. Remember the mantra: Read the Label! (See "How to Read a Label" on page 241–245.)

There are also many inviting recipes in this book, some using unique products designed for the person following a controlled carbohydrate regimen. Also see *Dr. Atkins' Quick & Easy New Diet Cookbook* and go to *www.atkinscenter.com* for even more recipes.

THE POWER OF FIVE

These portions contain roughly 5 grams of carbohydrates. Food groups are arranged in the general order in which they should be added.

Vegetables

¾ cup cooked spinach
½ cup red peppers
1 medium tomato
⅔ cup cooked broccoli
8 medium asparagus
1 cup cauliflower
⅓ cup chopped onions
½ California avocado
⅔ cup summer squash

Dairy

5 ounces farmer's cheese or pot cheese
5 ounces mozzarella cheese
½ cup cottage cheese
⅔ cup ricotta cheese
½ cup heavy cream

Nuts and Seeds

1 ounce of:
macadamias (approximately ten to twelve nuts)
walnuts (approximately fourteen halves)
almonds (approximately twenty-four nuts)
pecans (approximately thirty-one nuts)
hulled sunflower seeds (three tablespoons)
roasted shelled peanuts (approximately twenty-six nuts)

½ ounce of cashews (approximately nine nuts)

Fruits

¼ cup blueberries
¼ cup raspberries

½ cup strawberries
¼ cup cantaloupe, honeydew

Juices
¼ cup lemon juice
¼ cup lime juice
½ cup tomato juice

Convenience Foods
You can select from the variety of convenience foods (bars and shakes are the two most available), but be sure to determine the actual number of digestible carbohydrate in any particular product (see Chapter 8, page 77).

Time to Retest

Chances are you are feeling great, and you'll feel even better when you see evidence of the good things that are happening inside you. That's why I recommend you now repeat the blood and other medical tests you had done before you began Atkins (but not sooner than six weeks after your first tests). Do *not* repeat the GTT at this point.

What will you find? Your lipid profile should have done an about-face. If your total cholesterol was over 200, you should see a significant drop. If not, check for a dramatic increase in HDL (good cholesterol). You'll want to know your HDL and LDL (bad cholesterol) levels now, anyway, to see how they've changed. Your heart risk is dramatically decreased when your HDL has gone up relative to your LDL. The probability is that both will have moved in the proper directions. Relish these positive findings: A vast number of people in this country has to take medications with unpleasant side effects to get this kind of improvement in cholesterol levels.

Even more significant are your triglycerides. Elevated triglyceride levels, especially when combined with low levels of HDL cholesterol, have been shown in well-conducted studies to be the most important combination of heart-disease risk factors ever discovered.[1]

If your triglyceride level was originally elevated, or even high-normal (anything above 100 increases the risk of heart disease), it will have almost certainly plummeted dramatically. Drops of between forty and eighty percent are commonplace for someone doing Atkins, as they should be. After all, stored fat is made up of triglycerides, and Atkins focuses on burning stored fat for energy. If you don't get such a response, make sure you are doing the program correctly, or else repeat the test, making sure you wait fourteen hours after your last meal before the blood is drawn.

If your cholesterol has not improved to a level that represents reduced risk factors, yet you were satisfied with your weight reduction and other physical improvements, continue to do Atkins, take the cholesterol-lowering nutritional supplements outlined on page 309 (also refer to *Dr. Atkins' Vita-Nutrient Solution*) and repeat the test in a month. Continue to get retested every three months until the figures are satisfactory, then have them checked only annually.

Now that you've moved on from the simplicity of the Induction phase of Atkins, why don't you get yourself a little notebook and keep track of the food you eat daily? With more choices, you'll to some degree need to replace your willpower with your brains. The more you know about the carbohydrate quantities of foods you eat, or want to eat, the better equipped you will be to plan an effective weight loss strategy.

As Your Weight Loss Slows

As you keep raising your level of carbohydrate intake (and even if you don't), you'll notice a slowdown in the rate at which you lose weight. How soon you notice those changes is another major tipoff as to how great your metabolic resistance to weight loss is. During Induction (20 grams of carbohydrate), you may have been losing 5 pounds a week. In the first week to ten days some of that loss was water weight, since the program has a strong diuretic effect. If you continued doing Induction for a few more weeks, your weekly weight loss probably slowed down, as you were losing primarily fat, perhaps up to 3 pounds a week.

A couple of weeks later you begin OWL, and the first week you start eating an additional 5 grams a day, taking you to 25 grams. You are now losing 2½ pounds a week. Within a couple of weeks, during which you add another 10 grams daily of carbohydrate, you might drop down to a weekly loss of just under 2 pounds. And so on.

You may find that you can go up to 40 or 45 grams of carbohydrate a day—or even more if you are young, male and active—and still lose 1 pound a week. This would put you at an average level of metabolic resistance.

On the other hand, if you chose to leave Induction with 30 or more pounds still to lose, you may not be happy with a major slowdown. In this case, I would urge adding carbohydrate very slowly, staying for two or more weeks at each 5-gram incremental level. In either case, whether you are adding 5 grams each week or every other week or even less often, you'll increase your carbohydrate consumption steadily. When your weight loss begins to become imperceptible, you'll back down from that level.

The rate at which you want to lose is up to you. As long as the pounds are disappearing, and you're heading steadily toward your goal, why worry? Let's suppose, though, that you are rapidly coming to the conclusion that the extra 10 grams of carbohydrate don't mean as much to you as the extra pound per week of weight loss does. You may opt to stay at a lower level of carbohydrate and be satisfied with that knowledge. An additional fact—true of any weight loss program—is that the rate of loss will also slow down as you get closer to your goal weight.

That's why it's very important to plan to take two or more months to shed the last 5 to 10 pounds in the third phase—Pre-Maintenance. Pre-Maintenance is the last lap before the finish line of reaching your goal weight. It is mandatory if permanent weight loss is to be achieved, which I will explain to you in Chapter 16.

The Lucky Few

If you can go up to 50 or 60 grams of carbohydrate a day and still lose a little weight, you have a fairly low level of metabolic resistance. In all probability you weren't all that overweight, and staying permanently slim on Lifetime Maintenance will be a breeze for you. As you move through OWL you can experiment with adding healthy but higher-carbohydrate foods that most people cannot enjoy until Pre-Maintenance. But still be careful to add these foods slowly to prevent re-addiction and the emergence of cravings. If you're careful, and you find you don't go into a weight-gaining spiral, you may be able to have even an occasional potato and some wild rice.

Considering you're already consuming from one of the world's most luxurious nutritional plans, I predict a great deal of pleasurable eating ahead. But I do ask this question: If so little of your problem is metabolic, how did you become overweight in the first place? You should be on the lookout for a pattern of self-destructive behavior. It could be that that is a component of your weight problem. See Chapter 21 for more discussion of this possibility.

If Your Metabolism Is Stubborn

Others of you aren't so lucky when it comes to metabolic resistance. Those of you with a very high metabolic resistance to weight loss are most in need of this book. If you are unable to lose during Induction or had an initial loss and then stalled out while still doing Induction, you will have to adapt to eating not much more carbohydrate than 20 grams daily. You certainly will want to study Chapter 20 carefully.

Remember, if you're going to stay slim and healthy, a significant increase in the amount of exercise—which I strongly recommend for everyone—is absolutely essential for those of you with high metabolic resistance. Without it, losing weight may actually be hard for you. (See Chapter 22.)

Rules of OWL

- Protein and fat remain the mainstays of your nutritional regimen.
- Increase your daily carb intake by no more than 5 grams *each week*.
- Add new foods in the order listed in the Carbohydrate Ladder (see page 171).
- Add one new food group at a time.
- Eat a food group no more than three times per week to start. Then you may eat it daily.
- If new foods provoke weight gain, or return of physical symptoms lost doing Induction, or increased appetite or cravings, stop them immediately.
- Continue doing OWL until you have from 5 to 10 pounds left to lose.

Looking Forward

After OWL—having become as wise as that dignified night-roaming bird—you'll move up to the key phase of Pre-Maintenance, and then finally to Lifetime Maintenance. You're going to find that every one of these phases is one that you can comfortably personalize for your own needs, tastes and lifestyle. In the next chapter, before we get to Pre-Maintenance, we'll take a small detour to discuss the crucial subject of plateaus.

KEY POINTS!

- As you transition into OWL, your rate of weight loss will gradually slow. This is normal and intentional.
- The key to OWL is determining your personal Critical Carbohydrate Level for Losing (CCLL).
- By incrementally increasing your carbohydrate intake you can personalize an eating program that suits your individual needs, tastes and lifestyle.
- Individuals' CCLLs can vary substantially.

A FREQUENTLY ASKED QUESTION (OR TWO):

Are nuts and seeds okay on this phase of Atkins even though they have carbohydrates?

As you know by now, Atkins is not about eating *no* carbs. It is about controlling carb intake and eating those that are most nutrient-dense. Different nuts and seeds have different percentages of fat, protein and carbohydrate. I don't recommend eating them during the first two weeks of Induction. But now (in OWL), if you are continuing to lose steadily, you can try introducing some nuts (see "The Power of Five" in this chapter) and see if they fit into your Ongoing Weight Loss regimen. Note, however, that nuts and seeds may contain mold, which could trigger an allergic response.

I should tell you that nuts are one of the first foods I recommend my patients reintroduce in Ongoing Weight Loss—right up there with cheese. But I also remind them that nuts are notoriously hard to eat in moderation. One leads to another until you may have eaten several ounces. Try buying the one- or two-ounce packets so you won't be tempted to over indulge.

Can I drink alcohol now that I am in OWL?

The body burns alcohol for fuel when alcohol is available. So when it is burning alcohol, your body will not burn fat. This does not stop weight loss; it simply postpones it. Since the alcohol does not get stored as glycogen, you immediately get back into lipolysis after the alcohol is used up. But keep in mind that alcohol consumption may increase yeast-related symptoms in some people (see Chapter 25) and interfere with weight loss. If it does not slow your weight loss, an occasional glass of wine is acceptable once you are out of Induction so long as you count the carbohydrates in your daily tally. (A 3½-ounce glass of wine contains about 4.3 grams of carbohydrate.) Spirits such as Scotch, rye, vodka and gin are acceptable, but do not mix with juice, tonic water or non-diet soda, all of which contain sugar. Seltzer, diet tonic and non-aspartame diet soda mixers are permitted. If you have added alcohol to your regimen and suddenly stop losing weight, discontinue your alcohol intake.

TIPS:

- To raise your CCLL, increase your activity level.
- Keep a picture of "the old you," before Atkins, on your refrigerator.
- Pass up fried foods in restaurants. The batter is made with flour and the oil is often hydrogenated.
- Eat berries and other fruit with cheese, nuts or cream to slow down their impact on your blood sugar.

15

Engine Stalled?
How to Get Past a Plateau

You've been shedding pounds like a pooch drops fur in the dog days of summer, and then, suddenly, things come to a screeching halt. Don't be discouraged; you've hit a plateau and there are actions you can take to break through it.

A plateau—which I define as an inexplicable pause in weight loss that cannot be traced back to dietary misdemeanors or lifestyle changes—is not an uncommon occurrence. It usually happens in the later stages of weight loss, after the easy pounds have come off. Fortunately, plateaus are seldom permanent. I counsel a calm approach to the problem, followed, if necessary, by aggressive action. But first you have to figure out if you're really on a plateau.

The Definition of a Plateau

If a pause in weight loss is a genuine plateau, I require that it meet the following criteria:

- You have experienced no weight loss or loss of inches for at least four weeks. (Increased muscle mass will deceive the scale because muscle weighs more than fat—but inches will continue to disappear.)

- You have not started a new medication, such as hormone therapy, altered your exercise regimen or made any other significant lifestyle change.
- You have examined your physical state carefully and are able to conclude that you have no symptoms indicative of a diet-related disorder (see Chapters 24–27) or a thyroid problem.
- You can take a close look at your eating habits and honestly say that you've adhered to the same healthy, controlled carbohydrate eating plan that has brought you success up to now.

Now let's examine these criteria one by one.

Losing Pounds Isn't Everything

For too many of us, trying to lose weight induces a fixation on the bathroom scale. I have patients who get upset when the scale doesn't show a change for three consecutive days, so you can imagine how crazy they get when it doesn't budge for four weeks.

Remember two things: First, your body is not a machine. Nor is it a duplicate of anyone else's body. It has its own system, its own agenda, and its own timetable. In the long run, it nearly always responds to sensible management by the person in charge—you. But, in the short run, your body may decide to go its own way, for its own reasons, which perhaps we don't understand. Don't get mad at it. It's a good body or it wouldn't have gotten you this far. Be patient; you can afford to outwait it.

Second, loss of pounds is not the only way to measure success. Look at the other markers. Are you feeling better than you used to? Do you have the energy to do things you want to do? If so, then something is happening to your body. Do your clothes feel looser? Have you tried on those clothes that "felt a little too tight" just a few weeks ago? I hope you've followed my advice about measuring your chest, waist, hips, thighs, and upper arms. If you're losing inches, the scale will eventually catch up.

Did Something Happen?

If you're losing neither inches nor pounds and four weeks have passed, let's consider the next possibility.

People frequently get frustrated after a week or two without weight loss, when a little reflection would tell them what's gone wrong. Certainly if you've been put on some new medication—including hormone treatment or birth control pills—around the time you stopped losing, you'll need to consider its possible metabolic effects. Turn to Chapter 20 for guidance in dealing with this problem. Medications are a common and often formidable obstacle to weight loss, and I outline many of the problem drugs and chemicals in that chapter and offer alternatives that a physician may be able to prescribe for you.

Significant changes in your lifestyle also can alter the rate at which you consume energy daily. Maybe you've been hit with an urgent deadline at the office and you've been glued to your chair for three weeks. No more lunchtime walks, no more half-hour sessions at your health club and no more ten-block strolls with your spouse after dinner—because you've been eating too late.

If you've reached OWL (see Chapter 14) or Pre-Maintenance (see Chapter 16), changes like those could be enough to halt your loss for a few weeks. Not only are you burning fewer calories, but when you get less exercise, your metabolism tends to slow down (just as increasing exercise revs it up). Dear reader, from a health perspective, exercise is a beautiful thing. I just wish I could inject a love-exercise gene into all my patients—and readers. It would make their lives a lot easier.

Having mentioned lifestyle, I wouldn't want you to forget the obvious. Have you been living it up on a vacation, eating all sorts of foods of dubious carbohydrate content? Did the holidays come and, with them, four hors-d'oeuvre-laden parties in the past three weeks? And now you're blaming me? If so, I hope this makes you blush, and I hope you had a good time. Not guilty? Well, then, let's look at a more serious panoply of problems that might cause your weight loss to plateau.

Yeast, Food Intolerances and Thyroid Problems

Perhaps, as you have moved through the weight loss phases of Atkins, you have inadvertently added into your regimen a particular food that is triggering a metabolic reaction. This reaction can cause you to hit a weight loss plateau.

In Part Four, I discuss problems that I've long referred to as diet-related disorders. These aren't problems that arise from embarking on a weight loss program. I'm using the word *diet* in its larger sense, to signify, simply, the types of foods you eat. So let's take a quick look at some of those disorders to see if they might account for your plateau.

YEAST

If you've been eating a high-sugar diet for years, it's quite possible that your digestive tract has an overgrowth of an organism called *Candida albicans*. In addition to overgrowth of yeast in the gastrointestinal tract, most people also experience an allergic inflammation of the mucous membranes throughout the body. This can result from exposure to environmental mold (in your cellar, for example) or eating foods that contain yeast. Symptoms include constipation, diarrhea, gas, bloating, heartburn and even abdominal pain and rectal or vaginal itching. All are a sign of yeast overgrowth in the mucous membranes. Symptoms such as fatigue, depression, headaches (even migraines), post-nasal drip, brain fog and water retention are often signs of allergy resulting from exposure to environmental mold or mold in food products such as cheese and nuts.

In addition to its other annoying or painful symptoms, *Candida* overgrowth or allergy can keep you from losing weight by causing cravings for sweets. Indulging those cravings will cause unstable blood sugar and more carbohydrate cravings. *Candida* thrives on sugar, but with Atkins you've already sent all that wretched, tempting sweet stuff into deep Siberian exile. However, Atkins does allow cheese, nuts, vinegar, mushrooms and pickles—all of which are aged or fermented items—and will provoke symptoms. If you discover or suspect you have a yeast problem, those foods will have to go for at least some period of time to give your body a rest from exposure.

Here are some examples of how a yeast problem could lead to a weight loss plateau. Say you had always been sensitive to a food such as cheese, but were eating very little or none while you were on a low-fat regimen. When you started doing Atkins, you began to eat more cheese, which eventually triggered a yeast overgrowth or allergy. Another scenario: You were prescribed an antibiotic for a sinus infection, and that triggered an overgrowth of yeast. Yet another possibility is that the increased environmental mold typical of humid summer weather might have tipped you over the edge. Finally, hormonal changes can trigger yeast reactions. Any of these could cause your weight loss efforts to stall. Although the mechanism that links yeast to a plateau is not well understood, I have observed this to be a problem in many patients, and they had to address it to make progress in their weight loss efforts. If you feel you might be sensitive to yeast, take the "Yeast Symptoms" questionnaire on page 332.

If you have a major yeast problem, your engine will most likely stall out at some point in the program, so—even if your only concern is weight loss—take care.

FOOD INTOLERANCES

I believe that food allergies (more properly called *individual food intolerances*) to substances other than yeast can be a major roadblock to weight loss. Without knowing it you may have added to your meal plan a food to which you are allergic. Wheat and wheat products are frequently culprits. Other common problem foods include milk, cheese, eggs and soy. Eating a food to which you're allergic may cause symptoms such as gastrointestinal or respiratory problems, joint pain and skin eruptions.[1-2] From the point of view of someone trying to slim down, the most damaging aspect of eating a food to which you're allergic is its tendency to cause cravings, which, if indulged, can lead to unstable blood sugar. Your real challenge will be to discover that you have a food intolerance in the first place and then to determine which food is the culprit. Please read Chapter 26 carefully.

THYROID PROBLEMS

The other diet-related disorder that can cause a weight loss plateau concerns the thyroid gland. This remarkable little butterfly-shaped organ regulates the production of energy in our cells. If it becomes underactive—a condition called *hypothyroidism*, which is not uncommon as you age or develop hormonal imbalances—you will become sluggish and overweight. Whenever a person is incapable of losing weight on the best weight loss program available (namely, this one), my first suspicion is a thyroid problem.

If nothing I tell you here or elsewhere works for you, then turn directly to Chapter 20 and follow the detailed advice it contains on how to diagnose and treat an underactive thyroid (see pages 269–271). This is one problem for which you'll certainly need a doctor's assistance. Fortunately, treatments for hypothyroidism are straightforward and generally quite effective.

If you lost weight initially doing Atkins but now have plateaued, that does not necessarily exclude a thyroid explanation. Prolonged dieting (of any type) will sometimes cause reduction in thyroid function.[3] Your body, feeling a little disturbed at all the pounds you're taking off, is playing with your "set point," the weight level it thinks it ought to keep you at to prevent starvation. Heed the thyroid discussion in Chapter 20 and you'll get things back on track.

If you have any one of these three diet-related disorders— yeast, food intolerances or thyroid problems—you must seriously address it or in time it will make your life an utter misery.

Of course, I hope that your problems are simpler ones. Many of you, in fact, will find that your plateau is easily solved in the next section.

Carb Creep?

Could it be that you've gotten sloppy? Are you doing whatever weight loss phase of Atkins you are now in with the same rigor with which you began it? Or has success gone to your head?

Perhaps you're the victim of an innocent error. It may be that those 5-gram increases in your carbohydrate intake have gotten out of hand and you've done a lot more of them than you think you did. Search your memory, examine exactly what you've been eating over the past five or six days, and compare it to what you were eating a few weeks ago. I've seen people who, once they really put their noses to the carb counter, discovered that it was 30 grams and not 5 or 10 that they had added on. Keeping a food diary is an indispensable tool for keeping an eye on your food intake and connecting it with patterns that may hinder progress.

Is it possible that you may have forgotten some of the rules of Atkins? Let's run down the list of possible errors:

- Did you go to the supermarket and pick up *low-fat* foods? Always remember that manufacturers make up for the flavor missing in these foods by adding high-carb fillers and sugar. Not only do such dreadful artificial foods have no place when doing Atkins but most of them are spectacularly unhealthy. Pry open the lid on the garbage can and stuff them in. That's where they belong.

- Check for the hidden carbs in prepared foods. Many canned and dried soups, salad dressings, sauces and gravies and frozen vegetables in sauce contain thickeners such as cornstarch, fillers such as milk solids and even sugar.

- Watch out for condiments. Barbecue sauce, ketchup and sandwich spreads often have added sugar in one form or another. Teriyaki sauce? Three grams of carbohydrate in one tablespoon. If it's your passion, you need to count the carbs. A tablespoon of skim milk or lemon juice each has 1 gram of carbohydrate, a tablespoon of balsamic vinegar more than 2 grams. The numbers add up, especially if your "tablespoon" is more like a quarter-cup splash.

- Avoid aspartame. Although the cause is as yet unknown, clinical observations show that certain individuals find weight loss slows with excessive intake of aspartame, the artificial sweetener sold as NutraSweet® and Equal®.

- Stay out of the java jungle. Excessive caffeine (found not only in coffee but in tea, chocolate and many soft drinks) has been shown to cause a hypoglycemic (low blood sugar) reaction, which will provoke cravings and cause you to overeat.[4] Omitting caffeine may be a big sacrifice for you, but, in my experience, weight loss often starts up again as soon as people remove aspartame and caffeine from their regimen.

- Don't go whole hog on the cheese and nuts. These are acceptable foods, but they do contain some carbohydrates. If you've been munching without mercy, scale back the cheese and nuts. Then see what happens. Not much? Cut them out altogether for a week or two and see if that has an effect.

Breaking Free

If you've looked through all the suggestions I've just offered and found precious few clues to explain why your weight loss efforts are stalled, you may indeed be on a plateau. If you've been on many diets in your lifetime, you may be surprised to discover that you've plateaued at the same point in the past. These are the weights at which your body naturally starts to resist weight loss. It may be that your perception of what you should weigh is inappropriate and unhealthy. It's unlikely that at 45 you can be quite as slim as you were at 18. It may be that if you are unable to lose, it's because you are already where you should be.

And if that definitely isn't the case, you really should lose more. Don't panic—the fat-burning engine usually starts up again.

I recommend spending a week in close examination of what you're eating. You might want to keep that food diary I mentioned earlier. It's easy to forget one or two spots of indulgence. Try backing off your carbs slightly. Take away the last 5 grams of carbohydrate you permitted yourself. You may have slipped slightly above your CCLL.

If you have not been in lipolysis for a while and are now stuck, you may want to gradually lower your carb level by 5-gram increments until your lipolysis test strips turn purple again. If all else fails, it's time to go back to Induction. Three to five days in Induction will usually start weight loss moving again. Sometimes the body just needs a little nudge.

Then, when you move beyond Induction again, add on the carbohydrates a little more cautiously than you did before. It's quite possible that you have a fairly high degree of metabolic resistance.

If you're serious about following Atkins for life, I must reiterate that you have to invest some energy in exercise. Contrary to the messages our society generally sends us, your body was meant to move. Sitting around is unnatural. Working in an office is unnatural. A whole lot of modern life is unnatural. Parking in the far corner of the parking lot is not a mistake. It's where you should be, because exercise is not optional. It's an integral part of doing Atkins. It's often neglected and sometimes quietly scorned, but if you think you're doing the program and you're not exercising, you're not doing the program. This may be the time for you to read Chapter 22. Building exercise into your lifestyle is one of the most intelligent ways of cracking through a plateau.

Discouraging as a plateau may be, you can't let it beat you. It may comfort you to hear that some individuals lose weight in a pattern of plateauing for a month, then taking a dip of four or more pounds, plateauing again and so on. If you get discouraged and start to cheat before seeing results, you will sabotage your success. Read this chapter once, twice or three times if you have to, but be convinced. You will win out in the end.

KEY POINTS!

- A plateau is a halt in weight loss that lasts at least a month and has nothing to do with changes in food intake or lifestyle.
- Plateaus are natural and not uncommon in later stages of weight loss.
- Causes for plateaus include adding a new medication, reduction in activity level, yeast and thyroid problems and food intolerances.

- Getting sloppy about counting carbs or not being vigilant about watching for hidden carbs in condiments and other foods is different from being on a plateau.
- If a plateau does not come to an end, it may mean you are truly metabolically resistant and need to read Chapter 20.

A FREQUENTLY ASKED QUESTION:

My husband and I are both doing Atkins, but he zips along losing regularly even though he sometimes cheats. I follow the program religiously but have hit several plateaus. Do men have an advantage doing Atkins?

Yes, they do. Unfortunately, weight loss is not an equal opportunity activity. Gender and age play a role. There are at least three reasons that most men—particularly young men—tend to lose more easily than women—particularly older women. First, men generally have greater muscle mass than women so they burn more calories than women do. Second, a woman's body is much more subject to hormonal fluctuations, which can play havoc with your blood-sugar and insulin response. Finally, estrogen supresses thyroid function, which in turn slows your metabolism, making it more difficult to lose weight.

TIPS:

- A food diary and a carb gram counter are powerful tools to help you understand what may be blocking weight loss.
- Avoid aspartame and cut out all caffeine, candy (including sugar-free types), cheese, nuts and condiments and you may break through a plateau.
- Try reducing your carb intake by 5 grams a day; then, if necessary, by 10 grams. If weight loss is still stalled, go back to the Induction phase for three to five days.

16

Pre-Maintenance:
Prepare for Permanent Slimness

You're almost there! All your good work and healthy eating habits have paid off, and you now have only 5 to 10 pounds left to reach your goal weight. Give yourself a good pat on the back; you deserve it!

Having said that, I have to insert a note of caution. You may not like what follows, but it is vitally important that you hear it.

If you have been racing along the road to your destination, now is the time to put on the brakes. Much as it is tempting to say, "I can banish these last pounds in a few weeks now that I know how to do Atkins," I strongly advise you to do something that seems quite the opposite on Pre-Maintenance, the all-important third phase of Atkins. As you advance toward Lifetime Maintenance, my advice is to proceed so slowly that your weight loss is almost imperceptible. I know that this snail's pace can be excruciating when the end is in sight. But remember, getting to your goal weight is not your ultimate goal; your real goal is to *maintain* that magic number indefinitely.

Our focus is now different. There is little doubt you can and will reach your goal weight. The only doubt is whether you will stay at that weight for life. The purpose now is to create the optimal lifetime eating program—one that fits you so perfectly you will want to stay on it for life.

When you moved to OWL, you deliberately slowed down your weight loss by adding more carbs and more variety to your menus. Now I am going to ask you to slow things down even further. The more you learn about eating as you lose those last few pounds, the better. Your next assignment is to increase your carbohydrate consumption until you're losing less than a pound a week. The additional foods will provide increased nutrition and culinary enjoyment. Ideally, you should spend at least a month and preferably two or three in this phase.

There is method in what may sound like madness here. If you search for the level that achieves a small amount of weight loss, by the time you reach your goal weight you will, in effect, be on Lifetime Maintenance, at which time your weight loss will naturally slow to a halt. During Pre-Maintenance, you will both accustom yourself to your lifetime eating plan and get a good indication of what it will be like. Think of this phase as a learner's permit, like the one you had when you were just beginning to drive. You were allowed out on the roads, but only with a licensed driver by your side. Pre-Maintenance is like that. You're out there doing it, but you still need some more hours behind the wheel before it's safe to allow you on the highway all by yourself.

That's why it is crucial that you NOT make the assumption that Pre-Maintenance and Lifetime Maintenance must be pretty much the same thing because their names sound alike. Not true: One is a training program; the other is the rest of your life. If you have any misguided ideas about skipping this third phase and going right to Lifetime Maintenance, I implore you not to do so. In fact, I would go so far as to say that Pre-Maintenance is mandatory if permanent weight loss is to be achieved. Let me repeat that: If you omit Pre-Maintenance, you may well be doomed to failure when it comes to maintaining your weight loss for the long term.

When it comes to the last few pounds, slower is better. Here's why: When Madge O'Hara came to see me, she weighed 156 (on a five-foot two-inch frame), and she planned to slim down to 115. She lost 21 pounds the first month, and I surmise that 6 or 7 pounds of that was water weight. The next month she moved to OWL and lost 7 more pounds. She then moved on to Pre-Maintenance and peeled off the last 13 pounds over a leisurely three months. By the time Madge reached her goal weight, she knew exactly how she was going to eat for the rest of her life—and controlling her carb intake had become automatic for her.

What You Will Learn in Pre-Maintenance

Now that you understand that Pre-Maintenance is the phase that bridges losing weight and maintaining weight, let me spell out exactly what this crucial phase will do for you. During it, you will:

- find your new Critical Carbohydrate Level for Losing (CCLL) slowly, as well as your Critical Carbohydrate Level for Maintenance (CCLM).
- explore more food choices, while learning how not to abuse them.
- become aware of the foods or situations that can make you lose sight of your long-term goals.
- internalize your responses to food so that what used to be a struggle becomes a conscious choice, one that serves you for the rest of your life.
- find out how flexible Atkins is.
- learn how to deal with temptation.
- learn how to immediately erase the problems created by making unhealthy food choices to prevent "yo-yo" weight gain and loss.
- develop a style of eating for a lifetime.

It's a Lifestyle

Pre-Maintenance is crucial to getting your weight under control for good, but it is also about far more important things—the first, of course, being your health. To reduce your long-term risks for conditions such as cardiovascular disease, hypertension, and diabetes there is nothing more effective than maintaining a healthy weight. But I am also thinking about such things as your ability to make choices that are right for *you,* not for your spouse, your parents, your friends or even your doctor. When you realize you can be in charge of what you eat, how you look and how healthy you are, it empowers you in all the other aspects of your life. Instead of worrying about looking good to please someone else, you are likely coming to realize that what matters is how *you* feel about how you look and feel. You are learning the skills that allow you to take charge of your life.

Phil Monte couldn't agree more. What does a corrections officer in Maine do when he's 30 pounds overweight, eats a high-carb diet and keeps falling asleep after lunch in a roomful of noisy inmates? Well, first he tries a low-fat diet, filling up with plenty of pasta, bread, rice and potatoes. I leave the sad results to your imagination.

Then he listens to his brother who lost a ton of weight doing Atkins, and he picks up a copy of an earlier edition of this book. His menu plan changed—fast. "Now I have meat cooked on the grill with green vegetables," says Phil. "Another dish I make is a stir-fry with chicken, cabbage, garlic, green peppers, onions and soy sauce. Before I might have used cornstarch to thicken this dish and served it on rice, but not anymore."

Phil lost his 30 pounds and when his doctor saw that his HDL (good) cholesterol had gone up to 90, he said, "With numbers like these, Phil, you'll *never* get heart disease!" At 35 years old, Phil has become a diet guru for the people he works with; they call him up weekly to ask how to do Atkins.

Phil's self-confidence has gone through the roof, and, exploiting his avocation as a golfer, he's starred in two instructional videos and self-published a book. When he went to his sister's wedding, people he'd known all his life didn't recognize him. He thinks it's the biggest compliment he's gotten yet.

How to Do Pre-Maintenance

When you were doing OWL, you learned how to increase your carb intake in increments of 5 grams. In this phase, you can shift into a higher gear: Increase your daily carb count by 10 grams each week so long as you continue to lose. (See "The Power of Ten" on pages 201–203 and refer to the carbohydrate gram counter in this book.) If you introduce new foods slowly and increase your grams of carbs gradually, your CCLL should increase gradually. This new and higher CCLL will reflect the fact that you are now losing weight more slowly.

As you continue to make 10-gram incremental additions, you will rather quickly reach a point at which you will find that you are no longer losing. If you are at your goal weight, stay at that level for a month or so before you increase your daily carb consumption by another 10 grams to see if you can consume that level without gaining. Once you do begin to gain, drop back 10 grams and you should have established your Critical Carbohydrate Level for Maintenance (CCLM).

On the other hand, if after an incremental increase you find that you are gaining or are not losing and you are not yet at your goal weight, you need to back down to the previous level. The line between gaining, maintaining and losing is a thin one and you may have to "play" with your CCLL and CCLM for a while to understand what your body can handle.

While it may take as long as three months to drop the last few pounds and clearly establish your CCLM, I reiterate:

This leisurely pace is critical to your ultimate success. Continue to add new foods slowly and carefully so you'll be learning good eating habits at the same time. For example, you'll discover whether your metabolism can handle whole-grain bread, legumes, starchy vegetables and other potential "trouble" foods. (People with extremely low carb tolerance—meaning high metabolic resistance—won't be able to add many new foods and will find Pre-Maintenance similar to OWL or even Induction.)

Some Variations on the Rule

Another approach to Pre-Maintenance is to continue eating as you were at the end of OWL and to allow yourself a 20-gram carb treat two or three times a week. Add a piece of fruit or a starchy vegetable—a serving of brown rice or sweet potatoes, for example. You can also have a glass of white wine, a light beer or the white spirits. You could get more adventurous with some of the excellent controlled carbohydrate convenience foods that are increasingly available. Or, if your metabolic resistance is at the low end, you may be able to enjoy such treats more frequently.

Still another way to do Pre-Maintenance is to average out your carb intake for the week. This is how it works: If, for example, your CCLL is 80 grams, you might drop back to 60 grams on Tuesday, then deviate with a beef, potato and carrot stew the following night, pushing your daily total to 100 grams. (Up until now, when weight loss was essential, I have told you to spread your carbs out through the day. If you do have a heavy dose at one meal, make sure there is enough fat, protein and fiber in the rest of the meal to slow the glucose load on your system.) However, if you find such deviations create cravings, it is probably best for you to stick to a steady number of carbs spread evenly throughout the day.

But be careful! There are a couple of reasons why people sometimes get into trouble:

1. They don't recognize that this phase is still relatively restrictive of carbohydrates, compared to the way they were eating before they were doing Atkins.
2. They're startled to discover that without the wonderful advantage of deep lipolysis, appetite suppression has diminished.

Rules of Pre-Maintenance

- Increase your daily carb intake by no more than 10 grams *each week*.
- Add new foods one at a time.
- Eliminate a new food if it provokes weight gain, return of physical symptoms lost during Induction, increased appetite, cravings or water retention.
- If you gain weight, drop back to the next lowest level of carb intake.
- Be sure to continue eating adequate amounts of fat and protein.
- Continue to take your vitamin and mineral supplements regularly.

These reasons point out exactly why Pre-Maintenance is so important. This is the phase of Atkins during which you acclimate to the carbohydrate moderation you will need to practice for the rest of your life. Not only are you losing less weight and doing so at a slower rate, you are burning less of your body fat. Thus, the natural appetite suppression provided by lipolysis is reduced considerably. But as long as you are not skipping meals and continue to lose weight, you are controlling your blood sugar and burning fat, so your appetite should not be out of control.

If it is, you have gone too far and you need to go back a few notches.

As you may have inferred, while you are on Pre-Maintenance, in all likelihood you are no longer in ketosis. However, you are probably still burning fat rather than storing it—at least some of the time. As you increase your consumption of carbs, your body switches back and forth between lipolysis and glucosis, between burning fat and burning glucose from carbohydrate. You'll want to eat a bit more food, and a bit more is fine for most people. But heed the lessons you have learned about the difference between being satiated and being stuffed: This is no time to begin overeating. You have nothing to make up for. Unlike low-fat diets, this nutritional approach hasn't caused you any pain or deprivation.

If Addictions Recur

If addictions do reappear—in the form of food obsessions and cravings—you're probably indulging too much in the foods that got you into trouble to begin with. The vicious cycle of hyperinsulinism and resultant low blood-sugar levels, combined with the possibility of specific food allergies or intolerances, can create an addictive situation. When you go back to bread, fruit or fermented foods, you may suddenly discover that you *must* have these foods, that no day or meal feels right without them. Observe yourself carefully. You are engaged in a real battle for self-control as your defenses crumble. You'll notice that the need that develops is genuinely physical. It isn't simply that you know pasta tastes good, and you'd like to have it. No, your body absolutely roars with anxiety and passion for that pasta. You are under its spell. When this happens, you'll *know*.

Such addictions aren't shameful; they're physical, biochemical, metabolic—and that's precisely why you must avoid them. Most of you already know that for a significant portion of your life, excessive quantities of carbohydrates have been stronger than you. Don't trifle with them now.

As soon as you suspect your carbohydrate cravings are returning, you are confronted with a true health emergency that demands immediate action. You must cure them by returning to the Induction phase for several days until you get your cravings under control. Carefully doing Pre-Maintenance will help prevent you from once again being controlled by your cravings.

By the time you finally reach your goal weight, you are by definition officially in phase four, Lifetime Maintenance. As we move into this next phase of Atkins, you absolutely must *ease* into your Lifetime Maintenance regimen, rather than make an abrupt transition. The next chapter will explain how to do just that.

THE POWER OF TEN

The following portions each contain roughly 10 grams of carbohydrates. Food groups are arranged in the general order in which they should be added.

Nuts
½ cup almonds
¼ cup cashews
½ cup filberts
½ cup macadamias
2 ounces roasted shelled peanuts
¾ cup pecans
½ cup pine nuts (pignoli)
¼ cup pistachios
¾ cup walnuts
⅓ cup pumpkin seeds
⅓ cup sesame seeds
2 ounces sunflower seeds

Starchy Vegetables*

½ cup carrots
1 cup winter squash
¼ cup yams (or sweet potatoes)
½ cup peas, shelled
¼ cup plantain
¾ cup beets
⅓ cup parsnips
¼ cup white potatoes

Legumes*

¼ cup lentils
¼ cup kidney beans
¼ cup black beans
¼ cup navy beans
¼ cup lima beans
¼ cup great northern beans
¼ cup chickpeas
¼ cup fava beans
¼ cup pinto beans

Fruit

½ apple
12 cherries
1 peach
12 grapes
1 cup strawberries
½ grapefruit
¾ cup cantaloupe
1 kiwi
1 cup watermelon
½ cup fruit cocktail, canned in water
1 plum
⅓ banana

All figures are for cooked vegetables, starches and legumes.

1 guava
⅓ mango

Grains

¼ cup rice, long grain brown*
½ cup oatmeal*
¼ cup corn kernels*
1 slice whole wheat bread
⅓ cup whole wheat cereal*
¼ cup barley*
¼ cup spinach pasta*

KEY POINTS!

- The key to success on Pre-Maintenance is advancing slowly, losing less than a pound each week for two to three months.
- Nothing will have a more significant effect on reducing your long-term risks for cardiovascular disease, hypertension and diabetes than maintaining a healthy weight.
- Increase daily carbohydrate intake by 10 grams per week so long as you continue to lose, adding new foods slowly and carefully.
- The line between gaining, maintaining and losing is a thin one, and you may have to "play" with your CCLL and CCLM for a while to understand what your body can handle.

A FREQUENTLY ASKED QUESTION (OR TWO):

Why has my appetite increased, and what can I do to manage it?

Appetite can return when you are no longer in lipolysis. Or you may have added a food that may be causing your blood

---

All figures are for cooked vegetables, starches and legumes.

sugar to become unstable, contributing to hunger or the re-emergence of cravings. Examine what you've recently added and determine if it contains sugars or refined grain. Be sure that you are maintaining a regular intake of protein and fat and, if eating more of acceptable foods assuages your hunger, eat a bit more. If all else fails, stop the most recent additions until you get your appetite under control.

My weight varies by a few pounds every day. Is there any other way to determine when to stop increasing my weekly carb intake?
It's natural for your weight to vary from day to day, which is why I recommend you do not weigh yourself every day. But from week to week, you should be seeing a difference in the way your clothes fit. For some people, adding 10 additional grams of carbs each week to their daily menu may be too much. Try dropping back to 5-gram increments.

TIPS:

- Think of Pre-Maintenance as "driver's education."
- When eating in a restaurant, ask the server to replace your rice or potato with a serving of vegetables.
- Keep a controlled carb bar or ready-to-drink shake on hand to feed hunger pangs and keep you from being tempted by the snack vending machine.

17

Lifetime Maintenance

The bells should be ringing, the flags should be flying: You're there! You've arrived at the place where millions of overweight people have never been since they were children—at the weight you were meant to be. And the impact on every part of your life is enormous. Am I right?

Take a good long look in the mirror, try on your newly tailored clothes or climb into duds you haven't been able to shoehorn yourself into for years, and then—oh, bliss—listen to the comments people make. I'll bet you've taken center stage. Losing weight sure attracts attention! And who doesn't want to look his or her best?

Now let me interject a reality check. Have you won the battle of the bulge? Or have you only graduated from boot camp, in shape now for the battle ahead? I can personally attest to the fact that you have achieved the latter. Recidivism among people who have lost considerable weight is such a well-documented phenomenon that many cynical doctors advise their patients not to even bother trying to lose.[1] Fortunately with Atkins, such pessimism is unwarranted. This is not to say you don't need a lifetime maintenance plan accompanied by unceasing vigilance. This chapter supplies you with the former; the determination to succeed is your responsibility.

Before she saw me, Mary Anne Evans had given up. "I said to myself, 'I'm simply going to be fat for the rest of my life.' I weighed 209 pounds when I came to see you, and I had been putting on weight steadily for twenty years—especially after the birth of each of my kids."

At five feet five inches tall and 42 years old, Mary Anne's 200-plus weight load was a health hazard and a half, and I told her so. She had tried countless diets—low-calorie diets, including Weight Watchers, a hospital-based program that measured calories and a liquid-protein diet on which she had lost more than 30 pounds in three months and gained back, with interest, in four.

So what was the use? Besides, she hadn't come to me with weight loss in mind. Her problems were medical. Mary Anne's blood pressure was an abnormally elevated 160/100, she had a number of allergies, and her chief complaint was the extreme fatigue she had endured for the past several years. Add her excess weight to all that, and I knew she was heading into a difficult midlife physical crisis. I recommended and she agreed to do Atkins.

"By the second week doing Induction, I realized I felt really good," recalls Mary Anne. "I had a lot more energy than I'd had on my old diet, and I wasn't hungry."

After five weeks, she'd lost 21 pounds, and her blood pressure was a normal 120/78. It took nine months for her to get to 139 pounds. "I lost weight without any hassle," she says. "I was eating things I really liked to eat anyway. And the change in my life was incredible. Before, my favorite position had been sitting. Now I go out camping with my youngest son, and last summer I went horseback riding in the Rockies. The people at the lab where I work can't believe the new me. I go out to lunch with some of the other women who are on diets, and they can't seem to lose weight, and they're hungry. And I'm sitting there eating a juicy hamburger and a large salad."

Another two years have passed. Mary Anne's weight still hovers around 142. She has a glass of wine before dinner a couple of nights a week, and she eats two potatoes weekly. Her only other carbohydrates are plenty of vegetables and salads. She's on a luxurious regimen that she enjoys. She's full of energy, and her blood pressure is normal.

Is Mary Anne Evans ever going to fall off Atkins? Knowing her intense motivation, I have no doubt that she will enjoy long-term success. You need to have within yourself that same strength of conviction.

At the Finish Line

I would expect that as you traveled along the slow Pre-Maintenance path, one day you realized you were actually in Lifetime Maintenance: Your weight remained constant within a pound or two for several weeks. The decisions to move from Induction to OWL and from OWL to Pre-Maintenance were conscious choices on your part. But it is not always easy to define the moment at which you leave Pre-Maintenance and move to Lifetime Maintenance; the former segues naturally into the latter. But from now on, you will have conscious choices to make every day of your life. So, let me remind you of why it is worth making the right choices.

What Lifetime Maintenance Does for You

By now, you should know this by heart, but in this case a little repetition is a good thing. Adhering to Lifetime Maintenance will:

- provide you with a way of eating that allows you to stay slim for the rest of your life.
- allow you to maximize the amount of healthy carbohydrate foods you can eat while staying within 3 to 5 pounds of your goal weight.
- prevent re-addiction to foods that have gotten you in trouble before by helping you to avoid frequent exposure to them.
- teach you how to drop back to an earlier weight loss phase, when needed, to achieve lifetime weight control.
- teach you how to make the healthiest carbohydrate choices, which will allow you to continue to stay in control of your eating habits, feel your best and maintain improved blood-lipid levels, blood pressure and other lab test results, as well as optimize your blood pressure, energy and more.
- teach you how to adjust your carbohydrate consumption when metabolic circumstances change, before you find yourself regaining inches and/or weight.
- reduce your risk factors for cardiovascular disease, hypertension, diabetes, and other sugar metabolism disorders.
- give you a sense of accomplishment and confidence that spills over into the rest of your life.

How to Do Lifetime Maintenance—Correctly

Now that you've made it to your goal weight, you can continue to select from a greater range of foods and consume more carbs than you did in the two earlier phases of Atkins. But as I've said at every transition: No way is this a license to return to your old eating patterns. All too often, people win the battle of weight loss only to lose the war of weight control. To maintain your goal weight, you must know your metabolic needs. Your Critical Carbohydrate Level for Maintenance (CCLM) (see page 197), which you found during Pre-Maintenance, lets you know how many carbs you can eat each day to maintain your weight. Stay right at or around that number, and your weight should not fluctuate beyond the perfectly natural range of 2 or 3 pounds. (Hormonal changes and other daily fluctuations in your body account for a small seesaw effect.) Later, I'll tell you about why and how you may have to adjust your CCLM at various times in your life.

Carbohydrate Gram Levels and Metabolic Resistance for Maintaining

Metabolic Resistance	Approximate CCLM Range
High	25–40 grams of carbs per day
Average	40–60 grams of carbs per day
Low	60–90 grams of carbs per day
Regular exerciser*	90 or more grams of carbs per day

*In this context, a regular exerciser is someone who does vigorous exercise five days a week for at least forty-five minutes.

You also must conquer your former bad habits and learn how to cope with real-world challenges. Maintaining weight loss is as much a mental challenge as a physical one. For example, you need to eat right even under stress. How? By realizing that we tend to reach for sugar and starchy foods for comfort, when proper food choices can actually lessen the impact of stress on your body. Similarly, you'll need coping strategies for holidays and special occasions, as well as knowing how to get restaurants to serve you exactly what you know you should be eating.

Perhaps you can plan to "cheat" by cutting back for a few days before an event and then carefully choose a few indulgences. Or go back to a previous level of the plan prior to a vacation or holiday to give yourself some leeway. (For more coping techniques, see Chapter 19, "Eating in the Real World.")

As you did in the three weight loss phases of Atkins, make weight control a constant priority in your life. Re-create that attitude and you can continue your success. One good tool is to—once and for all—get rid of your "fat" wardrobe. When your clothes are getting tight and you don't have the next size in the closet to retreat to, you'll be forced to confront your weight gain sooner. By never letting your weight vary more than 3 to 5 pounds, you'll head off trouble and get off the weight roller coaster for good.

If your metabolism can handle it, I'm about to allow you, in moderation, many of the foods you used to enjoy. (The exception is sugar.) I have worked with too many over-weight individuals who have reached their goal weight four or more times, only to gain back the pounds every time. Their fatal flaw: always trying to return, as closely as they could without giving up Atkins altogether, to their old way of eating. I hope you have learned better on this odyssey.

Here's what I recommend to my patients when they begin Lifetime Maintenance: Promise to weigh yourself at least once a week. Choose a lifetime weight range of 5 pounds, the low number being your goal weight. The higher number will be your maximum allowable weight. Whenever you reach the higher number, you must promise that, within a week, you will begin the Induction phase and quickly switch to OWL until you again reach your goal weight. Do this and you will never have more than 5 pounds to lose.

The Nitty-Gritty of Maintenance

What you should be asking yourself is "What level of carbohydrate consumption do I feel best on?" That's a more rational goal than trying to find the highest number of carbs you can get away with. This may mean you actually stay slightly below your CCLM. Many people find they feel better on a low level of carbs—perhaps only 30 or 35 grams a day—than they do on the most liberal version of the plan. That might be two salads and a couple of helpings of other vegetables. Together with satisfying portions of protein and fat, such an approach could provide good nutrition if you were vigilant about opting for nutrient-dense foods.

Other people feel best on twice that amount of carbohydrate and have the metabolism to support it. That is why CCLMs can vary so greatly from one person to another. This is your opportunity to individualize a perfect eating plan for yourself. Remember, your best carbohydrate level is the one on which you can be happiest and healthiest without experiencing cravings and regaining weight.

Rules of Lifetime Maintenance

- Adhere to your Critical Carbohydrate Level for Maintenance (CCLM).
- Continue to eat natural, unprocessed, nutrient-dense carbohydrates.
- Exercise regularly.
- Continue to take nutritional supplements, modifying your regimen to meet your needs.
- Develop a strategy for dealing with temptation.
- Never let yourself get more than 5 pounds above your goal weight.

A Lifetime of Delicious Meals

What most of my patients discover by the time they reach the Lifetime Maintenance phase of Atkins is how endlessly varied, rich and satisfying this way of eating is.

Donna Miller, who came to see me a couple of years ago drained of all energy, beset with allergies and 30 pounds overweight, had always been a bread, bagels and pizza freak. In four months, she went from being a size 12 (almost bursting at the seams, as she admitted) to being a size 8. In addition, her energy returned almost as soon as we took her off of wheat, sugar and milk. But what was she going to eat?

She was a resourceful woman, and I hope her eating plan sounds as attractive to you as it does to me. For breakfast now she often eats smoked salmon and a small salad or two scrambled eggs with tofu. For lunch, she'll stir-fry or steam vegetables the way the Japanese do, and with them she'll have corned beef or a lean hamburger patty or some fish. For dinner, along with chicken, rib steak or salmon, she likes zucchini, eggplant or asparagus. She also finds she can have lentils, split peas and kasha (buckwheat groats) without gaining weight. She often has the kasha with cinnamon and a few apple slices.

Donna has been expanding her variety of salads, trying greens such as arugula, watercress and endive, since she started doing Atkins. She told me recently that she particularly appreciates the range of possible food alternatives, compared to the rather repetitive high-starch menu she used to be on. What impresses me the most is that every item in her new eating plan is wholesome, fresh and healthy. Frankly, I defy anyone to propose a tastier and more flexible eating plan—on which you can remain trim and healthy for a lifetime—than the Atkins program.

Dealing With Weight Gain

But even with flexibility and great food, you can come upon a patch of trouble. What if you're happily eating away and feeling great, and then suddenly you notice those awful pounds and inches are staging a revival? Since you are in Lifetime Maintenance, I know that you've reached your goal weight. Therefore, you're probably no longer in lipolysis, which, by definition, involves an element of fat loss. Newly slim people are no longer trying to shed pounds, and so they don't burn fat for fuel most of the time because they're above their CCLL.

But here's the catch that many people don't see: There is very little leeway before you break through your CCLM to the level at which you begin to gain. A typical male of average metabolic resistance may find he has a CCLM of 50 grams. As long as he regularly eats no more than 50 grams of carbs a day he will not lose more weight and become too thin. On the other hand, if he starts consuming 60 grams a day, he'll be above his CCLM and will start to regain weight.

At your goal weight, you are, in fact, pretty finely balanced in your carbohydrate intake. Nothing is exact, of course. Life has a way of changing and your weight will, in fact, constantly shift up and down by small increments. The most convenient way to maintain your best weight now is to not ever let that "up" get too far out of hand. If it does, you may find yourself sliding down an uphill path, to coin a phrase.

I recommend that you know your weight—after all, it's one aspect of your general health that you can easily keep track of. Getting on the scale at least once a week is a must for successful weight maintenance. When you find that you've gone 5 pounds or more over your maintenance weight or that your clothes are getting tight, you must put things back on their proper course. And you must do it without delay!

Protect Your Weight Losses

You have invested a lot of effort and psychic energy in the lessons you learned on your weight loss journey. Since you and I both know you have a tendency to put on the pounds, I want you to keep a sharp eye for any resumption of weight gain. Maybe Thanksgiving is coming up, or Christmas, or your birthday, or your spouse's birthday, or your vacation. By the time you celebrate any one of those with a bout of unrestrained indulgence, you may find that instead of being 5 pounds overweight you're 15 pounds overweight. Instead of waiting, act now!

Don't get depressed and give up. Even if you do temporarily get off track, continue to exercise and take your supplements. It's crucial that you don't surrender all control. Start with Induction and stay on OWL until you've reached your goal weight again, at which time you should ease back into Lifetime Maintenance. Exercising more vigorously after going overboard will also help get you back on the straight and narrow.

Remember, going straight back to the Induction phase is as simple as beginning Atkins in the first place. Do not go back to Lifetime Maintenance without first losing all you have regained. It's simple. A salad a day, a portion of veggies, plenty of protein and fat and, voila!, you've slashed your weight back in as little as six to eight days, or two or three weeks, depending upon your degree of metabolic resistance.

It's no news to anyone that as we get older, our metabolism tends to slow down a bit, making it harder to maintain the slim body many of us were blessed with in our youth. This means that the CCLM you had in your thirties may not be the CCLM you will be dealing with in your forties, and it is almost definitely not the CCLM you'll have in the decades after that. As you age, you may eventually have to control your carb intake a little more or increase your activity level—or perhaps even both—to maintain your goal weight.

Your strategy here should be very much like the base runner who allows himself to take a lead off first base, but never so far that he cannot scurry back to touch the base should the pitcher suddenly turn to pick him off. Your goal weight is the base you must touch between deviations, and the deviation must never be more than five pounds. Going back briefly to Induction allows you to get back to that number. Experience has taught me that people who regain weight after reaching their goal by doing Atkins—and then don't lose the weight—

are the ones who don't go back to Induction at a sign of trouble. The Lifetime Maintenance level they stick to isn't enough to get them back on track.

For consistent success, you must interpose the strict Induction phase between your weight gain and the eventual return to Lifetime Maintenance. This allows you to re-stabilize your blood chemistry and moderate cravings so you can be in control again.

Uses and Abuses of Induction

Induction not only jump-starts your weight loss, it is also a convenient refuge to which you can retreat whenever you need to get off a weight loss plateau or to get back on the program after a lapse. So if you've fallen off your Lifetime Maintenance program for whatever reason, you can return to Induction, and, like the ignition of an automobile, it will get your engine to turn over and start you down the road again.

If you reached your goal weight before slipping off the wagon for a brief period, you won't have to do Induction for long—just until you get back into lipolysis and the secondary process of ketosis. You'll know that has happened when you once again experience the ability to be in control of your appetite—the feeling that was such a revelation after the first forty-eight hours doing Induction.

These are perfectly appropriate uses of Induction. However, Induction can be abused and that abuse can ultimately threaten your ability to maintain a healthy weight. First of all, if you retreat to Induction every time you stray, you may begin to reinforce a dangerous pattern of behavior. By knowing Induction is there as a refuge, it may keep you from following the guidelines of the stage you are in. For a minor infraction or even a day of cheating, there is no need to go back to Induction. Simply drop down 5 or 10 grams for a couple of days, or go back to the previous phase. It is important that you learn how to eat properly as a way of life. Zigzagging back and forth between Induction and Lifetime Maintenance means you have not integrated this new, healthy eating pattern into your life.

Another more serious concern I have is the impact this back-and-forthing can have on your metabolism. (See "The Wrong Way to Do Atkins" on pages 223–225.) I have heard people say, "I love doing Atkins, because we can cheat on the weekends, then go back to Induction on Monday morning." While this behavior pattern may work for the short term, it will probably backfire in more ways than one. It's likely that your metabolism will adapt at a certain point—in a sense, developing a tolerance. People who repeatedly regain weight and go back to Induction sometimes find that they do not experience the dramatic and easy weight loss they initially enjoyed. Add in the fact that none of us is getting any younger and our metabolism's natural tendency is to slow down with passing years. Finally, your body pays a price healthwise if you dramatically switch back and forth repeatedly from a fat-burning to a glucose-burning metabolism.

If you keep retreating to Induction from Lifetime Maintenance, it becomes a form of yo-yo dieting. I'm not saying you shouldn't go back to Induction when you need it, I'm simply saying don't do it regularly, in the belief that it will always work the same way for you. You may be in for a nasty surprise.

The Bountiful World of Maintenance

Lifetime Maintenance may not be much different from OWL for people with high metabolic resistance. If you are one of the lucky folks with low metabolic resistance, you may be able to eat most vegetables—including starchy vegetables, fruit, legumes and whole grains such as oats, barley, millet, wild rice, couscous or buckwheat. You may even be able to handle an occasional potato. But, and this is a significant distinction, that does not mean you can eat all these things in one day. You still have to count carbs to stay at your CCLM. You can begin to use recipes, such as breaded veal chops, that contain some carbohydrate ingredients.

But the last choice, the truly hazardous indulgence, is sweets. Frankly, my suggestion to you is that you restrict your consumption of sweets made with real sugars to the occasional slice of birthday or wedding cake for really special celebrations. Those of you who have had a sizable chunk of your life made miserable by sugar may even decide, after graciously accepting them, to quietly deposit those pieces on somebody else's plate.

While you probably cannot convince your best friend to have her baker make a controlled carb wedding cake just to satisfy your needs, you can create your own personal world of sweets in your kitchen. In recent years, there have been more artificial sweeteners approved for use by the Federal Drug Administration. (See "Artificial Sweeteners" on pages 128–129 for more on sugar substitutes.) The recipe section at the end of this book will also introduce you to sugarless versions of many classic sweet treats.

Your Metabolic Tendencies Are Never Cured

They never are, you know. The fat you just sent to kingdom come was one symptom of a chronic metabolic condition. You do have and always will have a metabolic tendency to be overweight. The blood-sugar imbalance that I identified for you in Chapter 5 will not go away permanently because you have taken a nutritional path that circumvents it. All you have to do is go back to eating the way you once did, or even partially so, and you will arouse the sleeping demon. In very short order, your pancreas will once again secrete large quantities of insulin, and you'll suffer the symptoms of unstable blood sugar—jitters, brain fog, afternoon fatigue and the like. Then your insulin resistance will lead inevitably to the production of more insulin and that, in turn, to weight gain if your carb intake exceeds your tolerance.

Need I remind you that you don't want to go there?

But What About My Bad Habits?

If you want to be healthy and free of surplus body fat, then you cannot return to a perfectly random and careless pattern of eating. That's why one of the chief purposes of this book has been to build good habits into your lifestyle. Of course, we all have bad habits. Food is so confusing, so delicious, so psychologically essential even at times when it's not physiologically necessary. We all eat for pleasure and for reassurance, as well as for nutrition.

It may have been a hard week at work, and come the weekend you definitely intend to engage in some modest pigging out. I, too, enjoy the occasional binge. The question really is what type of binge. People usually binge on chocolates, desserts, cookies, ice cream and candy. Today there is a world of controlled carb products in all these taste-tempting categories, and I strongly recommend that they become part of your Lifetime Maintenance program so that you will enjoy the maximum eating pleasure. But even with these remarkable inventions, you could, by overdoing, still get into trouble. A controlled carb chocolate bar may have only 2 grams of carbohydrates that impact on your blood sugar compared to 17 to 20 carb grams in the sugar-filled variety of comparable size. But eat five of them and you could well be back to the same kind of destructive behavior that got you in trouble in the first place.

So you have two choices: You can use some of these delicious treats in moderation, *the way they are meant to be used*. Or, if you absolutely must binge, binge on protein/fat foods. I say that not because you can't gain a pound or two if you put away too many lamb chops, but because protein foods are fundamentally self-limiting. Most everyone has eaten thirty cookies at one sitting at some time in their life, and many carbohydrate addicts have done it hundreds of times, but how many people have eaten ten hard-boiled eggs at one sitting? Protein and fat foods satiate appetite quite quickly. It really isn't possible to go on munching them endlessly, and hardly anyone desires to. (Nuts and seeds may be the exception, but they are still better than cookies.) That doesn't mean a chicken breast doesn't make a delicious snack, and that, combined with a few other things, it couldn't constitute a delicious minor binge.

The crucial fact about protein foods is that they don't unleash a metabolic tidal wave in your body. Very few people get addicted to protein. Your blood-glucose level doesn't sharply rise and fall when you sit down to eat a Cobb salad. But it does just that when you chow down a slice of pie. That leads to the "need" for another slice and then another.

I don't want to scare you with the prospect of never eating another piece of Grandma's pumpkin pie. If you weren't an uncontrolled carbohydrate addict with an obesity problem that only this program has been able to cure, then you might cautiously see if you can indulge occasionally without causing noticeable aftereffects.

Trigger foods—ones to which you are addicted—are the ones you can't stop eating, and they are the very foods you should not add back. It might be peanuts, chocolate, potato chips or something else. If you find you are always planning when you can have your next portion of that food, cut it out altogether, or be sure to have it just once a week, perhaps as a Friday night treat. Only you know whether the first or the second strategy will work better for you. Remember, it's about what works! (For more on bingeing and strategies to minimize its damage, see Chapter 19.)

If you aren't addicted, then you have room to maneuver. The occasional slice of pizza or the ice cream cone just might be permissible. I don't recommend such compromises, I simply recognize that human nature demands them now and then. But be careful: Remember 5 pounds above your goal weight is the maximum; then take yourself firmly in hand and get back on plan. A firm resolution to deal with weight regain immediately will serve you well. An even better idea is to hold out for sugarless, full-fat ice cream.

And, don't forget, the way you're eating now is healthful. Junk food isn't, and it isn't going to make you feel good. After you've been off it for a while, the ice cream or the pizza go down nicely, but once you've eaten them, you may notice a temporary return of some familiar old symptoms. Many of my patients tell me that after not eating junk food for months while doing Atkins, the distress they experience when they do eat it has cured them of these urges once and for all.

Influences Beyond Your Control

As you have learned, a proper lifetime eating plan involves utilizing all four phases of Atkins. That's because, much as you may not want to hear it, maintaining your goal weight can provide a challenge or two. Factors independent of your appetite can influence it. No one's weight is constant. There will be times in your life when you gain some weight back. A change in activity level—a more sedentary job, for example—hormonal changes, the addition of certain medications and simply the passage of years can slow your metabolism.

Fortunately, you'll have developed the confidence to know that those small weight gains can be easily controlled. But such changes also mean that you may need to adjust your CCLM from time to time, in effect going back to OWL or to Pre-Maintenance or to Induction for a week or so. If you are eating just as you always have on Lifetime Maintenance and you suddenly begin to gain weight, try reducing your carb intake by 5 grams and see if your weight stabilizes. If so, that number is your new CCLM. Of course, you will then also want to trim off those extra pounds by temporarily dropping below that number.

Some Parting Recommendations

For those of you who have been successful, your nutritional voyage with me seems to be almost over. It will continue—indefinitely, I hope—but now you're driving the car. I want to leave you with eight basic principles for your lifetime doing Atkins:

1. Be food aware—remember that fresh meat, fish, fowl, vegetables, nuts, seeds and occasional fruits and starches are the foods nature intended you to eat. That packaged refined carbohydrate stuff in the supermarket puts money in somebody's pocket. And it puts garbage into your stomach. This is the only body you've got. Notice how good it feels now! Notice how much better it looks! Keep it that way!

2. Be wary—endlessly wary—of sugar and corn syrup, and white flour and cornstarch. Look at the labels of any packaged food you are considering and avoid (like the plague) those that contain sugar, corn syrup and honey. And read those labels for the carbohydrate content of the foods you want to eat.

3. Individualize your personal eating plan. Try new foods. Increase the variety of foods that you like and enjoy. It will help to prevent you from going back to eating foods that you have enjoyed in the past, but which simply aren't good for you. Use controlled carb alternatives as well as the recipes provided in the recipes section of this

book, or on our website at *www.atkinscenter.com*, or in my companion cookbook. I most strongly recommend that you develop a menu that's appealing, tasty and satisfying to you. Once you're happy with eating healthy foods, your nutritional future is almost assuredly going to be a healthy one.

4. Continue your already established and effective program of vitanutrient supplementation. I've told you some of what you need to know. Chapter 23 provides further details.

5. Consume caffeine and alcohol only in moderation.

6. Remember that addictions can be managed only through abstinence.

7. Take care of weight regain promptly and effectively by returning to the Induction and OWL phases for as long as it takes to get back to your goal weight. Swear that you will never allow yourself to be more than 5 pounds and two weeks worth of Induction away from your goal weight.

8. Make exercise a regular part of your life.

One final word. It is well known that virtually all individuals regain all or most of their hard-lost pounds within five years.[2] But when a program changes the composition of the diet, not the quantity, and when pre-maintenance teaching and the 5-pound rule are consistently applied, recidivism is a rare phenomenon, indeed. My experience resoundingly confirms this fact.

Instead of bouncing you back into the land of the fat, the four phases of Atkins welcome you permanently into the home of the slim.

The Wrong Way to Do Atkins

Over the years, I have been amazed at the way people ignore the advice in this book and devise ways to abuse the Atkins Nutritional Approach by doing it their own way. Here are nine of the most common misconceptions among Atkins abusers:

1. **Misconception:** Atkins can be used as a short-term or crash diet.
   Reality: If you do Induction for two weeks to drop 10 pounds and then go back to your old way of eating, you *will* be treating it as a crash diet. But that goes against everything I recommend, and will lead to problems in the long run.
2. **Misconception**: You can lose weight doing Atkins, then return to your old way of eating.
   Reality: Do this, and as with your past attempts, you will neglect to change those eating habits that ensure you always regain lost weight.
3. **Misconception**: You can focus solely on losing weight and minimize the maintenance aspects.
   Reality: Any weight loss program that does not segue into weight maintenance is doomed to failure. The eating plan you will follow during Lifetime Maintenance is likely to be somewhere between your menu during the Induction phase and the way you ate before you started Atkins.
4. **Misconception**: You can eat any food so long as you do not exceed 20 grams of carbs a day.
   Reality: If you eat junk foods or other nutrient-deficient carbohydrate foods instead of vegetables and other nutrient-dense foods, you will miss most of the benefits I write about and you certainly will not be fostering long-term health.

5. **Misconception**: You can use Atkins for weight loss, but you don't have to bother with exercise and supplements if you don't have any health problems.

   Reality: If you don't supplement with vitanutrients and exercise regularly, you may take off pounds, but you will miss out on important health benefits. And everyone needs exercise: It is not related solely to weight loss.

6. **Misconception**: You can just continue to do Induction until you lose all of your weight.

   Reality: You will lose weight more quickly if you continue doing Induction, but you won't learn how to keep that weight off permanently if you don't move through the four phases. More important, you will miss out on the benefits of the phytochemicals present in health-promoting carbohydrate foods.

7. **Misconception**: You can go back to eating your favorite foods after you lose weight.

   Reality: Your favorite foods may well be your problem foods. Unless you acknowledge and learn how to deal with your addictions, you are doomed to regain your weight and fall back into the dangerous cycle of high blood sugar and overproduction of insulin.

8. **Misconception**: You can do Induction during the week and binge on weekends and still lose or maintain weight.

   Reality: When you do Atkins during the week and then cheat on the weekends, for several days after your binge, you are no longer burning fat. At most, you could be in the fat-burning state for only three days each week. In addition, you may have overstimulated your insulin response, increasing the metabolic risk factors underlying your weight problem. Remember that when you burn fat, dietary fat is also being burned. However, if you combine high carbs with high fat—the typical American diet—you can be increasing your cardiovascular risks.

9. **Misconception**: You can do Atkins while following a low-fat regimen.

   Reality: To encourage your body to burn its own stores of fat, you need to reduce the amount of carbohydrates you eat, meaning you need to eat primarily foods rich in protein and fat. Remember that essential fatty acids play a role in normal metabolic function. Fat also plays a role in stabilizing blood sugar and increasing satiety. If fat intake is too low, you will not burn fat aggresively. Moreover, excess protein converts to glucose and can keep fat from becoming the primary fuel.

KEY POINTS!

- Lifetime Maintenance provides you with a way of eating that allows you to stay slim for the rest of your life.
- To maintain your goal weight you must know your metabolic needs.
- Don't stray more than 5 pounds from your goal weight.
- Don't be afraid to return to Induction, or OWL, for a few days if you need to restart your fat-burning engine.

TIPS:

- Stay away from foods containing sugar.
- If you feel the need to binge try eating a few hard-boiled eggs instead of chips or candy, or use many of the controlled carbohydrate products.
- Variety is the spice of life; try new foods.

18

A Regimen to Jump-Start Weight Loss

The heat is on. You've been invited to a friend's beach house two weeks from now. But you're spilling out of all your bathing suits; some of them look as though they might actually burst. Crying won't burn up enough calories to shed those pounds. You need a high-powered solution that will last a lifetime so you never have to repeat this misery.

Your problem is simple. You don't know how to start. Even though you've read everything in this book so far—you still want a bit of help to get going. Truly, I wish you could call me up or come see me, and we could work together to change your life. But we know that is not practical. So, in this chapter I give you some very specific information, and some very specific meal plans. Follow them to the letter and you will be well on your way to feeling good, looking good and being healthier. And well on your way to fitting into those bathing suits.

I've made the point many times in this book that Atkins is an individualized nutritional approach. But it has been my experience that certain people succeed much better if given a strict regimen to follow. It is likely that if you eat exactly what's presented to you here, you will achieve weight loss. So, at the end of this chapter is a week-long menu that spells out precisely what to eat. If you've opened the book directly to this chapter, the following instructions, before the menu, will be very important. For the rest of you, they will be a good review.

Remember, I don't advise losing more than one pound a day. (People with a lot of excess weight may lose more than a pound a day in the beginning. And you may very well lose water weight this fast in the beginning, and that is also okay.) That's about as fast as a normal human body can dump pounds safely and comfortably. Go faster, and you'll probably pay. Your metabolism won't have had time to adjust, you'll be losing an excessive amount of water and minerals and you may well feel fairly awful. Back off, for heaven's sake, and don't say I didn't warn you. Your body has its own wisdom, so listen to it.

And, just in case you actually did the unthinkable and skipped the beginning of the book to get to this chapter, let me repeat one important health warning: None of the weight loss phases of Atkins is appropriate for pregnant women or nursing mothers, and people with severe kidney disease should not do Atkins at all.

Ready . . .

I want to pause for a minute to remind you about the Atkins Nutritional Principles for weight loss. These points are so important I can't risk that you somehow skipped over them in our earlier discussion.

- During the Induction phase of Atkins your body switches from primarily burning carbohydrates to burning fat as its main energy source.[1-5]
- Controlling carbohydrate intake stabilizes blood-sugar levels, producing diverse and favorable physical effects. You will achieve these benefits by switching to the slower burning fuel found in proteins and fats.
- Typical results of these changes are a decrease in appetite, reduced sugar cravings and dramatic increases in energy.

Set . . .

As you jump-start your weight loss, remember that carbohydrate intake during Induction should be no more than 20 grams a day in the form of vegetables and other acceptable food choices. In this phase, you will be eating no breads, sugars, grains, potatoes, rice, pastas or fruits. Once your carbohydrate intake goes below a certain threshold, you will primarily burn your body fat for fuel. Since your body stores enough carbohydrate reserve to fuel it for approximately forty-eight hours, it will take that long for the process to start. You may feel hungry and out-of-sorts for the first two to three days. Be patient and persist.

Go!

1. Eat three meals a day. Stabilizing the blood sugar is the basic tool of controlled carbohydrate weight loss, and to achieve this you should not go longer than six waking hours without eating acceptable food. You can, however, eat four or five smaller meals a day, so long as you don't exceed 20 grams of carbohydrates.
2. You are permitted to eat liberal amounts of eggs, meat and fish, including beef, pork, chicken, turkey, duck, wild game, shellfish, veal and lamb. Eat until you feel pleasantly full, but do not gorge.
3. Liberal amounts of fats and oils are permitted. This includes butter, olive oil, mayonnaise and any oil that is liquid at room temperature. (Consume no hydrogenated oil or other trans fats—including margarine.)
4. Herbs and spices are permitted as long as they do not contain sugar.
5. Cheese (aged full-fat, firm, soft, semi-soft) is limited to three to four ounces daily. Fresh cheese, such as cot-

tage cheese and farmer's cheese, is too high in carbo-hydrates for Induction.

6. You may have up to three cups loosely packed (measured raw) salad vegetables each day. This includes all leafy green vegetables, mushrooms, celery, radishes, green peppers, and cucumbers (see also "Salad Vegetables" on page 125).

7. Other vegetables low in carbohydrates are limited to one cup daily. (If you have a cup of these veggies, consume only two cups of salad vegetables.) This includes the following non-starchy vegetables (see also "Other Vegetables" on page 126):

   - Artichoke hearts
   - Asparagus
   - Bean sprouts
   - Broccoli
   - Cauliflower
   - Eggplant
   - Kohlrabi
   - Okra
   - Onion
   - Pumpkin
   - Rhubarb
   - Sauerkraut
   - Scallions
   - Snow peas
   - Spaghetti squash
   - String beans
   - Tomato
   - Turnips
   - Water chestnuts
   - Zucchini

8. You may also include the following items in your daily carb count:

   - Olives (up to twenty)
   - Avocados (up to half a small avocado)

- Lemon/Lime juice (two to three tablespoons)
- Cream (heavy, light or sour, two to three table-spoons)

9. You must drink at least eight 8-ounce glasses of pure water daily. This can be filtered, mineral or spring water (not seltzer). You may also have unlimited amounts of herbal tea (without sugar), but these do not count toward your total of eight glasses.

10. Drink only decaffeinated coffee and tea and use only acceptable sweeteners (listed in #13 below).

11. Alcohol is not permitted in any form.

12. Treat aspartame (NutraSweet® or Equal®) with caution. Avoid whenever possible. This includes products sweetened with this ingredient, such as diet sodas and diet Jell-O. Check labels on other products that purport to be low or controlled carb.

13. You may use up to three packets of sucralose (Splenda®) daily. (More and more products are being made with Splenda® so if you use any, include those grams in your tally also.)

14. Exclude the following items entirely:
- Sugar (in any form, including corn syrup, honey and maple syrup)
- Milk and yogurt (cream is allowed in limited amounts)
- Fruit and fruit juice
- Flour products (breads, pasta, crackers, etc.)
- Grains
- Cereals
- Beans and legumes
- Starchy or high sugar-containing vegetables (potatoes, yams, corn, peas, parsnips, beets, carrots)
- Sweet condiments (such as most ketchups, barbeque sauce and balsamic vinegar)
- French dressing, Thousand Island dressing (check labels for carb count)

- Cottage cheese, farmer's cheese and other fresh cheeses
- Nuts and seeds

15. When eating out be careful that you're not consuming "hidden" carbohydrates in sauces or breaded products. Tell your waiter that you would like your food prepared free of sugar, flour and cornstarch.

16. Unless you are physically unable to do so, exercise every day, even if it's just a walk around the block. This is an important part of the program in all phases and will certainly increase the rate at which you lose weight.

17. Chapter 23 will give you extensive details on nutritional supplementation for the Atkins Nutritional Approach. At this stage you should, at a minimum, take a good daily multivitamin with minerals, including potassium, magnesium and calcium but without iron.

Time to Be Strict

Anyone who is committed to doing Atkins properly needs to follow these rules to the letter. Remember that it takes two to three days for the body to switch to fat burning. One cheat and you're back to a glucose-burning metabolism. You can lose the effects of two or three days of fat burning with one cheat. So if you have the misguided belief that you can do Atkins all week and then indulge over the weekend, don't expect to see dramatic results.

Let me emphasize two key points:

1. You may have heard that you can eat as much as you desire of the acceptable foods. This is *not* the case. If you stuff yourself with steaks and cheeseburgers, some of that protein will convert to glucose in your body. Instead, simply eat the amount that allows you to feel satisfied. If you have been overeating for years,

perhaps even decades, you may not know what being satiated feels like. Experiment and find that place where you say, "I could eat more, but I am satisfied." Know that you can have a snack in an hour or two if you wish.

2. Number 16, on page 231, with regard to exercise, was not put in there merely as decoration. Exercise is good for you, and it will help you lose. Moreover, it not only causes you to burn calories, but it accelerates your metabolism, increasing the speed with which every other part of a weight loss program works and keeps you on the road to better health.

Now to the meal plans. Follow this menu for the first week, then repeat it for the second week. Items with an * are included in the "Food and Recipes" section starting on page 367.

One-Week Induction Menu

MONDAY
Breakfast
Two scrambled eggs
Two turkey sausages

Lunch
Greek salad made with Romaine lettuce, half a tomato, feta cheese, olives and dill vinaigrette
Small can of tuna

Dinner
Veal Scallops with White Wine Caper Sauce*
Sautéed spinach
Gelatin dessert made with sucralose topped with whipped cream

Snack
Controlled carb strawberry shake

TUESDAY
Breakfast
Crustless Quiche*
Two tomato slices

Lunch
Chicken salad served over chopped cucumber, radishes and
   watercress

Dinner
Maple Mustard-Glazed Salmon*
Sautéed broccoli with red pepper
Small green salad with vinaigrette

Snack
Ten to twenty olives

WEDNESDAY
Breakfast
Smoked salmon and cream cheese roll-ups
Two hard-boiled eggs

Lunch
Homemade Chicken Soup*

Dinner
Broiled steak
Oven-Fried Turnips*
Arugula and Boston lettuce salad

Snack
Turkey, Romaine lettuce, mayonnaise roll-up

THURSDAY
Breakfast
Western omelette with green salsa

Lunch
Vegetable broth with shredded white radish
Shrimp salad over greens

Dinner
Turkey Cutlets with Green Peppercorn Sauce*
Cauliflower-Leek Purée*
Gelatin dessert made with sucralose topped with whipped cream

Snack
One ounce Swiss cheese

FRIDAY
Breakfast
Two ounces cream cheese sprinkled with cinnamon and
    flaxseeds
Two Bran-a-Crisp™ crackers

Lunch
Chef's salad with blue cheese dressing

Dinner
Pork burgers
Creamy Red Cabbage Slaw*
Broiled portobello mushrooms with sesame oil

Snack
Mocha granita

SATURDAY
Breakfast
Whitefish salad
Two tomato slices

Lunch
Ham, spinach and cheese omelette
Mixed green salad

Dinner
Herbed-Roast Chicken with Lemon*
Buttered green beans
Italian Almond Cream*

Snack
Celery stuffed with Roasted Garlic and Vegetable Dip*

SUNDAY
Breakfast
One-and-a-half slices Zucchini Nut Bread*
Two ounces cream cheese

Lunch
Broiled cheeseburger
Large mixed green salad with two tomato slices

Dinner
Cajun Pork Chops*
Sautéed kale with garlic

Snack
Controlled carb vanilla shake

Having seen how straightforward it is to get started, I have only one question: Are you going to read the rest of this book? There is only one answer: You must, because your health and well-being depend on it. But let me remind you: Two weeks won't get the job done—only a lifetime of health-oriented behavior will.

19

Eating in the Real World

There's a quote from Oscar Wilde that I love to paraphrase: There is only one thing that I cannot resist, and that is temptation. I think we have perfected the art of weight loss to the point where that is so true! And temptation wears many guises.

The biggest booby trap is called the "Real World." Here, sad events can upset us so much that we turn for solace to our old reliable friends, the foods that have always comforted us (see Chapter 21, "The Psychology of Weight Loss"). But happy times can also undermine our weight loss efforts. Vacations, holidays, let's-bring-out-the-champagne celebrations, family weddings and gourmet dinner parties are also challenges to overcome. Then there's business travel and entertainment, plus pit stops at fast food places. In all of these situations, those of us determined to shed excess pounds and inches must find ways to avoid pitfalls or, if we do succumb, ways to right ourselves and get back on course. With the tools in this book, you will be able to do just that.

Dealing With Temptation

The truth is that temptation lurks everywhere, unless you deny yourself a social and working life and the attendant pleasures of eating out. I believe that the best way to overcome temptation is not with willpower, which is so often in short supply, but with our brain power, a potentially unlimited resource.

Imagine that you're doing great, losing weight, feeling better than ever, thrilled with yourself, hearing compliments from friends and acquaintances—and then it happens! Despite all your good intentions, you're mightily tempted by a food you're not supposed to have. What to do? I'll tell you this: You'd better have a strategy ready!

Strategies you can employ are:

- Talking yourself out of your momentary passion so you can stay the course.
- Deliberately stopping the Atkins plan, but you must do so intelligently. Pick your poison. Don't throw all reason to the wind. Do you want that potato with your meal, or a glass of wine with your dinner, or a taste of your partner's dessert? Pick one and only one and be done with it. Then get right back to doing Atkins. Used *occasionally*, and I stress the word "occasionally," this strategy can be a useful technique.
- Finding an alternative that is low in carbs but gives the same taste sensations. Make or purchase controlled carbohydrate ice cream, mousse, bread, crackers, chips or chocolate sensation.

Let me explain something about cravings, because this point might allow you to continue with Atkins. Your craving appeared, most likely, because it was triggered by a drop in blood sugar. Your body perceived a need to halt the falling glucose level and transmitted a signal that it needed sweets. (This theory applies only when you crave some form of quick-fix carbohydrate.) Your solution, simply put, is to eat some rich food, high in fat and protein with very little or no carbohydrate. Such a snack will stabilize your blood sugar, and presto-change-o, no more cravings.

The best foods to head off cravings are foods that contain both protein and fat. I call macadamia nuts the Atkins follower's best friend. Almost as effective are walnuts, pecans or Brazil nuts. Other good foods for stopping cravings are cream cheese or such rich dessert cheeses as mascarpone. Another cravings buster is something sweetened with sucralose, along with heavy cream. My personal favorite is to whip three ounces of heavy cream with two-thirds of a scoop of controlled carbohydrate shake mix to create a chocolate, vanilla, strawberry or cappuccino mousse. Or you may opt for a diet gelatin dessert slathered generously with whipped heavy cream (not the pre-made, sugar-added type, of course). Some controlled carbohydrate bars are also excellent cravings busters. There are also controlled carb chocolate bars (appropriate only after Induction) that serve when only chocolate will satisfy your cravings.

Let me just remind you of the basic principle behind this kind of eating. Macadamia nuts, for instance, may be on every conventional diet's no-no list because they are so calorically dense, but what counts is the effect they have upon your body chemistry. Because macadamia nuts have such a high ratio of fat to carbohydrate, they help control your appetite and tend to result in your eating fewer calories. Moreover, let's not forget convenience—nuts and seeds can easily be kept in your purse or pocket. If your business or travel schedule forces you to miss meals or be frequently exposed to unacceptable meals, you've got a substitute or perfect tide-me-over at hand.

Another favorite of mine is the avocado, one of the few fruits that contains fat (yes, it is a fruit, not a vegetable). It is the beneficial monounsaturated-type fat, and the avocado provides a welcome taste departure for those who crave something fresh, natural and filling. You can make an elegant lunch by filling the big seed hollow with shrimp, crabmeat or tuna salad. Half a California or Haas avocado—the kind with a dark, textured skin—contains about 5 to 6 grams of digestible carbohydrate. You can also garnish your breakfast omelette with avocado. And then there's guacamole, just about everyone's favorite dip. You'll find my recipe on page 400.

But what if we're not talking about an addictive craving or a simple impulse that can be satisfied by a change in body chemistry? What if we're talking about long-term desire, something that has always been one of your favorite foods and now is on your no-no list? You know, things like pizza, bagels, tacos, egg rolls, pancakes, linguini and _____ (you fill in the blank).

Finding Substitutes for Favorite Foods

One of the best don't-fall-off-the-program techniques is to eat foods that substitute for a highly desired food. If you lust after any of the above, or for blintzes, lasagna, Yorkshire pudding or even chocolate truffles, ice cream, cheesecake or strawberry shortcake, the answer lies in using the ingenious substitutes for these foods I've provided in the recipe section or through our website at *www.atkinscenter.com*. Learn to use them. They can be just as much a part of your menu-planning as grilled chicken and tossed salad. (Remember: Not all these recipes and products are suitable for the Induction phase.)

Understand that controlled carb cheesecake is not the same as cheesecake made with sugar, and that controlled carb pizza is not the same as pizza made with wheat flour. Conventional foods can contain ten times more carbohydrates than those made with sucralose, soy flour or other controlled carb ingredients. Interestingly, calorie-restricted foods may legally be called low calorie if the calorie level is reduced by thirty-three percent, but acceptable controlled carbohydrate alternatives typically contain a mere ten percent of the carbohydrate of the standard fare. So although there is enough carbohydrate in a portion of regular pizza or ice cream to send your fat mobilizers and ketones to a screeching halt, controlled carb substitutes can be safely used—in moderation. But eat five slices of controlled carb pizza or a whole pint of ice cream sweetened with sucralose and you're right back to your excessive behavior.

Formed in response to needs voiced by thousands of Atkins followers, there is a variety of controlled carb food products available, including energy bars, breakfast bars, bake mixes, shake mixes, ready-to-drink shakes, ice cream, bread, bagels and even a chocolate bar. All products have negligible amounts of carbohydrate, and several come in a variety of flavors. Companies like mine have numerous other products in development, and each may provide a controlled carb alternative for your taste preferences.

Although many other commercial products may also be acceptable, I do want to caution you that all controlled and low-carbohydrate foods are not created equal. Thanks to the immense success of Atkins, other companies are producing products to serve the growing population of controlled carb followers. A word to the wise: Be sure products that claim to be low in carbs really are. Also make sure they do not contain aspartame. What can you do to protect yourself? Read labels carefully (see "How to Read a Food Label" on pages 241–245). If a product seems too good to be true, it probably is. When you try a new food product, test how you react to it before eating a full portion. If you find it sparks new cravings or disagrees with you in any way, your safest option is to eat no more.

There is also a food that contains so little carbohydrate

that it can raise your count only 5 or 10 grams: crisp breads. My personal eating pleasure improved considerably when I found something flat and crunchy upon which to pile my cream cheese or guacamole or to serve as finger-size appetizers at parties. These toasted rye or wheat-bran delicacies, based on a popular Scandinavian concept, are mostly carbohydrate, so unlimited use of them would interfere with continued weight loss. But, because they are baked so thin and provide so much crisp surface area per carbohydrate gram, they are quite an ingenious way to spend your carbohydrate allowance. There are many brands and each has a different carbohydrate content per crisp, ranging from 3 to 6 grams, some of which is fiber. Fiber is good for keeping you regular; moreover, it does not impact your blood sugar, and you can deduct it from the total carb count to get what I call "the carbs that count when you do Atkins." This means that if a wheat crisp contains a total of 6 grams of carbohydrates and 3 of those grams are listed as fiber, the impact on your blood-sugar mechanism is the equivalent of just 3 grams of carbs. But again, when the desire for something crunchy surfaces, have one or two, then put the box away!

I have a point worth stressing: Every food I suggest could be off limits for those of you who demonstrate intolerance to one of its ingredients, and wheat and rye are two of those foods that turn up rather frequently as problems. Also, some fiber breads contain sugar. (Stay away from them, even if the fiber content is high.)

How to Read a Food Label: Just the Facts? Not Quite!

To ensure that consumers know what is in the foods they buy, the Food and Drug Administration (FDA) requires that the packaging of every manufactured food product display certain information. For starters, ingredients must be listed—in descending order of weight. Labeling must also include a Nutrition Facts panel (see page 244). Although the intent is informational, such labels do not supply all the facts, especially when it comes to carbohydrates. But once you know the secret to figuring out how many carbs really count when you do Atkins, the labels will become easy reading.

Backing into a Carb Count

But, first, let me explain a few things. Almost everything displayed on the Nutrition Facts panel is based on specific laboratory procedures called *assays*, regulated by the FDA. The quantity of fat, protein, ash and water can all be directly and exactly assayed. (Water and ash need not be listed on nutrition panels.) Carbohydrates, however, are the exception. Instead, the amount of carbohydrate is arrived at only after the other four components are directly computed: In other words, what is not fat, protein, ash or water is called *carbohydrate*.

All Carbs Are Not Created Equal

To complicate matters still further, carbohydrates are comprised of several sub-groups, which include dietary fiber, sugar, sugar alcohol and "other" carbohydrates—a kitchen-sink grouping of gums, lignans, organic acids and flavenoids. (These individual items *can* be assayed.) The FDA requires that a nutrition label include the total carbohydrates. The amount of dietary fiber and sugar must also be listed. However, the law does not require that other carbohydrate sub-categories appear. Some manufacturers voluntarily include the sub-categories of sugar alcohol and "other carbohydrate."

Not all types of carbohydrates behave the same way in your body. For example, when your body digests table sugar, it turns immediately into blood sugar. So sugar and most other carbohydrate are what we call "digestible carbohydrate." Other carbs, such as sugar alcohols, have a minimal impact on blood-sugar levels; still other carbs, such as dietary fiber, pass through your body without having an impact on your blood-sugar level. To date, the FDA has yet to focus on these important biochemical differences and treats all carbohydrates alike.

The Impact on Blood Sugar

When you look at a food label, you do not see a number for the carbs that have an impact on your blood-sugar level, or what I call "the carbs that count when you do Atkins." Fortunately, you don't have to be a food scientist or math whiz to figure it out. To calculate the carbohydrates that "count," simply subtract the number of grams of dietary fiber from the total number of carbohydrate grams. That's right. A little simple subtraction, and you've got the number. Actually, this number is a conservative one because most labels don't give you the additional info you would need to do further subtraction, such as the amount of sugar alcohol grams contained in the product.

What Is a Serving?

Now, there is another rather sneaky aspect of nutrition labels. In the old days, when you were still drinking such things, you may have purchased a twenty-ounce bottle of flavored ice tea sweetened with corn syrup. That's one serving, right? Wrong! Look carefully at the Nutrition Facts panel and you will see that a single serving is calculated not as the twenty ounces in the bottle but as eight ounces. You are expected to share that bottle with another friend and a half! That means all those calculations about carbohydrate content, sugar content and calories are for only eight ounces, not the whole bottle.

So, whenever you check a label to make sure you are not going over your daily carb count, double-check the serving size as well. And if you are planning to have more than what is considered one serving, multiply the adjusted carb count by the appropriate number of servings.

Here is what you should be aware of on a nutrition label:

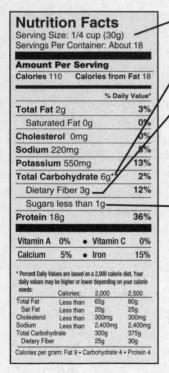

Serving size. If you have more than one serving, be sure to add in the carbs.

Total carbohydrates expressed in grams.

Amount of dietary fiber expressed in grams (subtract from the total number of carbohydrate grams to get "the carbs that count when you do Atkins").

Sugar expressed in grams.

Full Disclosure

At my food products company we try diligently to provide consumers with all the information they need to do Atkins. I believe you will benefit tremendously from the understanding about carbohydrates you have gained by reading this book. I would like to see all product manufacturers be required to present the important carbohydrate information right on the Nutrition Facts panel.

Let me give you an example of how it would work:

```
Food Product A
Total carbohydrate
     (as defined by the FDA)              15.0 grams
Non-caloric and/or
     non-blood sugar impacting carbs  12.5 grams
          (Polydextrose/Fiber  9.0 grams)
          (Glycerine            2.5 grams)
          (Sugar alcohol        1.0 grams)
Net carbs that count when
     doing Atkins                         2.5 grams
```

Now wouldn't that be helpful?

When Bending Becomes a Binge

Sometimes, of course, you might do more than just bend the amount of carbs you are supposed to be consuming each day—by eating a food that should be avoided altogether. The food in question may turn out to be the trigger mechanism for a craving. Then, look out! A full-blown binge usually begins right then and there.

Binges come in all shapes and sizes and can prove so disastrous that they turn a seemingly surefire weight loss success story into an instant failure. The weight regain is usually so profound it can be measured in pounds *per day*. Obviously, the longer you stay on your bender, the worse the results.

To stop a binge, your first responsibility is to know you're in trouble and immediately apply an effective technique. The best way I have found to do this is to take certain nutrients: chromium picolinate or chromium polynicotinate (400 mcg, three times daily for two days); L-glutamine (500 to 1,000 mg, three times daily); plus a single dose of vitamin B complex (50 mg). At the same time, overwhelm the cravings by instituting a high-fat, high-protein, Induction-level regimen: fatty fish, poultry, meat, cream cheese, shake mix or diet soda with heavy cream. Two days after you induce lipolysis and the secondary process of ketosis, the cravings should be gone, you should once again be in control and the weight gained so rapidly during the binge should already be falling to its previous level. And congratulations, you just dodged a bullet! But I stress again, you must do this quickly, a day or two after you went astray—and not after *weeks* of bingeing.

Once you are back in control again, you must figure out what food or food combination was the binge trigger. You certainly won't want to play with that "poison" again.

But there is a hardcore problem that arises when you discover there's something about my nutritional approach you don't like. Or, more specifically, that there's something you like too much, and you're not getting it. Naturally, you're thinking, Why did I promise that I would never have that food again? I'm no longer willing to keep that promise. Must *always* be always and never be *never*?

This important question has several answers. First, I ask you to consider the plight of a recovering alcoholic. Most of us realize that when an addiction such as alcoholism is the problem, it is far better that never *really* be never. So if your proposed carbohydrate deviation involves something you're addicted to, sadly I must give you that *never-never* advice. But if you are sure that your desire for a favorite food is for the sake of pleasure and not out of addiction, I guess I must allow you to try it and find out. It's better you have a small portion of that beloved food and feel satisfied than deprive yourself and later—in a moment of weakness—experience a full-scale blow out. Just keep your portion small, count the carbs in your daily tally and watch like a hawk to see if eating this food causes cravings or the return of other symptoms that vanished while doing Atkins. (Important: This kind of experimentation is not allowed during Induction.)

Outside Your Home

Actually, doing Atkins is easy in most circumstances. On weekends, in restaurants, on the job, when you travel a lot—unless someone imprisons you in a candy store—you really have nothing to worry about. Of course, the program is not completely adaptable to dinner parties given by people with fixed ideas about what everyone should eat. You'll need a little ingenious diplomacy to get you out of that situation. Let's examine possible scenarios one by one.

At work, you'll need to apply large doses of common sense. The coffee and Danish cart that circulates mid-morning and mid-afternoon smells so good! The bagels on the conference room table at the weekly staff meeting look so yummy. But not if you've had a three-cheese and mushroom omelette for breakfast and a filling lunch. Your resistance is at its greatest when you're satiated. Does the cafeteria or nearby luncheonette serve suitable food? Check it out, because if it doesn't, you'd better start brown-bagging it. Bring along some finger food—chicken drumsticks, hard-boiled or deviled eggs, slices of ham, cheese and steamed shrimp to have with your green salad.

Controlled carb followers will usually find restaurants to be much more friend than foe. They stay in business because of their ability to make food taste great and supply good service. However, fast food restaurants pose special challenges (see "Make Fast Food Friendly" on pages 254–255). Most main courses qualify as Atkins-acceptable. The trick is not to be seduced by all the extras. If it's at all possible, know what you're going to order before you walk in. And don't go for the carbohydrate extras just because they're right in front of you. You could safely eat all your weekly meals in a restaurant, as long as you become familiar with the possibilities of the menu and be alert for hidden pitfalls.

If the eating establishment is one you patronize often, talk to the waiter or the maitre d' and make it crystal clear that you're on a plan that permits no sugar in any manner, shape or form. This way you can root out "hidden" sugar in salad dressings or even in such prepared dishes as tuna fish salad. Sometimes fruit juices are used in cooking as a sugar substitute, which are equally unacceptable.

Go right down the menu and make sure your appetizer, main course and salad all qualify as controlled carb. Avoid sauces, breading and flour as a thickener. Such carbohydrate ingredients can be hidden in surprising places. There may be flour or grain in your hamburgers, or breadcrumbs in your crab cakes. Be alert. Otherwise, one meal can destroy your weight loss program for the day and set it back for the week.

Finally, engage the server with all the determination and finesse you can muster, and tell him or her what you can't have in your food. Don't hesitate to inquire firmly and insistently about what is in a particular dish. Very few waiters are offended if you make it clear how important this is to you. After all, you're the one who's going to tip him at the end of the meal. I've been told by many people that when they make their controlled carbohydrate preference clear, the waiter often tells them about his own success doing Atkins. Don't be surprised—millions of people have succeeded on this program in the last few years alone.

The fun comes when you discover restaurants that do great things with the acceptable foods you can eat freely. It shouldn't be too difficult to find a good cut of meat, fish or fowl with the right seasonings, prepared well and without carbohydrate. I've eaten thousands of wonderful restaurant meals—one hundred percent in compliance with Atkins. I know where to get the best lobster, roast beef, rack of lamb, crispy duck and poached salmon in my hometown (Manhattan). But I also know the best trout with a macadamia nut crust, the best veal a la Triestina, saltimbocca a la Romana, Chinese shrimp, Mexican guacamole, and chiles rellenos. Ladies and gentlemen, this is the true gourmet's delight. I always say, "If you're going to lose weight, you might as well do it with satisfying quantities of fine food."

The trick in restaurants is to not start eating until the appetizer or main course arrives. Or ask for a celery and olive tray in lieu of bread. If your companions want bread on the table, move the breadbasket to the far end of the table so it won't be under your nose. Remember, too, never save room for dessert.

Dinner parties can be real obstacle courses. At a pasta party, for example, there is a possibility that you may find nothing acceptable to eat. Let me warn you again that going off program for just one meal could set you back for nearly a week in regard to weight loss. The better policy is to let your host(ess) know beforehand that your doctor has prescribed a certain diet and politely ask what is being served. If the meal does not qualify, simply have a high-protein/high-fat entrée and a salad before you leave home. Or, if you fear that protein food will be in short supply—at a buffet, perhaps—make sure you bring something along—those macadamia nuts, for example.

Then there are the airlines—the Final Frontier of Junk Food. Your first line of defense is to call in advance and ask for a special meal. Tell them you're on an eating plan that is low in carbohydrate. It never hurts to ask because the more people who ask, the more likely airlines are to add this option.

If none of the airline options available is acceptable, bring your own food with you. But make sure that you have enough. Plan ahead. Don't allow for even the slim chance that you might be hungry enough to turn to the carbohydrates on board. It would be ironic if your ironclad willpower evaporates in the one place universally considered to provide the worst possible food. For more on the challenges you may encounter while traveling, see "On the Move" below.

On the Move

Whether you are traveling by plane, train or car, travel is inherently unsettling. Suddenly you're without your familiar routines and resources. Not only are you confronted with temptations you would never allow in your house, you're exposed to them precisely when you're most vulnerable. (Just think about those ubiquitous cinnamon buns that perfume every airport.) As if such factors weren't hazardous enough, traveling in and of itself can bring on stress, which in turn may cause cravings for unhealthy foods.

The key to remaining disciplined when on the road is a combination of mental and physical preparation. The following tips should help ensure that you don't leave your progress behind when you travel:

- Think big picture. Don't use your trip as an excuse to go off the program. Remember, if you continually make "detours" from your planned route, you'll never reach your destination.
- Take food with you. When you miss a flight or a meeting runs late, be prepared. Take along some low-carb snack foods like one-ounce portions of cheese in plastic wrap. If you're traveling by car, consider taking a cooler packed with cold cuts and cheese. You can even bring along salad in a plastic bag with dressing on the side. Or stow away a few controlled carb bars and some shake powder to use as meal replacements.
- Eat first. Start out on the right foot by eating a well-planned, satisfying meal before you leave home.
- Go a little nuts. If you're past the Induction phase, you can snack on nuts and seeds. Macadamias, almonds, walnuts, pecans, filberts and sunflower and pumpkin seeds are all good choices because they're high in protein and fat. You'll feel more satisfied and in control of your appetite after eating a handful.
- No skipping allowed. Tempted to pass on lunch

and make better time? Don't do it. Omitting a meal could make you ravenous, out of control and more likely to grab anything edible that's handy.

- Fly right. If you're on a flight where a meal will be served, call ahead and ask what's on the menu. You may be able to find a seafood salad or other dish that is acceptable.
- Drink up. When you're traveling, consume lots of water. Staying hydrated will help you feel satisfyingly full. Stay away, however, from caffeine and diet sodas full of aspartame—both increase carbohydrate cravings.
- Pack your pills. If you've gotten into the habit of taking nutritional supplements, congratulations! Now make sure you continue this part of your lifestyle when you're on the road. Once one element of your routine gets upset, other good habits tend to slide as well. Even if you make some mistakes with your food choices, staying on the vitanutrient program will help you focus on getting back to eating properly.
- Speed counts. If you do slip off Atkins for a day or more, get back on ASAP. The longer you're off, the harder it may be to resume.
- Be ready to compromise without quitting. If you find that your food options on the road or in the air are all really poor, adhere to the program as closely as you can. For example, if you find that you need to increase your consumption of salad and other vegetables beyond your usual allowance, it doesn't mean you might as well eat bread and pasta. It's better to deviate a little than to throw the whole program out the window.

Training Those Special People

Even if you overcome your temptations and the challenges of eating in places other than your own kitchen table, one of the obstacles you may find in the real world is people—the very same people upon whom you normally rely for advice and support. I'm talking about your spouse, family members and well-meaning friends, all of whom may have been so influenced by the media's fixation on low fat that they are certain Atkins has no validity. "Oh, that's a high-fat diet. It can't be good for you" may be the reflex response, said without any knowledge of the solid scientific research supporting the lipolytic approach to weight loss.

Although a particular person's advice may have been valuable in the past, you must reply that he or she can't know something until it has been examined thoroughly. If your naysayer is someone you live with or must deal with every day, then you know you need total cooperation as much as you need your own single-mindedness. If I were you, I would start by suggesting that the person read this book. You might say, "Since I need your support, why don't you study Dr. Atkins' arguments and his backup carefully and see if you can poke holes in the material?" If the naysayer refuses to read the whole book, insist that he or she at least reviews the impressive list of research papers in the reference section starting on page 503. This can be a particularly effective approach with a doubting physician.

You must gain the cooperation of everyone in your immediate environment because resisting temptation is a lot easier if you don't see and smell your favorite carbohydrates. I've mentioned the problem with nonbelievers, but what about those who basically say, "Losing weight is your problem; eating is my privilege"? Here you must apply the pragmatic take-charge motto: "If you can't lick 'em, get 'em to join you." My recommendation is to get your significant other involved in doing Atkins. If that person is also overweight, you will have a very good selling point—the prospect of painless weight loss. But if he's locked into the low-fat-will-do-it fairy tale, you may suggest: "Why don't we try both approaches and see what is best suited to our metabolisms?" Make it into a friendly competition. I guarantee you that when you compare results your naysayer may quickly change his mind. (Results should include not just weight loss but disappearance of symptoms and whether the other program provides a feeling of satisfaction that will allow you to keep the weight off permanently.)

Now suppose you're in the situation where you're the only one who has to lose weight. You might suggest that your significant other follow Atkins along with you—by eliminating sugar, white flour, other nutrient-deficient carbohydrates, hydrogenated fats and processed foods from his regimen. His menus will include extra portions of veggies as well as whole grains, some of the starchy vegetables and moderate amounts of fruit. Chances are he will feel so much better that within a few weeks he'll be convinced.

One more very important message: Suppose that temptation takes the form of sugar-laden junk food that's in the house "for the kids." You're not doing them any favors by allowing them to eat this food. In my opinion, the most dangerous food additive on the planet is sugar in all its forms. Proper nourishment is one of the lifetime gifts you can give your children, so perhaps you should rethink your position. Who more than little ones with virtually their whole lives ahead of them stand to be damaged by a substance that helps provoke diabetes, hypertension and heart disease? Allowing kids to eat according to the pleasure principle and not according to the principle of health maintenance is probably not the kind of parenting you wish to do. So, make the resolution now: Sugar is *not* going to enter my home! Your whole family will benefit.

Make Fast Food Friendly

There's no need to avoid those fast food joints that dot the roadside—so long as you know your way around the menu. Here's a quick road map:

- **Burger chains:** Sandwiches are usually a good bet. Yes, even the bacon cheeseburger! Just toss the bun. Mayo and mustard are permissible but beware of ketchup, which often contains a lot of sugar. Watch out too for special sauces, as they also often contain sugar. Slices of tomato and lettuce garnish are fine. Steer clear of anything advertised as "low fat" because this label often translates to "high carb."

- **Sandwich shops:** Chicken or tuna salad is a good choice. In sub shops, bring on the turkey, roast beef and cheese; try to steer clear of salami, bologna and other meat products preserved with nitrates. Ask for your selection on a plate instead of on a roll, and you're all set.

- **Salad bars:** Select acceptable vegetables as a base, top with protein foods such as hard-boiled eggs, turkey or chicken and the like. Avoid cole slaw, which may contain sugar. Pass up that pasta salad. Use oil and regular red or white wine vinegar instead of a prepared dressing. Commercial dressings and balsamic vinegars often contain sugar. Baked stuffed potatoes are an absolute no-no.

- **Fried chicken joints:** Avoid anything barbecued or breaded. Barbecue sauce is typically full of sugar, and even if you remove the skin from the chicken, the sugar has probably seeped into the meat. Dry-rubbed meats are fine, or look for roasted chicken and acceptable side dishes such as salad. If there's a grilled-chicken fillet sandwich available, grab it! Discard the bun, and you've got a pretty good selection. Or scrape the breading off a fried chicken breast.

- **Avoid at all costs!** Mexican-style fast-food restaurants, doughnut shops, and yogurt/ice cream parlors. If you wind up in a pizza parlor, order a salad. Or if absolutely necessary, order a pizza and eat only the cheese and fixings and leave the crust. It's messy, but you'll avoid the nutrient-deficient high-carb crust.

Finally, remember who's boss. You are absolutely in control of what goes in your mouth at all times—even when you're not in your own home. When dining out, ask how things are prepared and give instructions. After all, you're paying for it. Even in a fast food restaurant, you're entitled to "have it your way." After all, why should some stranger get to influence the success of your program—and your health?

TIPS:

- Remain in control of what goes into your mouth at all times.
- Traveling can bring on stress, which sometimes induces cravings. Be prepared by bringing acceptable foods with you.
- The best foods to neutralize cravings contain both protein and fat.
- Stop a binge by doing Induction within a day or two of going astray (waiting longer may curb your success).
- At a restaurant, take the time to explain your way of eating to the wait person.

- At fast food joints, toss the bun and avoid the ketchup.
- Stock up on controlled carbohydrate food alternatives, including bars, ready-to-drink shakes, shake mixes, syrups, bread and ice cream.

PART THREE

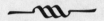

Understanding Health and Well-Being

20

Metabolic Resistance: Causes and Solutions

This chapter is dedicated to all you tortured souls who have been told that the only reason you are overweight is because you eat too much. What this statement ignores is the well-documented fact that people who are significantly overweight may also have metabolic disorders. Such conditions not only *cause* weight gain, but also make it difficult to *lose* the accumulated weight.

Part of the obesity epidemic we face in the United States may be due to the misconception that those of us who are overweight are simply gluttons or lazy couch potatoes. For most of the last century, the majority of doctors involved in treating obesity did not accept extreme metabolic resistance as a possible explanation for their patients' plight, but rather chose to believe that they were being untruthful about what they ate.

This chapter is about *extreme* difficulty in losing weight and will help you understand why certain ways of eating that *should* lead to weight loss simply do *not* work.

The inability to burn fat or lose weight, the phenomenon called *metabolic resistance to weight loss*, is not uncommon. In my clinical practice, I have been called upon to treat hundreds if not thousands of patients who simply could not reach their goal weight no matter what weight loss program they tried. But my co-practitioners and I were determined to help, and ultimately we did!

How to Overcome Metabolic Resistance

There are four major categories of problems that contribute to metabolic resistance:

1. Excessive insulin and insulin resistance, usually accompanied by high triglycerides.[1-4]
2. The use of prescription drugs or hormones which impede weight loss.
3. Underactive thyroid (hypothyroid) function, which can be present even when blood tests indicate no abnormality.
4. Overgrowth of the yeast organism *Candida albicans*.

There are a multitude of other problems, as well, but they occur rarely and aren't within the purview of this book. Instead, I will go into greater detail to show you how the Atkins Nutritional Approach and complementary medicine can successfully help overcome these four most common obstacles to weight control.

When Insulin Is Out of Whack

We've discussed the issue of excessive insulin output— what the medical profession calls *hyperinsulinism*—and the inefficiency of insulin usage—what is called *insulin resistance*. There can be no question that overweight individuals whose weight control difficulties are caused by hyperinsulinism respond best to the Atkins controlled carbohydrate nutritional approach. Even the majority of people who do not lose weight on a 1,000-calorie low-fat diet will lose weight on an 1,800- to 2,000-calorie meal plan—if carbohydrates are limited to 20 grams per day.

The vast majority will lose weight, yes, but not absolutely everyone.

For those individuals who have not lost weight during the Induction phase of Atkins, nutritionally oriented medicine offers ways to break through this last barrier. In conjuction with Induction, certain vitanutrients can assist in breaking up weight loss logjams.

In my experience, the leading nutrient to accomplish this fat-busting feat is L-carnitine. When carnitine is deficient, the conversion of burned fat to ketones is impaired.[5-7] The mechanism for carnitine's effectiveness is that it has the ability to ensure that fat converts to fuel. But very high doses of carnitine are often necessary. I start most of my patients off with 500 mg, three times daily (taken before meals), but frequently the dose must be increased, to perhaps as high as 5,000 mg in divided doses before meals. Often, more effective responses occur with the use of aceytl carnitine, a compound that helps focus the carnitine action.

Co-enzyme Q_{10} (CoQ_{10}), another vital nutrient necessary for fat to serve as fuel,[8] may also require large doses, often in excess of 300 mg daily. Both CoQ_{10} and carnitine are extremely valuable for other reasons, such as preserving heart health. You should read more about them and other nutrients in *Dr. Atkins' Vita-Nutrient Solution*.

Other nutrients capable of overcoming slow weight loss include chromium, alpha lipoic acid, glutamine, phenylalanine and the combinations of inositol, choline and methionine. To get the optimum benefits of these vitanutrients, you should work with doctors experienced in their use to combine them with the Induction phase of Atkins.

The Role of Prescription Drugs

As much as metabolic abnormalities can cause a true inability to lose weight, an even greater number of people are stymied because of prescription medications they are taking. The shocking truth is that the vast majority of these weight loss-stymied victims are completely unaware that the drugs are holding back their weight loss. The breakthrough answer lies simply in getting off the medications that inhibit weight loss. One of complementary medicine's greatest contributions to good health is its ability to find safe and effective alternatives to many pharmaceuticals with unacceptable side effects.

Of the numerous prescription drugs that are frequently found to slow or prevent weight loss, these are the most common:

- Estrogens and most synthetic hormone replacement therapies (HRTs), including birth control pills
- Anti-depressant drugs
- Insulin and insulin-stimulating drugs
- Anti-arthritis medications (including steroids)
- Diuretics and beta-blockers

Let's study them, item by item.

IF YOU ARE ON HORMONES

How many of you on HRT are now realizing that weight gain coincides with the period during which you have been taking these powerful drugs? I'll wager that the doctor who prescribed HRT for you did not warn you it might cause weight gain. Many standard hormones also increase blood-sugar imbalances, causing cravings and the inability to control intake of carbohydrate foods.

Your objective, once you learn that HRT has been inhibiting weight loss, is to find the lowest dose of HRT that keeps menopausal symptoms under control. Your doctor will have to work with you to achieve this goal. The first consideration is to optimize the balance between progesterone and estrogen. The majority of women with menopausal symptoms (even those who are not on HRT)—and certainly those on HRT—have a significant dominance of estrogen over progesterone, and estrogen is a fat-producing hormone. Also be aware that the progesterone usually prescribed (Provera) is a synthetic version, which also tends to promote obesity. Natural progesterone, which does not lead to weight gain, should be prescribed, and frequently can stand alone (without estrogen) in relieving menopausal symptoms.

Among the vitanutrients that have proven invaluable to ease the symptoms of estrogen withdrawal is the B vitamin folic acid, but it does require prescription dosages of 20 mg or more. To my knowledge, no one has ever published or performed a study on what effect folic acid has on hormone levels. However, since I was taught to use it by my mentor, Carlton Fredericks, PhD, one of the twentieth century's most highly regarded nutritionists, I have prescribed it for thousands of women. I found it not only to be as safe as all the other B vitamins, but to also consistently enable a significant lowering of estrogen dosage without bringing on any symptoms that indicate estrogen deficiency.

Another useful nutrient to allow reduction in HRT dosages is the mineral boron, which serves as a building block for the liver to manufacture natural estrogens. Boron, which is valuable for preventing and reversing osteoporosis, is usually recommended in the 6- to 18-mg-per-day range. You will get additional benefits by bringing the normal precursors of the sex hormones, such as DHEA and pregnenolone, to the levels considered normal for a 30-year-old woman.

Once the above nutrients and natural hormones are provided, I am usually able to reduce the HRT dosages by seventy-five percent—sometimes more, sometimes less.

ANTI-DEPRESSANT DRUGS

Another drug category that matches HRT in providing obstacles to weight loss is the anti-depressants, particularly those which are in the SSRI (selective serotonin reuptake inhibitors) category. Strangely enough, these drugs—such as Zoloft, Prozac, Paxil and Celexa—were originally touted as drugs that would accelerate weight loss, but a reality check soon put an end to those misleading statements. In general, these drugs have certainly been overprescribed, and many people who suffer from depression would get great benefits from metabolically innocuous, natural anti-depressants. Many of the older psychotrophic drugs (tricyclic anti-depressants) are also known to cause weight gain.

The Atkins Approach to Depression

Serotonin drugs are effective because this natural neurotransmitter helps the brain function, relieves depression and relaxes the mind. But the drugs work by blocking the body's normal ability to destroy serotonin once it has been created. Blocking agents block other normal chemical functions as well, resulting in such unwanted side effects as diminished sex drive and performance, dry mouth and constipation, to say nothing of slowed metabolism, which, of course, can stall weight loss.

The safe way to build up the serotonin level is to enable the body to manufacture its own serotonin by taking the immediate precursor to serotonin. This natural substance does not block a reaction, but simply enables a reaction to take place. The precursor to serotonin is a chemical called tryptophan; its immediate precursor is 5-hydroxy tryptophan, a popular vitanutrient available in health food stores.

Other natural substances for depression include N-acetyl tyrosine, S-adenosyl methionine (SAMe), St. John's Wort, acetyl L-carnitine, phosphatidyl serine and most of the B complex vitamins. These supplements relieve anxiety, as do inositol, GABA (gamma amino butyric acid), kava kava and valerian.

It would be inappropriate to go into full detail about how to determine dosages to replace anti-depressant pharmaceuticals with safe, effective natural substances. It takes considerable experience to individualize the dosage and combination of therapies. But do know that you can get off anti-depressant pharmaceuticals with the help of a complementary physician experienced in managing depression and anxiety.

DO DIABETICS NEED INSULIN AND OTHER DRUGS?

A large number of diabetics are overweight because they put out too much insulin. As you might imagine, nothing would be more inappropriate than to give insulin to these overweight diabetics, who already put out excessive insulin and have elevated blood sugar resulting from insulin resistance, rather than lack of insulin.

Are you a Type II diabetic taking insulin, or one of the oral drugs called sulfonylureas, which work by increasing your insulin levels? And do you seem to be metabolically resistant to weight loss? Then chances are a hundred to one that you are a diabetic who is simply a victim of a poor assumption on the part of your physician. My approach with those already diagnosed diabetics on oral medications and/or insulin who come to me is to determine if they can produce insulin on their own.

Here's how you find out if the insulin you are taking is necessary or not: Have your doctor run a test of insulin levels (as well as glucose levels) both before and ninety minutes after a typical low-fat/high-carbohydrate breakfast (including perhaps a blueberry muffin, cereal with skim milk and eight-ounce glass of orange juice). Make sure you take no long-acting insulin after 6 P.M. the evening before and no diabetes medications of any kind the morning of the test until after the second blood sample is drawn. (The blood drawn after eating or after drinking a glucose solution is called a *post-prandial reading*.)

Here's how to interpret the results: If the second insulin level is 10 or more points higher than the first, it means your pancreas is working and that you *probably* can get off insulin if you are willing to follow the Atkins Nutritional Approach. If it is 20 or more points higher, it is almost a *certainty* that you can do so.

The Induction phase of Atkins is essential to accomplish this feat, as is a program for gradually reducing your dosage level of insulin (and sulfonylurea drugs), as I discuss in Chapter 24. My staff and I have taken hundreds of diabetics off insulin and thousands off oral medications, all without any ill effects. **Do not discontinue medication, however, except under the care of a doctor.**

In Chapter 24, you will also learn that the only drug useful for overweight, insulin-resistant, but not insulin-dependent, diabetics is metformin. And that chromium, vanadium, alpha lipoic acid, zinc, biotin and Co-enzyme Q_{10} can also help individuals who are insulin resistant.

ANTI-ARTHRITIS MEDICATIONS

If you cannot lose weight and are taking powerful arthritis medications known as NSAIDs (non-steroidal anti-inflammatory drugs), it's time for you to consider getting off the drugs. The story is simple. Virtually all drugs known to be effective in controlling the pain and discomfort of arthritis may lead to weight gain. Some do so more than others, but no one has ever funded a study to find out which drugs had the most impact on weight gain. The best solution is for you to try to recall whether any of your weight gain coincided with the use of one or more arthritis drugs.

The good news is the truly impressive number of vitanutrients documented in scientific journals that can relieve arthritic symptoms. When arthritis has an inflammatory basis (the painful joints get red and swollen and a blood test shows your sed rate is high), the most effective natural therapies are MSM (methylsulfonylmethane), cetyl myristoleate, copper, bromelain, ginger, turmeric and pantethine (vitamin B_5). For the non-inflammatory type (osteoarthritis), natural therapies include glucosamine sulfate, chondroitin, sea cucumber, fish oil, niacinamide and the B complex group of vitamins.

Using vitanutrients to substitute for drugs in the case of arthritis is somewhat more direct than the previous examples. For dosages of natural therapies for arthritis symptoms, refer to *Dr. Atkins' Vita-Nutrient Solution*. Since reducing the quantity of pharmaceuticals is the objective, the dose of alternatives should be on the liberal side. Since most pharmaceutical drugs do afford pain relief, I tell my patients to determine what is the lowest dosage they feel comfortable with and settle for that. Any significant dose-lowering will probably allow for weight loss to resume.

Steroids such as prednisone are powerful medications that can be lifesaving but have a definite metabolic downside, especially if used for long periods of time. They are often prescribed for arthritis as well as for autoimmune disorders, inflammation of the bowel and any other inflammatory condition. These drugs actually cause water retention and weight gain. They can also damage the kidneys and pancreas and cause diabetes. The same nutritional supplements that can relieve arthritis are safer alternatives that will not hinder weight loss.

DIURETICS AND BETA-BLOCKERS— HIGH BLOOD PRESSURE MEDICATIONS

For your sake, I hope that your inability to lose weight dates from the time you were put on anti-hypertension drugs. The reason? In my experience, no medication has proven easier to get off than blood pressure drugs. And, if you can get off of them, since most widely used medications carry considerable side effects, there is an additional motivation to wean yourself.

At the top of the no-no list are the *diuretic medications*, which work by preventing your kidneys from doing one of their most important jobs: reabsorbing the minerals your body needs. Blocking the kidneys' ability to reabsorb sodium and chloride takes salt out of the body and lowers blood pressure by lowering the fluids that stay in the body. But those blocked kidneys also lose their ability to retain valuable minerals: not only potassium, but magnesium, calcium, chromium, zinc and many others. Prescription diuretics induce mineral deficiencies that can cause many problems. Numerous studies demonstrate that diuretics aggravate diabetes, elevate blood sugar and increase insulin levels, triglycerides and body mass index (the measure for obesity).[9-11] For all these reasons, I insist that my patients on diuretics discontinue them and replace them with L-taurine, the natural amino acid that is a powerful diuretic but has no ill effects on kidney function.

The other types of anti-hypertension drugs that aggravate all of the above are *beta-blockers*. If you are on a beta-blocker, you have little cause for concern about discontinuing your medication. In the first place, the controlled carb lifestyle that you are adopting lowers blood pressure itself. In addition to L-taurine, you may control blood pressure with magnesium, hawthorne, Co-enzyme Q_{10}, carnitine and garlic. Because Atkins will naturally lower your blood pressure, continuing to take pharmaceuticals could put you at risk for an overdose. **Again, speak to your doctor before discontinuing any medication!**

HOW MANY OTHER DRUGS DO IT?

I'm sure you are beginning to see how frequently the very drugs that people take for granted as necessary are in fact problematic. Safer, more natural options exist, and even people with no weight problem should consider using them.

There are probably hundreds of other drugs, certainly including psychotropic drugs and lithium, which also create difficulty in losing weight. If I were to go into full detail, it would require an entire book. So let me give you some general advice. If you have been on medication for any length of time, try to recall whether weight gain, increased appetite or lack of responsiveness to weight loss efforts might have co-incided with the time frame in which you began that drug. If so, you probably will be able to find a set of nutritional alternatives in *Dr. Atkins' Vita-Nutrient Solution*, which lists therapies for about sixty different conditions.

REPLACEMENT TECHNIQUES

How do you replace a drug in question with a natural alternative? In most situations, you begin the vitanutrient program that will replace the drug and work with your doctor to gradually lower the drug dosage by some ten to fifteen percent each week, as long as the condition that the drug is meant to control does not worsen. Combining vitanutrients with the personalized eating regimen this book describes has allowed me to reduce the intake of medications by virtually all my patients.

The Role of the Thyroid

Your thyroid gland's main purpose in life is to regulate the speed of your metabolism. So it is not difficult to understand that if it is underactive—the medical word is *hypothyroid*—your slowed metabolism makes you more resistant to weight loss. Among other things, your thyroid gland regulates your body temperature. In fact, sensitivity to cold is one of the first signs that you may have a sluggish thyroid. Like other hormones, thyroid production naturally diminishes slightly with age; in fact, easily twenty-five percent of adults suffer from low thyroid function. The swings of estrogen production in perimenopause or menopause can also throw thyroid function off.

To ascertain whether you have hypothyroidism, your doctor will do blood tests to evaluate your production of thyroid hormones T4 (also known as thyroxine) and T3 (your body converts T4 to T3), as well as another hormone called TSH (thyroid stimulating hormone), which is produced by your pituitary gland. I do tests on free T3, T4 and TSH levels. However, these clinical tests do not catch all cases. First think about whether you are experiencing any of the signs of an underactive thyroid—which include the aforementioned sensitivity to cold, as well as weight gain or inability to lose weight, hair loss, fatigue and lethargy, depression, dry skin, chronic constipation, poor nails, poor memory and elevated cholesterol levels. If so, there is a simple way—the Barnes technique of basal metabolism—to ascertain if you are hypothyroid. It doesn't even require a trip to your doctor.

Simply take your temperature orally four times a day (before each meal and before you go to bed) for four days. Average your temperature each day, and if it is consistently below 98 degrees Fahrenheit, you are likely to have hypothyroidism. If it is significantly lower, you almost definitely do, and you should bring this information to the attention of your physician. (Be prepared: Not all doctors take basal metabolism as seriously as they should.)

Occasionally, the reason for an underactive thyroid is the deficiency of the amino acid tyrosine and the mineral iodine, both of which help make T3. Zinc and selenium help produce the enzyme that converts T4 to T3. But nutritional deficiency is rarely the cause of hypothyroidism. There are other causes, one of which can be an autoimmune response.

The major reason for hypothyroidism that I'd like to address is simply the body's own attempts to preserve the status quo while on a weight loss program.

I use the therapeutic trial to treat thyroid problems. I start patients with a very low dose of a prescription thyroid hormone replacement and build up gradually and very carefully. In most cases, when we reach the right dose, patients start to feel dramatically better, with a much better overall sense of well-being and increased energy and vitality. Best of all, they start to lose weight!

The solution is to take thyroid hormone—both T3 and T4 preferably—in a natural form (rather than the synthetic type). I prescribe the synthetic kind of thyroid hormone only in cases of an autoimmune disease, when your own immune system might destroy the natural kind.

Candida

There is one other potential reason for blocked weight loss: *Candida albicans*, known as yeast. *Candida* is so important that it merits its own detailed discussion in Chapter 25. If you think this problem may be interfering with your weight loss, please consult that chapter.

None of the Above?

I expect close to one hundred percent success in achieving weight loss with my patients, but there are still exceptions. Certain individuals are so metabolically resistant that only more intense dietary restrictions prove successful. Read on, and I'll explain what I mean.

Once medications, thyroid problems and *Candida* are brought under control, we can quite logically expect that almost ninety-nine percent of overweight people who do Atkins diligently will lose and keep off weight. But since there are 150 million overweight Americans, even the remaining one percent means that there are one and a half million metabolically resistant people who still need help. For that group, I suggest something more than the Induction phase's 20-grams-of-carbohydrate-a-day meal plan.

I have treated hundreds of these people—all of whom were depending on me to help them—and I had no intention of letting them down. So I asked myself, "What is the most effective weight loss eating pattern ever described?" There can be no question what that is. You read about it in Chapter 7 in the discussion of the metabolic advantage. British researchers Alan Kekwick and Gaston Pawan developed it, and Frederick Benoit and his team confirmed its superiority in burning off fat, compared to an absolute total fast. This extreme diet consists of 1,000 calories, ninety percent of which is comprised of fat. No other weight loss regimen, before or since, has matched its ability to burn off stored fat.

The Fat Fast

The rationale behind the Kekwick diet is crystal clear: It forces the body into lipolysis so it burns its stores of fat. Lipolysis cannot take place if there is a significant source of glucose. Since all carbohydrates and some protein convert to energy by way of glucose, eliminating almost everything but fat from the diet forces even the most resistant body into lipolysis. That explains the ninety percent dietary fat component of the Kekwick diet. Lowering the caloric intake accelerates the need to burn up body fat—thus the 1,000-calorie limit.

When I wrote the first edition of this book years ago, I realized that a small but intensely suffering segment of my readers would need to know how to overcome metabolic resistance. So I decided to make the Kekwick diet as enjoyable as possible. But no matter how I tried, the quantities were simply too small and the selection too limited to meet the satiety and tastiness criteria that I had been demanding for people following my program.

I gave it the name "Fat Fast" because it contained virtually no food except for fat. I tried it on scores of patients and was not surprised to observe how often it worked for those who were unable to lose in any other safe, drugless way. Nor was I surprised to hear that none of my patients relished the idea of staying on it. But ten more years of experience with the Fat Fast has taught me how to make Kekwick and Pawan's brilliant concept a truly useful technique with which to combat metabolic resistance.

The Fat Fast is one controlled carb program where you do

have to count calories, I am afraid. You'll eat 1,000 calories a day, with seventy-five to ninety percent fat. Since frequent "feedings" prevent hunger better than three meals a day, I recommend five feedings, perhaps one every four hours, comprising 200 calories each. Because of the high fat content and frequent feedings, very few people on the Fat Fast experience much hunger. The stumbling block for some people is the absence of meals as we know them.

Let's look at some choices for a Fat Fast 200-calorie feeding. Each item equals approximately 200 calories:

- One ounce of macadamia nuts or macadamia nut butter
- Two ounces of cream cheese or Brie
- One ounce of tuna or chicken salad with two teaspoons of mayonnaise served in one-quarter of an avocado
- Two deviled eggs made with two teaspoons of mayonnaise
- Two ounces of sour cream and two tablespoons black or red caviar
- Two and a half ounces whipped heavy cream topped with sucralose zero-calorie syrup
- Two ounces of pâté (check label for fat content)
- Two egg yolks (hard-boiled) with one tablespoon of mayonnaise

When to Do the Fat Fast

Let me make it clear that the Fat Fast is actually dangerous for anyone who is not metabolically resistant. For people who lose weight fairly easily, the rate of weight loss is too rapid to be safe. But it carries very little risk for people who can barely lose on any other regimen. The reason why I ask such people to try the Fat Fast is to let them know that it is possible to lose weight.

I ask them to try the regimen for four or five days to see if they achieve what the Fat Fast is capable of doing—weight loss, curbed appetite, positive lipolysis testing strips and improved well-being. If these results occur, most people are willing to stick with it for a few days, even if the food selections are unfulfilling.

Modifying the Fat Fast

If increasing the fat-to-carbohydrate ratio and cutting the calorie count works, *any dietary change in that direction* might get the job done. Next, you can try four meals a day of roughly 300 calories for a total of 1,200 calories. That should work too, and what it allows is definitely more appealing to the taste buds:

- Two ounces of beef chuck (do not drain fat) cooked in two tablespoons of olive oil
- Two scrambled eggs with two strips of nitrate-free bacon
- Two tablespoons of full-fat sour cream with a tablespoon of sugar-free syrup
- One-quarter cup chicken or tuna salad made with two tablespoons of mayonnaise
- Three ounces of pâté (check fat content)
- One-and-a-half ounces of macadamia nuts

Try the 1,200-calorie regimen for a week, then go back to Induction. Or simply follow the concept of increasing the ratio of fat to protein. No one should have to feel that losing weight is hopeless. Sometimes the key to achieving your goal weight permanently is quite difficult to adhere to, but rarely is it simply impossible! With a clear-eyed approach to the factors that may be standing in your way, you should finally be able to slip into clothing a size or two smaller.

21

The Psychology of Weight Loss: Behavioral Changes for a Healthier Life

In this chapter, I'm going to show you how to prepare yourself to deal with behavior that may undermine your otherwise sterling efforts at weight control. It is said that fortune favors the prepared mind. If your past history gives you the slightest reason for thinking you might give up on the most effective and satisfying weight loss plan you've ever tried, read this chapter carefully.

Is it possible that part of your weight problem is emotional? You may be using food as nurse, mother or comforter, as well as a source of nutrition. Many people use food for far more than mere sustenance. Okay, I'll be honest, we all do—*some of the time*. But there are individuals—not infrequently, people with serious weight problems—for whom food is a major pillar and support of their emotional life. If this sounds familiar, you may have already considered the psychological components of weight loss.

I also know that right now a few of you are saying, "Dr. Atkins, you told me that being overweight may be due in part to a metabolic problem. I don't want to hear about emotional issues; I prefer the simple answer you already gave me." I did give you that answer, and if you're already doing

Atkins, you've probably discovered how real my claims were. Yet, sadly, there is a small percentage of people who try to do Atkins and discover it isn't metabolically suited to them. I'm talking about the folks who lose perfectly well and feel perfectly fine—but give up anyway. Their situation really troubles me.

Mapping the Patterns of Your Life

Have you failed on weight loss plans before? You won't have forgotten my criticisms of low-fat and low-calorie diets. It may seem natural to fail on those programs. But, if your pattern goes back a long way and represents a lifelong tendency to gain and lose, gain and lose, then you may be in the grip of what I call *emotional eating*.

At this point in the book, you may be doing Induction. Are you staying disciplined on this important phase? Then, perhaps all is well. But if you tend to have meals here, there and everywhere, when you eat what you shouldn't, you may need to address other issues.

Emotional Eating

The air conditioner is broken, the repairman didn't show up and the thermometer stands at 96 degrees in the shade. Or the dinner date you've been anticipating all week has just been canceled. To console yourself when you're sad, lonely or have just had a really bad day, you pull out the chocolate-chip cookies and dive into the rocky road ice cream, right? It is so easy to use food to comfort yourself when things aren't going well.

If you do, though, you not only won't feel better for very long, but after your blood sugar goes awry and the post-binge guilt takes over, you'll feel really awful. There are other ways to deal with a bad day, and some tricks you can use that will help you do so in a healthy way.

So let me offer a few practical responses to situations in which you need to assuage an emotional hurt or alleviate big-time stress:

- Treat yourself to an acceptable food. This isn't the best answer because it reinforces the idea that eating is a way to remedy emotional pain. But at least it won't leave you with the guilt of a bad binge to deal with on top of everything else.
- Log onto our website at *www.atkinscenter.com* or the many other Atkins-friendly sites and chat rooms on the Internet and interact with someone who understands your situation. Looking to another person for emotional support is much better than looking to a bowl of ice cream for it!
- If you're at home and feeling lonely, go out to a movie (ignore the concession stand), a friend's house or the local bookstore. Getting involved with something interesting or entertaining can cheer you up or at least distract you from the compelling urge to eat.
- If you like to cook, make yourself an Atkins treat (see the "Food and Recipes" section starting on page 367) and put it in the refrigerator where it can save you when temptation strikes in the future.
- Call up a friend and talk. This is when an "Atkins buddy" can be a godsend.
- Get some exercise! Are you groaning? How I wish I could teach you the emotional payoffs of exercise. Simply walking, for instance. On a day when life has thrown you some punches, go out for a brisk walk. I guarantee that when you're done, your problems will seem more manageable. By walking fast, you lower your levels of adrenal chemicals, you oxygenate your system and you release brain-soothing endorphins.

These natural chemicals actually relieve stress, stabilize your appetite and thereby minimize cravings.

- Recite the principles of the Atkins Nutritional Approach. Remember them from Chapter 1? You *will* lose weight. You *will* maintain your weight loss. You *will* achieve good health. You *will* lay the permanent groundwork for disease prevention.

That last suggestion deserves a more extended discussion.

Teach Yourself, Lecture Yourself, Habituate Yourself

You must have found this book's arguments convincing or you wouldn't still be reading. Now let's use your new insights to alter your way of life. I want you to figure out exactly how doing Atkins has benefited you; then I want you to use that knowledge as a form of self-empowerment. A conscious realization of how important your health is can actually overcome your old, bad habits. In the game of life, good reasons *can* trump old habits.

Settle down in a nice comfortable armchair with a pencil and a pad and ask yourself this short series of questions:

- What did I want to achieve by doing Atkins?
- Am I getting there?
- Do I feel good?
- Do I understand why Atkins makes me healthy?
- Is it worth controlling my carb consumption for a lifetime to maintain the weight control and get the health advantages I'm experiencing?

Let's assume your answers are largely favorable. Turn them into a list of positives. For instance:

- I'm losing weight steadily without starving myself.
- I'm enjoying the foods I'm eating.
- I feel more energetic and more focused than I have in years.
- I no longer suffer mood swings, afternoon fatigue or _____ (fill in your own symptoms). Look at the "Blood-Sugar Symptom Test" on pages 150–151; it may remind you of some irritating symptoms you've already put behind you.
- My lab tests show that doing Atkins is good for my cardiovascular health.

The list that *you* draw up should reflect *your* answers to the question of what you believe Atkins is doing for you. Now don't lose those answers. Ponder them. Refine them down to a short list that you thoroughly understand and believe in. If I were you, I'd recite that list daily, a sort of morning mantra, even before your first bite of the day—perhaps while you're putting on your makeup or shaving. Would so much conscious preparation embarrass you? It shouldn't.

It's by consciously preparing yourself for the challenges of the day that you outflank the powerful world of habit. If you know *why* you're doing things differently, you'll have a far better prospect of doing them long enough so that they, in turn, become habitual. Once doing Atkins is a habit, you will really be able to bask in your success. Until that happy day arrives, those of us who are all too familiar with weight loss failure must use our brains to survive.

Remember my suggestion to continually visualize yourself at your goal weight. Think about how much you deserve to look and feel good, to enjoy the happiness, health and sense of well-being that will come with weight loss. Eating healthily is something you're doing for you—a *gift* to yourself, not a punishment. Value yourself and you'll be able to enjoy and succeed at this endeavor.

Finally, don't be afraid to get help from a counselor or psychotherapist. The reasons we all overeat are so complicated and challenging that the emotional support and insight a professional can offer can be invaluable.

Ask People to Respect Your Needs

This conscious approach has another use. It helps to keep you focused on your health. Isn't that what's really important? If you can convince yourself that it is, you'll be ready to stand up for your own needs. Many people find it hard to assert, "What I need for myself is important." Women in particular—perhaps because they function so often as caregivers—have trouble saying, "My needs are essential, too."

If your spouse or significant other is giving you a hard time about your doing Atkins, that calls for self-assertion. You simply must make it clear that this nutritional approach is a need that you won't compromise. Even the most sweet-natured and unassertive people have areas in their lives in which they won't allow interference.

Time for Realism

I've just advised you to work out your own version of what Atkins does for you. Now I want you to apply a touch of realism to that grand scheme. Don't be trapped by expectations. This is a typical vulnerability found in people who repeatedly fail at weight loss. They have a preconceived version of how a weight loss plan should progress and demand perfection, or, at least, a steady and predictable progress that can't necessarily be achieved—even by doing Atkins.

Your experience will not be like your sibling's or your parents', and certainly not like your spouse's. You have a body that's unlike any other, with a unique history, and as you advance in years it will not behave exactly the way it did when it was 18. And sad but true, that "bod" may never be a "perfect 10."

But you can make it the best body possible if you don't fall into the trap of demanding a perfect figure and weight loss schedule that exists only in your head. You can succeed only if you forgive yourself your missteps, rather than calling the game a failure and withdrawing to the sidelines. The same goes for the fact that you'll hit plateaus, lose a little ground or sometimes lose more slowly than you'd like. I can assure that you will most likely succeed by doing Atkins, but each one of you will succeed differently, at a different pace.

Here are three more ways to defeat yourself—and I'm telling you about them only because I want to encourage you to avoid the pitfalls.

1. Getting on the scale four or five times a day is a form of slow torture. Even the most effective weight loss plan (this one) can't produce a change every few hours, nor even guarantee that you'll lose weight each day. The human body doesn't work that way. By doing Atkins, you're making highly favorable changes to an immensely complicated system. Your metabolism will decide how quickly you lose. There is, unfortunately, no little Dr. Atkins inside you ordering your metabolism to take off precisely three-quarters of a pound a day. The ultimate proof the plan is working is that you see a steady loss over a significant period. And, as I've said many times before in this book, you may notice a change in the fit of your clothes before you see it on the scale. You simply must not demand mathematical exactitude.

2. To think that the present will be just like the past is another mind trap. Alarm bells ring when I hear someone say, "But I'm not losing the way I did ten years ago." It isn't ten years ago, Ace. I wish I were ten years younger, too. The normal pattern of human aging is that we find it easier to stay slim when we're young,

and it gets harder as the decades pass. Unfortunately, this rule applies to you, too.

3. The same thing goes for exercise. Sometimes people with a fair degree of metabolic resistance find that to lose at a decent speed they have to exercise (which I urge you to do anyway). Then they tell me, "But back in 1994, I lost 20 pounds in two months without exercising." Get real. It's not 1994. Send all complaints to Father Time, Box Office Eternity.

Remember how individual your body is, and you should be forearmed against any other personal mind traps that I neglected to mention.

This is heavy stuff psychologically, and we all face it. Yet a high percentage of people do succeed doing Atkins—permanently. How?

Create Good Food Habits

You've already learned some new eating habits and I would like to see you extend that ability further. You can learn not just *what* to eat, but *how* to treat food in general.

We are all plugged into our habits. If you can discover your bad connections and disconnect them, you will start to change. If you can learn new and improved connections and solder them into place, you'll do even better. Try these steps and see if they make your nutritional life easier:

• Eat slowly and extend the meal to give your brain time to signal satisfaction before your stomach is distended and you feel stuffed.
• Don't eat as much as you can; eat as much as you need.
• Don't finish something just because it's there.
• Establish food rituals that slow down the process of eating. For example, set the dinner table—even when you

are eating alone—and don't eat standing up at the kitchen counter.

- Don't eat meals in front of the television set or computer, especially not snacks that you could eat great quantities of while distracted without even realizing it.
- Try not to eat while talking on the phone.
- Don't cruise the kitchen during the commercials.
- Eat three meals a day—or four or five smaller ones. Skipping meals leads to unstable blood sugar and cravings, which might allow your bad habits to kick in.
- If you're not staying on the program as perfectly as you should be, start a food diary and carry it around with you. This is an excellent way to bring your eating behavior to the forefront of your conscious mind.

Keep Control or Else Regain It

Maybe everything I've told you will make you perfect. But so far I've met very few perfect people, and it's quite possible that you will slip and slide now and then. Or else you'll go through a short period of rebellion and cheat with a vengeance. Here are a few ways to create a strategy for lifetime success:

- Try to keep the control you've won; don't re-addict yourself.
- If you do slip, be realistic—no one's perfect one hundred percent of the time. Above all, recover immediately; don't wait until tomorrow. One slice of pie may have limited ill effects. A late-night debauch could send you off in the wrong direction for a month.
- If you've slipped up badly, don't tell yourself there's no use trying. Learn to live in the gray area when you're not being perfect! A mistake in eating doesn't mean you should stop taking nutritional supplements or exercis-

ing. Quite the contrary—everything good you can do for yourself makes it that much easier to get firmly back on the right track.

- Be on your *best* behavior during Induction, the phase in which you break your bad habits and addictions and establish healthy eating patterns.

- If you're bound and determined to cheat, at least do so in the least harmful way. If a fruit will satisfy your craving for something sweet, it's better than a cookie or candy bar.

- Adjust your aims to your realities. If you're going on vacation and you know you won't be able to comply perfectly, don't make continued weight loss your goal. Instead, go on the Lifetime Maintenance phase and aim to maintain your weight and stay in control of your food choices. When you return, go back to the appropriate weight loss phase.

- Give yourself a cushion. If there's a special occasion on the horizon, why not drop down to an earlier phase of Atkins a few weeks before the event?

- Learn from your experience. If you slip up and go off plan, ask yourself why. Did you give yourself permission? How did you *think* you would feel after? How *did* you feel? How should you deal with a similar situation in the future?

- If Atkins works for you, don't let other people vote on your health. It's your life, not theirs.

What if you've muffed it and you have to start over? Don't be embarrassed! Don't let those naysayers say, "I told you so." Just pick yourself up and start over again with Induction. And at the same time, you should ask yourself a series of soul-searching questions about what happened. This is especially true if you're a person for whom overeating and being out of control have been ongoing problems. Think about the situations and circumstances that led to the problem and creatively change your life to avoid them in the future. Try to teach yourself new ways of responding to the challenges.

I wouldn't have written this chapter if I didn't believe that nearly everyone could succeed doing Atkins. I want you to believe in the immense power of human adaptability. Do a conscious appraisal of why you've chosen Atkins, and then *adapt* with all the willpower and energy you possess.

Don't Go There!

Here are some mind traps you must learn to avoid:

- Using food as an emotional comfort.
- Quitting the program altogether if you've cheated.
- Eating less than three times a day.
- Doing what other people want instead of what's right for you.
- Being afraid to ask family and friends—or even a psychotherapist—for support.

22

Exercise: It's Non-Negotiable

Calling all couch potatoes: If you're not getting regular exercise, you aren't following the Atkins Nutritional Approach. It's that simple. You must make a commitment to physical activity as well as change the way you eat—and take nutritional supplements. Doing one without the other is like riding a bike with flat tires. It's a lot more difficult.

Why Exercise?

In case you need convincing, I'm going to build the case for how important exercise is and how integral it is to your new lifestyle. First, you should know that being active is critical to your good health. A report from the Global Burden of Disease project—a massive research effort that studied disease and death around the globe—included physical inactivity *among the most important risk factors threatening global health*.[1] The second thing you should know is that regular physical activity has been proven to contribute significantly to each of the Atkins principles: weight loss, weight maintenance, good health and disease prevention. And, now, I submit my evidence. We'll look at the first two together.

Weight Loss and Weight Maintenance

It's one of the basic laws of the universe: If you use more calories than you consume, you lose weight. (You sharp-eyed readers might say, "Whoa, I thought we didn't have to worry about calories." That's true, but it's a great way, here, to illustrate an important point.)

For example: Without changing the way you eat, say you burned an extra 250 calories per day, which a 150-pound person could accomplish by walking for about forty-five minutes at a pace of three miles per hour. If you did this for two weeks, you would create a deficit of 3,500 calories and thereby lose 1 pound of body weight. In addition to enabling weight loss, exercise keeps the pounds off. Research shows that most people who maintain weight loss exercise regularly, while most people who gain weight back do not.[2]

Exercise is like a buy-two, get-one-free proposition. Not only does it elevate your metabolic rate while you're exercising, but it keeps your calorie-burning meter cranked up for significant periods after you're through. This means that you continue burning calories at a good clip even though you've stopped moving. Similarly, when you increase your muscle mass, you increase the amount of energy your body naturally expends just to keep functioning—even at rest.

Good Health

By building endurance, flexibility and muscle strength, regular exercise contributes to the health of your muscles, bones and joints, in addition to improving your cardiovascular health. All of this means you'll be less likely to injure yourself and you'll have greater energy and stamina. In the long term, it will help to ensure greater self-sufficiency in later years.

It also increases your likelihood of living into those later years. One important study, called the College Alumni Health Study, followed graduates of Harvard University and the University of Pennsylvania for thirty-eight years. They found that men between the ages of 45 and 84 who expended just 1,000 calories a week—engaging in activities ranging from tennis to gardening—had a twenty to thirty percent reduced risk of dying from all causes when compared to those with less-active lifestyles. And those who had even greater calorie expenditures reduced their risk still further.[3]

Exercise comes with another subtle but powerful health benefit: By now, you understand the dangers of insulin resistance and the importance of curbing the overproduction of insulin. (If you don't, refer to Chapter 5 for a refresher.) Regular exercise results in a more efficient use of glucose at the cellular level, and this in turn reduces the output of insulin by the pancreas. It's just plain healthy to get moving.

Finally, many studies have shown that regular exercise appears to elevate mood and reduce depression and anxiety. In a Swedish study of thirty-four hundred people, those who exercised at least two to three times a week showed significantly less depression, anger, "cynical distrust" and stress than did people who exercised less frequently or not at all. The frequent exercisers also showed higher levels of coherence and stronger feelings of social integration.[4] Sounds good, doesn't it? And as if those benefits aren't enough in themselves, think about how often those feelings of depression or anger are the ones that lead you to overeat. You'll kill two birds with one stone if you can reduce them.

Disease Prevention

Physical activity has important positive effects on virtually all of the body's systems: musculoskeletal, cardiovascular, respiratory and endocrine. These effects result in reduced risks of coronary heart disease, stroke, high blood pressure, colon cancer and Type II diabetes. As more exercise and disease research accumulates, we'll likely find many other conditions that may be prevented with regular exercise.

Probably the most compelling evidence out there has to do with exercise's ability to help our hearts: In the famous Honolulu Heart Program study of twenty-six hundred men ages 71 to 93, researchers found a fifteen percent decrease in risk of heart disease for every half mile walked per day. *The men who walked one and a half miles or more per day had less than half the rate of heart disease compared to those who walked less than a quarter mile per day.*[5] Other studies have had similarly amazing results.

Have I made my case? So why is it that sixty percent of us don't get regular exercise? Here are some of the excuses I hear most often:

- **"I don't have time."** Oh, how often I've heard this one. Listen, folks, if you sleep eight hours a night, you have sixteen waking hours a day. Subtract eight hours for working and two for eating and personal hygiene and you still have six hours left. In those six hours, there is no way you can't find half an hour for exercise. For other things that are important to you, you simply find or make time, and this should be the same!
- **"I'm too old."** If you're over a hundred, call me for a special consultation to discuss the possibility of your not exercising. The rest of you, get up out of your rocking chairs!
- **"I'm not in good health."** This is a reason to begin slowly and proceed cautiously. An exercise program can be tailored to any condition, and even the frailest person can start at a level appropriate to his or her condition. If you still have the use of your limbs, you can exercise.
- **"I'm too lazy."** This is usually the real reason, and I can hardly criticize you with a straight face since, for much of my life, I've been guilty myself. The solution for you may be what worked for me: Find an exercise you really like (in my case, tennis) and build your fitness program around that. I even find it easier to do some things I don't like at all—such as jogging and weight-training—because I tell myself they'll help my tennis game. If you find the sport or activity you enjoy, you'll look forward to doing it instead of thinking of it as a chore.

Transforming Your Inner Couch Potato

Here are ten great tips to make being active an ever-present part of your life:

1. Park far from the entrance to the mall, grocery store, your office or friend's house.
2. Don't leave your shopping cart in the parking lot; return it to the store.
3. Contract and relax all your muscles when you sit down.
4. Use music to pep you up during exercise and household chores so you'll pick up the pace and get your blood pumping.
5. Lay out the next day's workout clothes every night before going to bed.
6. Keep a log of all your activity—including household chores and walking.
7. Have an exercise plan for rainy days and when traveling.
8. For the first few months, do less than you think you can. It will keep you coming back for more while also helping you avoid injury.
9. Get in the habit of taking the stairs instead of the elevator or escalator.
10. Dance with your spouse, with your kids, with a friend—or even by yourself when you're alone in the house.

How Much Exercise Do You Need?

It may not be as much as you think. The Surgeon General's 1996 report on physical activity and health states: "Physical activity need not be strenuous to achieve health benefits."[6] The report recommends that people of all ages get a minimum of thirty minutes of physical activity of moderate intensity (such as brisk walking) on most, if not all, days of the week. The report also says that, for most people, it's even better to exercise harder and longer.

I recommend that your daily minimum of thirty minutes of physical activity take place all at once because it will get your fat-burning engine into a sustained mode. However, for those of you who absolutely cannot or will not do it all at once, the following provides some benefits, although results will take longer to achieve: Try three ten-minute sessions (or two fifteen-minute sessions) of moderately intense activity. For example, do ten minutes of sit-ups, leg lifts, stretching and arm exercises in the morning; take a brisk ten-minute walk at lunchtime; rake some leaves and do a bit of vigorous house or yard work for ten minutes before dinner and . . . *you've done it!* (See also "Transforming Your Inner Couch Potato" on page 290).

Another way to organize your exercise is to count the calories you burn (you know I'm not going to ask you to count the calories you consume!) According to renowned researcher and founder of the College Alumni Health Study Ralph Paffenbarger in his book *LifeFit: An Effective Exercise Program for Optimal Health and a Longer Life*, you should expend 1,500 to 2,000 calories per week for the greatest health benefit.[7] Check the calorie expenditure tables on pages 298–300 and draw up your plan.

An important note: The American College of Sports Medicine recommends that you include weight-bearing exercise in your workouts two to three (non-consecutive) days a week. It's recommended that you do one set each of eight to twelve exercises that address most of the major muscles in the body. The correct amount of resistance for you is that which will cause fatigue at eight to twelve repetitions. Once you can do twelve reps, step up the amount of resistance. If you don't have access to a gym, you can use inexpensive, lightweight dumbbells or resistance bands. If you go this route, get yourself a book or video that shows proper form for exercising with free weights (or bands), so you don't injure yourself and get the most out of your workout.

Two Kinds of Exercise

The best exercise programs combine aerobic and anaerobic activity.

- **Aerobic exercise** is any activity that increases your heart rate and causes you to consume more oxygen. Every cell in your body requires a constant supply of oxygen, and if you've been a couch potato for years, many of those cells are being deprived. This is why I can assure you: *Once you accustom yourself to a regular routine of aerobic exercise, you will begin to feel better than you did before.*

     If it's been a long time since you did any vigorous activity, I urge you to get some professional advice, from both your doctor and a certified fitness expert. It's important that you start slowly and learn how to stretch, warm up and cool down in order to avoid injury. You also may want to try an exercise trampoline. This is a gentle way to increase the stress on your bones and send a signal to the vertebrae to lay down more calcium along the stress-bearing planes.

     Exercise such as walking, golf, doubles tennis, horseback riding, ping-pong and dancing may only mildly increase the pumping action of your heart, but they are still tremendous improvements for a former non-exerciser. If you fall into that category, walking is the best way to begin. I know many of my readers are people who haven't walked more than two blocks in years. These are the individuals who will notice the greatest change in how they feel. Walk five blocks. Then try six. If it's hard on you today, take comfort in the certainty that the stiffness will ease, your breathing will improve and relaxing endorphins will be released into your body. And before you know it, you'll be walking a mile. Moving can and will feel good—it's actually what your body was built to do and wants! Remember, Mother Nature did not design us for our sedentary modern lifestyle.

- **Anaerobic exercise** is any type of physical activity that isn't significantly aerobic. This includes exercise that builds muscle mass, such as weight-lifting and other types of training such as resistance and isometrics. Building muscle mass does not mean becoming one of those bulging body builders. If you keep at it, you will begin to notice a gradual sculpting taking place under your skin—and I guarantee you're going to like how it looks. But if vanity doesn't drive you to take up some weight-bearing exercise, maybe the fear of frailty will. It is this type of exercise that helps stave off the loss of bone density that accompanies aging. This is why resistance training is so important to prevent osteoporosis.

The Myth of Carb-Loading

You've probably heard of marathoners and other elite athletes inhaling gargantuan amounts of pasta before big endurance events, often referred to as "carb-loading." It turns out that "fat-loading" may be more effective. More scientific research is required; however, studies on both animals and humans have suggested that a fat-rich diet may increase endurance. A 1994 study compared the effects of a high-carb/low-fat diet and a high-fat/low-carb diet on two groups of trained cyclists. During high-intensity exercise, the groups performed equally well; during prolonged, moderate-intensity exercise, endurance was significantly enhanced among the cyclists on the high-fat/low-carb regimen.[8] Two other studies on humans suggest that increasing dietary fat from fifteen percent to forty-two percent increases maximum oxygen consumption and endurance capacity.[9-10] My review of the published research suggests to me that increases in dietary fat may be beneficial—not only for general health, but also for physical endurance.

How Your New Eating Habits Will Help

On low-fat and low-calorie diets, people can do serious harm to themselves by overexercising. When the body isn't getting enough protein from food, it turns to its only source of non-dietary protein: muscle. The body will actually begin to consume its own healthy muscle tissue. If you think this happens only to starving people in developing countries, you're wrong. Do you know someone who eats half a bagel and fruit for breakfast and a salad and diet soda for lunch? And then goes to the gym right after work? Where is her body going to find the protein to fuel her for those forty-five minutes on the stair-climbing machine? It will turn to the very muscles she's trying to build and tone—not to the fat cells she thinks she's burning.

The other benefit of a controlled carb nutrition program is that your metabolism won't go into starvation mode when you start exercising. Consider this: When you restrict calories and increase exercise, your body reacts just as it would when we were cavemen. As far as your body knows, it thinks there's a famine going on out there and—by unfortunate coincidence—some bear must be chasing you at the same time. Your body goes into survival mode and wisely sends out an all-systems alert to conserve resources. It literally turns your metabolism down a notch.

If you instead give your body all the protein and fat it desires, your body will know that food is plentiful. It will then accept your running, walking, stair-climbing or bicycling and leave your metabolism to hum along, and maybe even step up its pace.

Find Your Comfort Zone

Before you embark on any new exercise plan, be sure to consult your physician. That done, review these plans and find the one that describes you best. Or work up an individualized program with your physician or a certified fitness trainer. You'll need to learn how to measure your pulse as well as calculate your Target Heart Rate (THR) zone. (See "Find Your Target Heart Rate Zone" on page 298.)

PLAN 1: JOHNNY GO LIGHTLY

Criteria:

- You are over the age of 50.
- Your body mass index (BMI) is greater than 35 (check the BMI chart in Chapter 13).
- Your current level of physical activity is either none or very little.
- You have been diagnosed with heart disease, diabetes, hypertension, severe asthma or severe arthritis. (Again, you must get a physician's approval before beginning this exercise plan. See also "Safety Counts!" on pages 297–298.)

Choose one or more activities from or similar to the ones listed below and do them for ten minutes each, two days a week.

- Walking on a flat surface
- Leisure bicycling
- Basic stretching
- Yoga
- Light swimming
- Beginner water aerobics

Increase your workout time by three minutes each week, and add a third day when you reach week three.

PLAN 2: LIGHT 'N' LIVELY

Criteria:

- You are 35 to 50 years old.
- Your BMI is greater than 30 but less than 35 (check the BMI chart in Chapter 13).
- Your current activity level is minimal.

Choose one or more activities from or similar to the ones listed below and do them for fifteen minutes each, three days a week.

- Brisk walking
- Lap swimming
- Training using an elliptical trainer
- Low-impact aerobics
- Hiking
- Tennis
- Beginner martial arts
- Dancing
- Roller skating/ice skating

Increase your workout time by three minutes each week, and add a fourth day when you reach week four.

PLAN 3: GO FOR THE BURN

Criteria:

- You are under 35 years old.
- Your BMI is less than 30 (check the BMI chart in Chapter 13).
- Your current activity level is moderate.

Choose one or more activities from or similar to the ones listed below and do them for twenty minutes each, three days a week.

- Basketball
- Jogging
- Racquetball
- Squash
- Inline skating
- Jumping rope
- Cross-country skiing
- Spinning

Increase your workout time by five minutes each week, and add a fourth day when you reach week four.

Note: The end goal is the same for everyone. Work up to thirty minutes of moderately intense physical activity most days a week. (Forty-five minutes is even better.) Your muscles need rest and recovery time, so the optimum frequency is five times a week.

Remember, exercise is the natural companion to weight loss. If you increase your muscle mass, you can also eat more.

Safety Counts!

- **Caution:** Whatever your physical condition, you must see a doctor before initiating a new exercise program.
- **Check your pulse** frequently so you do not exceed your maximum heart rate, and make sure you can talk at all times during your workout. If you find you cannot speak without a great deal of effort, decrease your intensity.
- **Warm up and cool down.** Start and end your workout gradually, with a reduced-intensity version of whatever activity you're doing.

- **Stretch** all your muscle groups as part of your warm up and your cool down.
- **Stay hydrated.** The heavier you are, the more water your body needs, especially before, during and after exercise. Drink *before* you feel thirsty.
- **Don't exercise on an empty stomach.** But don't eat for one hour before light exercise or for two hours before strenuous exercise.

Find Your Target Heart Rate Zone

Here's how to calculate your Target Heart Rate zone: Subtract your age from the number 220, then take sixty and seventy percent of that number. Mathematically, the formula works out as follows: (220–age) × .60 and (220–age) × .70 = THR zone.

So the sample calculation for a 58-year-old woman would be:

$$220{-}58 = 162 \times .60 = 97 \underline{\text{ and }} 162 \times .70 = 113$$

This woman should keep her pulse between 97 and 113 beats per minute while exercising. Very overweight people should be especially careful because they may reach the high end of their zone quite quickly.

Calorie Expenditure

Take Your Pick. Each of the following activities done for the stated time periods burns about 150 calories:

- Washing/waxing a car for forty-five to sixty minutes
- Washing windows for forty-five to sixty minutes

- Playing volleyball for forty-five minutes
- Playing touch football for thirty to forty-five minutes
- Gardening for thirty to forty-five minutes
- Wheeling oneself in a wheelchair for thirty to forty minutes
- Walking one and three-quarter miles in thirty-five minutes at a rate of twenty minutes per mile
- Basketball (shooting baskets) for thirty minutes
- Bicycling five miles in thirty minutes
- Dancing fast (social) for thirty minutes
- Pushing a stroller one and a half miles in thirty minutes
- Raking leaves for thirty minutes
- Walking two miles in thirty minutes at fifteen minutes per mile
- Doing water aerobics for thirty minutes
- Swimming laps for twenty minutes
- Playing wheelchair basketball for twenty minutes
- Playing basketball (a game) for fifteen to twenty minutes
- Bicycling four miles in fifteen minutes
- Jumping rope for fifteen minutes
- Running one and a half miles in fifteen minutes at ten minutes a mile
- Shoveling snow for fifteen minutes
- Stair-walking for fifteen minutes

Note that the number of calories burned is based on men and women of average size with average muscle mass. A smaller person or one with less than average muscle mass will burn fewer calories.

Source: "Physical Activity and Health: A Report of the Surgeon General," July 1996.

Number of Calories Burned in 30 Minutes

Your weight in pounds	110– 115	120– 125	130– 140	145– 150	160– 165	170– 175	185– 190	200– 205	210– 220
Basketball	210	230	260	280	310	330	360	380	405
Gardening (digging)	190	215	235	260	280	300	325	350	370
Gardening (raking)	80	90	100	110	120	130	140	150	160
Golf	130	145	160	175	190	205	220	235	250
Ironing	50	55	60	65	70	80	85	90	95
Running (11-min. mile)	205	230	250	275	300	325	350	375	400
Running (8-min. mile)	325	355	395	425	460	495	530	570	600
Swimming	255	285	315	345	375	405	435	465	500
Tennis	165	185	205	220	245	260	285	300	320
Walking	120	135	150	160	175	190	205	220	230
Weight-training	175	195	215	235	260	280	300	320	345

Source: www.healthology.com, "Weight Loss and Physical Activity," by Bruce Rector, MD.

TIPS:

- Find an exercise buddy.
- Rotate activities.
- Do not exercise more than five times a week.
- To avoid boredom, keep your brain occupied with a book or music.

23

Nutritional Supplements: Don't Even Think of Getting Along Without Them!

A growing trend—and one in which I believe I have played no small part—is that more and more doctors are treating their patients (whenever possible) with vitamin and mineral supplements in lieu of pharmaceuticals. Over the last two decades, thousands of physicians and more health practitioners have learned how to practice such nutritional pharmacology.

"Complementary Medicine" combines the best of conventional and alternative medical care. Its basic tenet is that all the healing arts can and should complement one another. And its primary principle is to always select the safest therapies, which inevitably brings the nutritional approach to the forefront.

Harry Kronberg, Mary Anne Evans, Gordon Lingard and many of the other people whose case histories you've read about here were my patients. In each case, I prescribed appropriate vitamins, minerals, herbs, essential fatty acids and other nutritional agents—the group I call *vitanutrients*.

Vitanutrients can benefit even people at the peak of health who eat an excellent diet. (Unfortunately, no matter how well we eat, our depleted soil no longer provides all the nutrients fresh produce used to yield.) I would go so far as to say that vitanutrients could extend one's lifespan. I'll cite just one example to prove my point: The antioxidant group of nutrients has consistently proven to protect the body from damage by free radicals—those destructive electrons that have been implicated in cancer and heart disease as well as in accelerating the natural aging process. Even a person who eats the best possible food is not living in a perfect environment. Moreover, air pollution, tobacco smoke and other environmental toxins assault our bodies daily. Consequently, a person can maintain good health longer by taking effective doses of such antioxidants as vitamins A, C and E, plus selenium, glutathione, CoQ_{10} and bioflavonoids.

However, actually ingesting adequate amounts of vitanutrients can be problematic. Scientific studies seeking the maximum effective doses of all the essential nutrients could lead you to conclude that you should take over one hundred vitamin pills a day. Clearly that is not practical, so I have devised a system of nutritional prescribing that I call *targeted nutrition*. This allows me to prescribe, and individuals to select, a variety of formulations that target certain conditions. For instance, if a person is subject to frequent colds and viruses, he might opt for an acute infection formula such as the one we at Atkins Nutritionals call Cold & Flu. This formula contains the antioxidant vitamins C and A, plus zinc, bioflavonoids and the B complex constituents. All are nutrients that published studies have shown to make a difference in our ability to handle such microscopic invaders. The nutritional agents are not directed against a specific disease or condition; rather, they provide support, allowing the body to defend itself to the best of its ability against disease.

Which Nutrients Should I Take?

I would like to provide you with a basic supplementation plan to follow now and after you've reached your goal weight. Certain nutrients can aid in weight loss, so I have devised a basic formula that is integral to the Atkins Nutritional Approach. This formula is also perfectly appropriate once you've reached Lifetime Maintenance. I'll list its contents, so you won't necessarily have to get them from Atkins Nutritionals (in which, of course, I have a financial involvement). You can simply provide yourself with a collection of vitamins that provide the equivalent nutritional support.

Atkins Basic #3 Formula contains all the ingredients in my basic multiple vitamin, known as Basic #1, although in somewhat different dosages (see table beginning below). Basic #1 is a good formulation when weight loss is not an issue. Basic #3, on the other hand, is designed to be taken as three tablets daily, one with each meal. Compared to Basic #1, it contains greater amounts of certain nutrients—including chromium, pantethine, selenium, vanadium and biotin—all of which play a role in regulating blood sugar and insulin, as well as in burning fat. We've also included additional amounts of antioxidants. Although you will certainly be able to find a good multivitamin that contains most of the ingredients in Basic #3, you may choose to purchase separately the individual substances I've just cited so you can take them in the desired amounts. Basic #3 is formulated with intestinal flora, which helps your body use the nutrients more easily. It contains the following:

Atkins Basic #3 Formula

Three tablets daily give you:	Amount Per Serving	Daily Value
Vitamin A (as acetate)	4000 IU	80%
Vitamin A (as natural beta-carotene with mixed carotenoids)	7500 IU	150%
Vitamin C (as calcium ascorbate)	360mg	600%
Vitamin D-3 (as cholecalciferol)	200 IU	50%
Vitamin E (as d-alpha tocopherol succinate)	150 IU	500%
Vitamin K (as phytonadione)	5mcg	6%

Three tablets daily give you:	Amount Per Serving	Daily Value
Vitamin B_1 (as thiamine HCL)	25mg	1666%
Vitamin B_2 (as riboflavin)	25mg	1470%
Niacin (as niacinamide)	20mg	100%
Vitamin B_6 (as pyridoxine HCL)	25mg	1250%
Folate (as folic acid)	600mcg	150%
Vitamin B_{12} (as cyanocobalamin)	200mcg	3333%
Biotin	150mcg	50%
Pantothenic Acid (as d-calcium pantothenate)	60mg	600%
Calcium (as phosphate/ ascorbate/citrate)	250mg	25%
Phosphorus	76mg	7%
Magnesium (as glycinate)	125mg	31%
Zinc (as zinc monomethionine)	10mg	67%
Selenium (as sodium selenite)	50mcg	71%
Copper (as glycinate)	1mg	50%
Manganese (as glycinate)	5mg	250%
Chromium (as polynicotinate)	300mcg	250%
Molybdenum (as glycinate)	30mcg	40%
Potassium (as citrate)	10mg	<1%
Pantethine (a co-enzyme A precursor)	20mg	*
N-Acetyl-L-Cysteine	60mg	*
Inositol Hexanicotinate	50mg	*
Para Amino Benzoic Acid	50mg	*
Citrus Bioflavonoids (20% bioflavonoids)	50mg	*
Quercetin	50mg	*
Green Tea (20% polyphenols)	40mg	*
Choline Bitartrate	21mg	*
Grape Seed Extract	20mg	*
Boron (as calcium borogluconate)	200mcg	*
Vanadium (as bis-glycinato oxovanadium)	40mcg	*

Daily Value not established.

Let me point out the merits of some of the nutrients in Basic #3 that specifically deal with weight control, so you get a sense of why supplementation is also important for weight loss and maintenance:

- **Chromium**, which deserves the most attention, helps activate the uptake of insulin at its receptor sites. It is best assimilated in the form of chromium polynicotinate. A spate of studies has shown that chromium will build muscle, decrease body fat and lower cholesterol levels.[1] Basic #3 contains 300 mcg, which is sufficient for most individuals. Others may need up to 800 to 1000 mcg per day.
- **Pantethine** (vitamin B₅) is a remarkable nutrient that helps control cholesterol, supports the adrenals and produces "friendly" bacteria in the intestine, making it a valuable tool in preventing yeast overgrowth.[2] Basic #3 contains 20 mg of pantethine, which is the precursor of pantothenic acid, and another 60 mg of the latter. This dose should be sufficient for most people; those who are metabolically resistant in the extreme may need to take an additional supplement.
- **Selenium** is a powerful antioxidant. It may also play a beneficial nutritional role in preventing diabetes. Basic #3 contains 50 mcg.
- **Vanadium** (vanadyl sulfate) is a trace mineral that dramatically aids diabetics, apparently by helping cells to absorb blood sugar more effectively and thereby decreasing the need for insulin. Basic #3 contains 40 mcg; people with diabetes or pre-diabetic conditions may require as much as 100 mcg daily. However, without medical supervision I do not recommend exceeding the amount found in Basic #3.
- **Biotin** is an unsung B vitamin whose nutritional role was emphasized by a study that noted a significant drop in diabetics' blood-sugar levels after taking the supplement.[3] Basic #3 contains 150 mcg of biotin.

More Basic Support

Once you've decided on an appropriate vitamin and mineral formula along the lines of Basic #3, there is another vital nutrient group that should be part of any permanent plan. Ever wonder why your doctor advises you to take one baby aspirin a day? It's because it thins your blood and helps it flow more easily through your veins, carrying nutrients to your cells and brain. It also protects your arteries from forming plaque.

Well, the essential fatty acids (EFA) do the same thing, without the side effects of aspirin. EFAs also keep your hair, skin and nails healthy. The typical American diet tends to be deficient in EFAs, particularly omega-3s. You won't find them in a multiple vitamin/mineral because oils don't mix well with the dry powders that are pressed into tablets.

There are three types of EFAs: Omega-9 fatty acids are readily available in olive oil, but you need supplements to get adequate amounts of omega-3 and omega-6 oils. The former come from animal sources (fish and marine mammals primarily) and vegetable sources, such as flaxseed oil, which provides alpha-linolenic acid (ALA). Omega-6, also known as gamma linolenic acid (GLA), is contained in borage oil and black-currant oil. I usually suggest one capsule of borage oil, one of fish oil and one of flaxseed oil. My Essential Oils Formula contains all of the above, and the minimum dose is two per day.

Other Weight Loss Assistance

Occasionally, a nutritional shortcoming can lower your metabolism and increase your resistance to weight loss. If you're unable to lose weight or your progress is slow or nearly nonexistent, you may want to consider certain nutrients that can help break up a weight loss logjam.

The first is L-carnitine, which is involved in fat transport. When carnitine is deficient, overweight people have difficulty getting into lipolysis and the secondary process of ketosis. As a nutrient, carnitine has been used to correct cardiomyopathy, help stabilize heart rhythm, lower triglyceride levels and increase HDL (the good cholesterol).[4] For these conditions, the dosage ranges between 1,000 and 2,000 mg daily. For weight loss, a typical dose is 1,500 mg.

Another weight loss aid is Co-enzyme Q_{10} (CoQ_{10}), which plays an important role in heart function. I often prescribe it to people over forty, usually in a dose of 100 mg a day. Since it works in collaboration with carnitine and chromium to mobilize fat, it is also useful for someone aiming to slim down. One Belgian study by Dr. Luc Van Gall reported on obese patients with deficient levels of CoQ_{10} who experienced significant weight loss after taking the nutrient. Van Gall used 100 mg daily in that research.[5]

So the basic supplementation during weight loss phases of Atkins (and if desired in Lifetime Maintenance) consists of:

- Basic #3 Formula—three times a day.
- Chromium—up to 1,000 mcg daily, **but be sure to count the amount of chromium contained in your dosage of the Basic #3 Formula**.
- Essential oils—three a day, either in a multiple, or individual fish oil, borage oil and flaxseed oil capsules.
- L-carnitine and CoQ_{10}—if you feel that your metabolic resistance to weight loss is high (see above for dosages).

Additional Advantages

Now that I've laid out the basic framework of supplementation, I'd like to discuss specific nutritional solutions to common problems. This information will help increase your knowledge and awareness of the benefits of complementary medicine. However, these dosages are general recommendations and not specific prescriptions. If you suffer from one of these problems I'd truly love it if you came for a consultation so that you could be provided with a personalized supplementation protocol. Since that probably isn't possible, please visit us at *www.atkinscenter.com* for other options.

- **For constipation:** My preference is psyllium husks. Start with one tablespoon in a large glass of water and increase or decrease the dose until the desired result occurs. Or sprinkle one or two tablespoons of oat bran or wheat bran (if you're not allergic to wheat) over your vegetables or salad. Increased exercise and increased water consumption also help relieve constipation.
- **For sugar cravings:** 500 to 1,000 mg of L-glutamine before meals and/or when cravings are greatest.
- **For hunger not assuaged by being in lipolysis:** 500 mg of L-phenylalanine or 500 mg of N-acetyl-L-tyrosine before meals.
- **For fluid retention:** 50 to 100 mg of pyridoxal 5 phosphate, plus 1,500 to 3,000 mg taurine daily.[6] Asparagus tablets also are effective.
- **For fatigue:** 5 to 10 mg of octacosanol, three to six sublingual tablets of dimethylglycine, one to three sublingual B_{12} tablets or one to three (50 mg) B complex tablets per day.[7]
- **For nervousness:** 500 to 2,000 mg of inositol, daily. Herbal teas, such as camomile, valerian and passion flower, are also effective.
- **For insomnia:** Before going to bed, take either of the above vitanutrients or herbal teas suggested for nervousness, plus 3 mg of melatonin. Calcium, magnesium, niacinamide, pantothenic acid, valerian or 5-hydroxy tryptophan may also be useful.

Nutritional Approaches to Health Problems

The most common health complications faced by over-weight men and women are complications that arise from the risk factors associated with blood-sugar disturbances, such as hypoglycemia and diabetes, and cardiovascular disease. For these conditions I commonly prescribe the nutrients described below. Again, I remind you that these dosages represent what I often prescribe and might in fact prescribe for you if you suffer from one of these complications:

- **For hypoglycemia:** Basic #3, my Blood Sugar Formula, plus chromium (800 to 1,000 mcg per day), L-glutamine, zinc, selenium, magnesium, all of the B complex vitamins and extra biotin. Alternatively, I use Atkins Formula HF-12.
- **For diabetes:** Basic #3, the Blood Sugar Formula, plus extra chromium, zinc, selenium, inositol, CoQ_{10}, biotin, vanadyl sulfate, magnesium. Alternatively, I use Atkins Formula DM-17.
- **For lowering cholesterol or reduction of elevated cholesterol:** Lecithin granules, chromium, pantethine, niacin (inositol hexanicotinate) and other B complex factors, garlic, vitamin C, GLA (borage, primrose, or black-currant oils), EPA (fish oil), beta-sitosterol, guggulipid, glucomannan, guar gum, pectin, psyllium husks and oat bran. Alternatively, I use the Vita-Nutrient "Cholesterol" Formula or Cholesterol Gold plus the Essential Oils Formula.
- **For elevated triglycerides:** Similar to the list for cholesterol, except that L-carnitine and Omega-3 oils are emphasized. Also, because of the correlation of triglycerides and hyperinsulinism, the nutrients helpful in diabetes will also prove helpful here.[8-9]
- **For hypertension:** Magnesium (preferably as orotate, taurate, arginate or aspartate), taurine, pyridoxal 5

phosphate or pyridoxine, garlic, essential fatty acids (GLA and EPA), CoQ_{10} and potassium. Alternatively, I use Atkins Essential Oils Formula and Blood Pressure Formula.[10–11]

- **For coronary heart disease:** The abovementioned magnesium compounds, L-carnitine, vitamin E, CoQ_{10}, bromelain, garlic, and chromium polynicotinate. Alternatively, I use formula CV-4[12–15] and Essential Oils Formula.

Note: In *Dr. Atkins' Vita-Nutrient Solution*, I supply the breakdown of all the Atkins formulas, the exact quantities of nutrients and greater detail on what these important substances can do for you.

I hope I have convinced you to learn about vitanutrients. While controlling your intake of carbohydrate gives you a metabolic edge, similarly, the targeted use of nutritional supplements arms you with another kind of edge. Learn about them and how to use them properly. When you do, you will enjoy a double health advantage.

PART FOUR

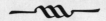

Disease Prevention

24

The Perilous Path to Diabetes

From the standpoint of saving lives, this chapter should prove to be the most significant one I have ever written. Here's why: For the past two decades, two illnesses have escalated so rapidly that they are considered twin epidemics—obesity and Type II diabetes. I might go so far as to say they are Siamese twins.

Obesity and Type II diabetes are actually two aspects of a single illness, characterized by insulin resistance (insulin not doing its job in your body) and hyperinsulinism (excess production of insulin). The overlap between the two is impressive. Over eighty percent of Type II diabetics are obese.[1] And in my experience, the vast majority of obese people have the identical problems that lead to diabetes. The most convincing connection of all is that these twin epidemics escalated at exactly the same time, coinciding perfectly with dramatic changes in the American diet. During the generation in which these conditions reached unprecedented heights, the intake of dietary fat fell from forty to thirty-three percent of total calories consumed. But, predictably, the intake of refined carbohydrates, including both sugar and flour, went up by an even greater amount.

Type II diabetes is caused by a genetic predisposition to the disease and/or a diet filled with refined carbohydrates combined with an overall decrease in physical activity. Let me call your attention to one of the most important books ever written, *Saccharine Disease: The Master Disease of Our Time*. By British Surgeon Captain T. L. Cleave, MD, the book examined nearly a dozen cultures in which diabetes (and coronary heart disease as well) simply never occurred until twenty years after the people in that culture began to consume significant amounts of refined carbohydrates (a further discussion of Cleave's findings appears in Chapter 27).

Cleave's logic has been confirmed with a worldwide epidemic of diabetes. United Nations researchers have stated that by the year 2025, our planet is likely to have three hundred million diabetic residents, the greatest number of which will be from nations that had very few cases of diabetes until they supplemented their indigenous diets with excessive amounts of refined foods.[2]

I am not alone in my concern that diabetes is a looming national health crisis. The American Diabetes Association (ADA) has redefined its standard for diagnosing the illness, enabling physicians to identify it at an early stage, when treatment can be more effective. In 1997 the Centers for Disease Control estimated that almost sixteen million adults in the United States had diabetes.[3] Almost eight hundred thousand new cases are diagnosed yearly. Direct and indirect costs of the illness were figured at ninety-eight billion dollars annually in 1997![4]

Even children are now at risk for Type II diabetes—although it has generally been referred to as adult onset diabetes. A Cincinnati study was typical of many that are currently being published—researchers found that the incidence of children and adolescents between the ages of 10 and 19 diagnosed with Type II diabetes had increased tenfold from 1982 to 1994.[5] All evidence indicates that this disturbing trend is continuing. Further, African-Americans, Latinos and Native Americans are at a significantly higher risk for diabetes than non-Hispanic whites, a statistic that presumably has a close relationship to their higher rates of obesity, although there may be a genetic component as well.[6]

The Answer

We know that the first key to unlocking the solution to this epidemic is the acknowledgment of a well-established scientific fact; the second key is the implementation of treatment based on understanding this fact. For my money, there are still far too many health professionals who acknowledge the fact but don't put the solution into practice. The simple fact is that the earliest diagnosable state of Type II diabetes is associated with the production of *excessive* amounts of insulin.

In such a condition, the body does not allow insulin to do its job (hence, the term *insulin resistance*); therefore, the glucose level in the blood remains elevated. High insulin levels cause additional health problems, including obesity, high blood pressure and two major cardiac risk factors: high triglycerides and low levels of HDL (good cholesterol). Scientists continue to uncover even more difficulties attributed to hyperinsulinism, including polycystic ovarian syndrome and an increased death rate from breast cancer. And I fear that, as time goes on, the list will grow.

I pray that if you get nothing else out of this book, you get fixed in your mind the answer to following question: *What causes a life-threatening elevation of insulin levels?*

The primary cause is eating too much of the wrong kind of carbohydrates. To a lesser degree eating excessive amounts of protein can affect blood-sugar levels; however, when protein is used for its primary function of building muscle mass, insulin is not produced. And, most significantly, insulin is not required to metabolize either our stored fat or the fat in the food we eat.

Now that you know how to do Atkins, you know it bypasses the problem of excessive insulin by switching the body to a primarily fat-burning metabolism. All the millions of early-stage diabetics who are eating meals high in carbs and taking medications that may stimulate insulin production are quite innocently on a path to self-destruction. They may think that their present diet will protect them, but if those people are limiting their carbs by limiting their calorie intake, it is likely that after a while they will become bored or frustrated by their restrictive diet. Then they are likely to revert to consuming too much of the wrong kind of carbohydrate, putting them back on the high-insulin pathway to trouble. But individuals who are doing Atkins control their carbohydrate intake and eat foods with so little glycemic impact that they can normalize their blood sugar and become latent diabetics. (This term applies to those people with the disease who are able keep it under complete control.)

The Benefit of Experience

What a dramatic difference! In my clinical experience—reading food diaries kept by patients—I have seen time and time again that a diabetic following a high-carbohydrate, low-calorie diet with the emphasis on fat restriction will usually find that such a meal raises his or her blood-sugar level an average of 100 points if tested about ninety minutes after the meal. That same person will note that a steak or rack of lamb or a broiled half chicken plus a tossed green salad with Italian dressing will raise the blood-sugar level no more than 20 points, if at all.

I have looked extensively but have not found a single scientific study showing that the higher-carbohydrate diet achieves better control over diabetes than the controlled carbohydrate nutritional approach that is Atkins. Certainly my clinical experience supports the position that the Atkins Nutritional Approach is the preferred nutritional treatment for Type II diabetes.

The Two Types of Diabetes

At this point we should take one step back to clarify that the two types of diabetes are truly so different that they should be considered two quite different illnesses. This chapter addresses only Type II diabetes.

- **Type I diabetes** typically occurs in childhood or early adulthood and is unrelated to dietary habits. It appears to be an autoimmune disorder, in which the body mistakenly attacks the pancreas, largely or totally destroying its capacity to produce insulin. Only five to ten percent of all diabetics are Type I.
- **Type II diabetes** is caused by a genetic propensity for the disease combined with improper eating habits. The research done by Cleave (referred to on page 314) showed that certain genetically predisposed races and cultures do not get Type II diabetes until exposed to significant amounts of refined carbohydrates. (I should point out, however, that it is possible to be at risk for Type II diabetes even if you don't have a family history of the illness.)

The great majority of people who suffer from Type II diabetes actually produce more insulin than do those who don't suffer from the illness. The reason the diabetics have elevated blood-sugar levels is not due to lack of insulin, but rather to insulin resistance. Therefore, insulin and insulin-stimulating drugs usually make matters worse. Only in the later stages of Type II diabetes does a person's insulin output decline.

Don't Underestimate the Danger

I fear that many of you think of diabetes as a rather innocuous condition that requires very little self-denial. "Oh, well," you may say, "if my blood sugar is out of control, I can take a pill to control it." Or if you are further along the path to diabetes, you might even say, "I'll just have to take insulin and watch the way I eat." Don't flirt with that radically incorrect viewpoint. Diabetes can be an innocuous condition all right, but only if you eat appropriately. If you don't, diabetes can be a heartbreaking scourge. It's the largest single cause of new cases of blindness in the United States. It's also the leading cause of kidney failure, a giant stepping-stone toward heart disease, and can so severely damage the circulatory system that eighty-six thousand Americans yearly suffer amputations.[7] I won't catalogue any more horrors. Instead, heed my many years of clinical experience: If you are at risk for diabetes, you have to make a lifetime pledge to stay away from those foods known to turn it into a grim collection of maladies. I can think of few illnesses I would sooner avoid.

Diabetes May Be Creeping Up on You

Traditionally physicians have diagnosed diabetes in people in their fifties and sixties. According to a recent survey,[8] however, the average age of onset in the baby boomer generation is now 37!

The crucial point is that whether you get this illness in your thirties or in your fifties, you've been building up to it over decades. Type II diabetes never springs forth out of nowhere. We eat our way toward it, three meals a day, a thousand meals a year, ten thousand meals a decade.

Type II diabetes is:

- frequently diet-induced.
- almost always completely preventable.
- almost always convertible to a latent condition if caught early enough.
- virtually always improvable and partially reversible, even late in the illness.

It is only partially reversible because, once you have it, proper eating habits may keep it under control, but such eating habits cannot necessarily heal all the damage that has already occurred.

Diabetes is insidious. It exists as pre-diabetes, usually for several decades. It is during this period that a simple glucose-tolerance test (GTT) can establish its presence. Although the ADA currently estimates that one diabetic in three is unaware that he or she has the condition,[9] we find, by doing GTTs on patients with symptoms and/or a family history, approximately three pre-diabetics for every one with established diabetes.

The Path to Diabetes

Let's outline the journey that diabetes typically takes.

As you now understand, the modern American diet is grossly tipped toward refined carbohydrates such as sugar and white flour, both of which comprise most junk foods and rank high on the glycemic index. Your caveman body is totally befuddled by such foods. When you eat them, so much blood sugar gets poured into the bloodstream that your pancreas has to pump out insulin as if it were handling an emergency.

When you were 18, the superb efficiency of your body may have meant that you hardly noticed any symptoms resulting from this flood of blood sugar and resultant insulin overload. Later the symptoms pile on, just as for many of us the pounds do. You should already have taken the Blood-Sugar Symptom Test and be aware of any blood sugar-related symptoms you might have. The vast majority of overweight people on a high-carbohydrate diet display an extensive range of symptoms, the by-products of unstable blood-sugar levels.

A significant number of people who are overweight are insulin resistant. It may be that in most people, insulin resistance precedes hyperinsulinism, but either way, because insulin in not effective in doing its work, the pancreas reacts by pouring forth ever-increasing quantities of insulin. People who are both obese and pre-diabetic often have insulin levels some twenty times higher than the norm. The massive amounts of insulin cause blood sugar to drop to an inappropriately low level. The adrenaline the body releases to correct the blood-sugar level when it has fallen too low also produces many of those symptoms.

Blood sugar/insulin difficulties become aggravated over the years. When the insulin response exceeds normal levels—up to 20 units fasting; 100 units one hour after a standard glucose load for a GTT; and 60 units two hours later (the thresholds we use at my clinical practice)—it may be called *hyperinsulinism.* When obesity, high blood pressure, high triglycerides and unstable blood sugar are found, we can be certain that hyperinsulinism is the common denominator.

Ralph deFronzo, MD, one of the nation's leading diabetic specialists, removes the confusion that leads to a delayed diagnosis by pointing out that there are five stages of diabetes.[10] The first three stages precede the actual diagnosis of the illness. That is because conventional medicine does not routinely recommend the GTT with insulin levels, so people at risk are rarely found in the early stages of the disease. I truly believe that early diagnosis could bring the diabetes epidemic to a screeching halt, so much so that I fully intend my next project to be a definitive book on how we can do just that, and, as a result, eliminate diabetes.

The stages are:

Stage 1—Insulin Resistance (IR) only.
Stage 2—IR, plus hyperinsulinism (HI).
Stage 3—IR, HI, plus abnormalities in a GTT.
Stage 4—Type II diabetes, with high insulin levels.
Stage 5—Type II diabetes, with low insulin levels.

The road to diabetes is a continuum, with no sharp curves and no steep ascents. You just keep trudging along until you get there. You take the high-carbohydrate trail, and you may, after many years of unstable blood sugar and excessive insulin release that you are not even aware of, finally arrive at that unpleasant destination. Since insulin is the body's premier fat creator, most of us will have picked up significant extra pounds along the journey.

Then, after you actually become diabetic, your blood-sugar level ceases to oscillate; it is now consistently high. Massive insulin resistance has been preventing insulin from effectively doing its job (Stage 4), or your pancreas will have exhausted itself after years of overproduction and will not be able to make enough insulin (Stage 5). Either way, you've waited a little too long to make the diabetes go away, but not too long to achieve a useful level of control.

This means that if you have not dealt with pre-diabetes, you are now in full-blown diabetes. You're in trouble! Blood sugar that cannot be transported by insulin into your cells (and liver) now spills over into your urine, wasting vital energy (Stage 4). Once your insulin has been reduced to impotence (Stage 5) you start losing weight inexplicably. Heavy urination leads to constant thirst. Your body burns anything it can find to fuel its daily operations, putting you in a state of ketoacidosis. You now know that something is very wrong.

I took you through this scenario so you could attend to the early warnings long before *you* hit this juncture. To do that effectively, you need to know where you stand in the range of risk. A competent physician should be able to help you, but it is up to you to determine whether your doctor fits that definition.

An Important Test

You must remember how vigorously I encouraged you in Chapter 10 to have a GTT with insulin levels. This test demonstrates how your body reacts to receiving a fixed dose of glucose, the substance most readily convertible to blood sugar. Obviously, if your metabolism has been dealing with any of the assaults I've just described, the signs of such metabolic malfunction will be clearly evident on a GTT with insulin levels. I advocate that everyone take this test. However, if you are overweight, have diabetes in your family tree, have high blood pressure or high triglycerides, or have symptoms that appear when you are hungry and clear up when you eat, I must insist that you get a GTT.

Be sure to get a five-hour GTT with insulin levels. Here is what will happen: Blood will be drawn so that both your glucose and insulin levels can be determined. After an overnight fast (with no food in your system for twelve hours) the first blood will be drawn so that your fasting levels, or baseline glucose and baseline insulin, can be determined. You will then swallow the glucose solution, and the practitioner will plot out the schedule for drawing your blood over the next few hours. Blood will be drawn thirty minutes after you drink the glucose, again at sixty minutes and so on during the remainder of the test. Your glucose level is checked each time blood is drawn. Your insulin level is checked at the one-hour and two-hour marks only, because insulin levels peak within two hours after you drink the glucose solution.

How to Understand the Readings of a Glucose-Tolerance Test

Depending on your glucose level at baseline, you fall into one of three categories:

Range	Category
70–109 mg%	Normal
110–125 mg%	Impaired Glucose
126 mg% or higher	Diabetes

Beyond your baseline level of glucose, note that your peak glucose level measured within the first two hours after drinking the glucose solution should not exceed 160 mg%, and your nadir glucose (after two to four hours) should be between 60–90 mg%. The delta (the difference between the lowest and highest reading) should be 30–80 mg%.

If the delta is higher than 80 points and you are overweight, you most probably have hyperinsulinism. If the delta exceeds 100 points, the probability is very strong. If it exceeds 125 points, you unquestionably have hyperinsulinism.

The first number, your fasting—or baseline—glucose level, is a standard criterion for determining if you have diabetes. The ADA now regards 126 mg% as the number at which diabetes should be diagnosed, and considers 110 to 125 as a measure of impaired glucose tolerance (Stage 3). One to two hours after you drink the glucose solution, the highest normal reading is 160 mg%. Between 160 mg% and 200 mg% shows a clear indication of the progression to diabetes, and anything higher than 200 mg% indicates certain diabetes.

What Do Your Results Mean?

You add the first four glucose readings (at fasting, thirty-minute, one-hour and two-hour intervals) of your GTT together. This is called your glucose-tolerance sum. If the total (in mg%) is below 500, you are normal. If the total (in mg%) is above 800, you are considered diabetic.

The gray area, between 500 and 800 mg%, is called *impaired glucose tolerance*, and nearly half of the significantly obese fall into that area. The closer your total approaches the 800 mg% mark, the more probable it is that you will eventually be classified as a true Type II diabetic. But there is still some good news for you: Even if you are well into the diabetic range and are heavy, normalizing your weight by permanently controlling your carbohydrate intake can get you within—and keep you in—the normal range for life.

Clearly these lab results could show you whether you have diabetes, but more likely they will show whether you're on the road toward it. If you have a pre-diabetic finding and especially a weight problem, you have an urgent reason to follow a controlled carb eating plan—in other words, to do Atkins—with diligence.

What Is the Nutritional Answer to Diabetes?

Earlier in this chapter I pointed out that I have yet to see a study that showed that a high carbohydrate level in a diet is more helpful to diabetics than is Atkins. But I didn't tell you why. Even though the controlled carbohydrate approach was the standard diabetic therapy until 1950, the ADA abandoned it without ever doing a single test comparing it with a controlled carbohydrate eating plan that followed the Atkins approach.

Most studies that have been conducted were done with diets too high in carbohydrates to be consistent with the controlled carbohydrate approach that is Atkins.

Here is a small sample of the research done over the last seven or eight years. In the mid-1990s, researchers began to compare the effects of high monounsaturated-fat diets with the effects of high-carbohydrate diets in diabetic patients. A study by Dr. Abhimanyu Garg at the University of Texas Southwestern Medical Center showed that compared with the high-fat diet, the high-carbohydrate diet increased risk factors for heart disease—in the form of triglyceride levels and VLDL (very-low density lipoprotein) cholesterol levels—by twenty-four and twenty-three percent respectively. The high-carb diet also increased glucose and insulin levels by ten and twelve percent.[11] The numbers are less impressive than we usually see in our clinical practice because, in the high-fat diet studied, the level of carbohydrate consumed wasn't low enough to trigger lipolysis.

In a somewhat similar Australian study, researchers noted that "the currently recommended high-carbohydrate, low-fat diet" produces unfavorable effects on both glucose levels and cholesterol levels in people with mild and severe cases of diabetes.[12] By 1996, researchers at the University of Rochester in New York were testing a high-ketogenic, very low-calorie diet in comparison with a low-ketogenic, very low-calorie diet for diabetics. The high-ketogenic diet turned out to be considerably more effective in controlling blood-sugar levels.[13]

All these studies indicate the superiority of almost any form of carbohydrate control over regimens comprising up to fifty-five percent carbohydrate foods. In Chapter 27, I'm going to show you in detail how formidable the evidence has become to indicate that the control of carbohydrates is not only heart-safe but also heart-protective. This is crucial to the diabetes question, for diabetes is a major risk factor for heart disease. Indeed, it's fair to say that if you have diabetes, you may also have heart disease. The damage done to the cardiovascular system by high insulin levels over decades is tremendous. Combine that damage with the health problems of being overweight and having high blood pressure, and you have what has become a new buzzword in medicine: Syndrome X. Turn to Chapter 27 for a thorough discussion.

The study closest to evaluating the effects of a controlled carbohydrate approach such as Atkins to diabetes control was done at Sansum Medical Research Foundation. There, diabetic subjects were put on a dietary regimen that contained only twenty-five percent carbohydrate for eight weeks. They were then switched to a regimen that contained fifty-five percent carbohydrate for another eight weeks. On the controlled carbohydrate segment, the subjects' glucose values improved, their diastolic blood pressure went down and they lost weight. When they were placed on the high-carbohydrate segment, one of the indicators for diabetes got worse and none of the improvements seen on the controlled carbohydrate segment occurred.[14]

Appropriate research in which the level of carbohydrate intake results in lipolysis, as compared to a higher intake of carbohydrates, is finally in progress (although not yet published). When these studies are published, the evidence that the standard dietary approach to diabetes should be changed will undoubtedly be compelling. The fact that by controlling carbohydrate intake one controls glucose and insulin is hardly surprising. When you add to this the fact that a controlled carbohydrate nutritional approach is outstandingly effective at decreasing the risk factors for heart disease, the medical world needs only to exert common sense and a little courage to overturn the standard clinical approach that has been so harmful to so many people for so many decades.

Can the Course of Diabetes Be Reversed?

If you want to know why I am so certain that the comparison testing will prove Atkins to be so effective, it is because in our clinical practice we have treated over five thousand Type II diabetics. Of those taking insulin-stimulating drugs (sulfonylurea) we were able to get the vast majority off those drugs. And of Type II diabetics taking insulin, more than half were able to cease their injections. Here is one of thousands of exciting case histories.

Janet Drake credits doing Atkins with saving her life and her leg. Only 47 years old, she had been diabetic for seventeen years. When she got a blister on one toe, it turned into cellulitis, with a red line extending up her leg to her knee. One of the doctors at the hospital where she then worked as a nurse warned her that she might have to have the toe or the whole leg amputated if she didn't get her blood sugar down fast. Janet knew that her glucose level was around 290, far too high despite the fact that she gave herself insulin injections two or three times a day and had been prescribed both Glucophage and Glyburide, oral medications that help control diabetes.

The next day she went to see her eye doctor because she had been having headaches. He told her about an earlier edition of this book. Janet went directly to the mall, bought the book, came home, put her foot in a tub of Epsom salts and water and started to read.

"I started doing Atkins that day at lunch," she recalls. "By Friday my foot was healed, my headaches were gone and my blood sugar was down to 190. I dropped 16 pounds by the end of the second week. A week later my blood-sugar level was consistently 150 and my doctor took me off insulin. When I had lost 30 pounds, I was able to stop the oral medications as well."

Janet's numbers tell the whole story. Before doing Atkins, her blood pressure was a frightening 180/90. It now stands at 110/70. Her glucose level of 290 is now 114—well within the normal range. Her total cholesterol has gone down 30 points to 180. Her HDL (good cholesterol) is up 6 points. Her triglycerides are now normal. Her weight has fallen by 49 pounds. Janet has gone from being a diabetic woman who was probably entering the final decade of her life to being a fit and healthy woman who recently started her own wellness center to counsel people—particularly diabetics—about nutrition and its role in health. Many of her patients are sent to her by doctors who were as impressed by her experience as she was.

The Atkins Nutritional Approach is not only the most effective treatment for diabetes currently available in the United States, but it is also a certain way to put an end to the epidemic nature of the illness. Modesty may not be my strong suit, but I would be a traitor to mankind if I said anything else.

Nutrients for Correcting Imbalance

Doing Atkins is a crucial first step to dealing with glucose/insulin disorders, ranging from unstable blood sugar to full-blown diabetes. There are also many supplements that can assist. First and foremost is chromium, which is an essential part of the glucose-tolerance factor (GTF). This compound has such a profound effect on correcting sugar metabolism that I consider it essential for anyone who is overweight. Chromium (both chromium picolinate and chromium polynicotinate are effective forms for the assimiliation of this mineral) has an added benefit: It helps lower total cholesterol levels and raise HDL (good) cholesterol. The effective dose range of chromium is 200 to 1,000 mcg per day.

The second most important nutrient for individuals with blood-sugar/insulin imbalances is vanadium. Most research, done with vanadyl sulfate, has shown benefits in combating both insulin resistance and lack of insulin.[15–17] A typical dose range of vanadyl sulfate is 30 to 60 mg daily. Vanadyl is one of the very few nutrients that may place stress on the kidneys, so I always recommend that kidney function be monitored when using it.

The third most important mineral for blood-sugar disturbances is zinc.[18] Other minerals probably advantageous for diabetics include magnesium, manganese and selenium.

Vitamins, especially vitamin C and the B complex group, are also important for diabetics and should be a liberal part of the nutritional supplement plan. Other promising nutrients are Co-enzyme Q_{10}, alpha lipoic acid and the essential fatty acids GLA and EPA (fish oil). To learn more about these and other diabetic control supplements, you may refer to *Dr. Atkins' Vita-Nutrient Solution*.

As for the pharmaceutical approach, I have long opposed the unrestricted use of drugs such as insulin and the insulin-mimicking sulfonylurea type of oral anti-diabetes medications. Since the majority of Type II diabetics produce too much insulin, those drugs simply make matters worse. It is necessary to gradually lower the insulinlike medication dosage beginning the day carbohydrate intake is lowered to prevent abnormally low blood sugar so as to avoid a possible overdosage of the drug.

One currently available drug, however, has special merit, for it works to overcome insulin resistance, and to the extent that it's successful, lowers both blood-sugar and insulin levels. This is metformin, a pharmaceutical that also has positive effects for weight loss and can improve blood-lipid levels. If you have diabetes, you may want your doctor to consider it.

Prevention First

Of course, the best approach to diabetes is never to get it. The Atkins Nutritional Approach is your best insurance. The food you eat when you do Atkins is surprisingly close to what our primitive ancestors ate. Meat, fish and fowl; nuts, seeds and berries; vegetables and salad greens—Mr. and Mrs. Caveman would have recognized most of those things. They certainly wouldn't have known what to make of all those boxes filled with sugar, white flour and salt in the middle aisles of the supermarket—and neither does your bewildered body.

If you have been doing Atkins for several weeks, the symptoms you used to suffer and that you recorded on your Blood-Sugar Symptom Test should be alleviating or disappearing now. Your blood sugar is normalizing and so is your insulin level. Unless you came to this nutritional approach too late, you have escaped diabetes, and momentum in that direction has been halted. In my opinion, you've been darn lucky.

Grim Glycation

In the last twenty years, science has discovered that elevated blood-sugar levels appear to play a significant role in the aging process itself.

Naturally, diabetes provoked these investigations; it is startling how this disease's effects on organs and tissues mimic the effects of aging at an accelerated pace.

Why should high blood sugar damage the skin, the nerves, the eyes, the joints and the arteries?

Part of the answer appears to lie in glucose's propensity, as it floats around in your bloodstream, to attach itself to proteins. That attachment is called *glycation* (or *glycosylation*). Scientists at Rockefeller University and other research centers have demonstrated that the process leads to irreversible cross-links between adjacent protein molecules. Cross-linking significantly contributes to the stiffening and loss of elasticity found in aging tissues.

If you want to know whether your blood sugar is generally elevated, ask your doctor to order a Hemoglobin A1c (glycosylated hemoglobin) laboratory blood test for you. It measures your blood-glucose control over a six- to eight-week period.

Dr. Anthony Cerami, the pioneer in this field, gave the new protein structures formed from this chemical collision an appropriate name: Advanced Glycosylation End-products, or AGEs.[19] Collagen, the flexible connective tissue that holds your skeleton together, is one of the first proteins to be affected. As collagen's flexibility is destroyed, your skin sags and your organs stiffen. And your arteries also take a major hit, which explains in part the connection between diabetes and heart disease. AGEs attach themselves to LDL (bad) cholesterol, and these LDL molecules then become more oxidated, causing severe damage to any arterial surface to which they become attached.[20]

AGEs are truly a main contributor to aging; therefore, I advise you to keep your blood sugar well down in the normal range so those glycating sugar molecules don't gain a foothold on your body.

25

Yeast Reactions

What could produce a metabolic slowdown hazardous to your weight loss program? What could require you to temporarily drop cheese, mushrooms, vinegar and other fermented foods from Atkins? The answer to both questions is a one-cell fungus called *yeast*.

Candida albicans, the culprit's medical name, is one of four hundred species of indigenous organisms residing in the human intestinal tract. In other words, *Candida* is a normal part of us, and, in healthy competition with our other intestinal flora, it serves us well. *Candida*, however, is an opportunistic organism and at the first sign of stress it has a tendency to spread inappropriately. When it does, you have a yeast overgrowth—and, very often, yeast sensitivity. The symptoms are extremely common: One in three people may be subject to them.

This might seem far from the subject of this book, but since you're preparing a lifetime eating plan, yeast reactions will affect the foods you can eat. When people with a predisposition to yeast and mold problems show characteristic symptoms doing Atkins, it's very often because they have started eating cheese again after denying themselves this pleasure while on a low-fat diet. Thus I can't ignore this topic.

A Wild World of Symptoms

Nor would I want to ignore it. Many physicians treat yeast only in the form of oral thrush or vaginitis. But it can be a far more extensive problem. People with yeast can suffer from a long list of complaints (see "Yeast Symptoms" below). I've seen thousands of people who exhibited many of these symptoms and eventually found out that the large majority were affected by overgrowth of yeast.

Yeast Symptoms

- Do you suffer from gas, bloating, heartburn, constipation, diarrhea or abdominal cramps?
- Do you suffer from sinus headaches or nasal congestion?
- Do you have a runny nose or post-nasal drip?
- Do you often feel "spaced out" or "foggy"?
- Are you bothered by odors such as perfume or chemical fumes?
- Do you feel worse on damp, humid days?
- Are you often depressed, low or irritable?
- Do you crave sweets and certain other foods?
- Do you retain water or get puffy?
- Is your energy low, even when you get enough sleep?
- Do you get skin eruptions, hives, rashes and such?
- Do you get rectal or vaginal itching?
- Do you experience PMS, low sex drive, irregular menses or impotence?
- Do you suffer from recurrent vaginal, prostate or urinary symptoms?
- Are you susceptible to a variety of infections?

A Set of Provokers

Yeast overgrowth occurs most commonly in individuals exposed to one or more of the items on the following list:

- A diet high in sugar and refined carbohydrates.
- Repeated courses of antibiotics (a total of more than twenty weeks in a lifetime—or more than four times in one year—would make *Candida* overgrowth likely).
- Birth control pills, fertility drugs or other hormone therapies.
- Prednisone and other steroids.
- Chronic and excessive emotional stress.
- Any immune suppression condition.

With a list like this, it's hardly surprising that millions of Americans suffer from yeast overgrowth—and most of them don't realize they have it.

Clearly, you know my thoughts on sugar and carbohydrates. As for antibiotics, they can be life-saving but are often overprescribed. Birth control pills, HRT and steroids are drugs whose importance to your life I cannot judge without knowing you. If you do have a yeast overgrowth, you may have to make a difficult decision regarding these drugs. All alter the balance of beneficial bacteria in the intestine— which keeps *Candida* in check.

To understand how yeast can interfere with your success doing Atkins, you should hear about one of my patients. Laurie Yule was just 5 feet tall and weighed 134 pounds before doing Atkins. Her goal was to reach 118 pounds. She got down to 122 quite easily. Then after getting severe bronchitis, she was placed on antibiotics by another doctor. Laurie soon began to feel bloated and had difficulty losing any more weight. Essentially, the antibiotic had disturbed the balance of her intestinal flora and she was experiencing a yeast overgrowth, which had stalled her weight loss. Once I took Laurie off yeasty foods, the bloating vanished and she moved beyond her plateau to lose another four and a half pounds in a month.

What You Eat

I cannot point to published research that proves diet can actually *cause* yeast. But my clinical practice has convinced me that the wrong foods can and will encourage the continuation and expansion of a *Candida* overgrowth.

The worst offender is sugar. It is the major growth factor for yeast, and *Candida* patients are invariably warned to stay away from ice cream, candy, pastry, corn syrup, maple syrup, molasses, etc. If you're doing Atkins, there's certainly no possibility you're eating any of that. You'll also be avoiding the natural sugar in fruit juice and lactose in milk.

However, if you do have a yeast overgrowth, there is another category of food that you will need to avoid: yeast- and mold-containing foods. This includes cheese (except for mozzarella and cream cheese), vinegar, soy sauce and other fermented condiments, plus mushrooms, sauerkraut, sour cream, peanuts, cashews and pistachios (all nuts are subject to mold but these last two often contain the greatest amount). The list also includes smoked or cured foods, yeast-containing vitamins (make sure the label says they are yeast-free) and wine, beer and spirits.

The Allergic Connection

You may wonder why I mention mold. If you have allergies, be aware that yeast and mold are co-reactors—meaning that if you react to one you react to the other. Therefore, if you have a yeast problem, you should do your best to avoid not only yeast and mold in food but also places that harbor environmental mold. This includes office buildings with "sick building syndrome," your damp basement and bathrooms with poor ventilation.

If you are subject to hayfever or other seasonal allergies, such as those stemming from ragweed or pollen, your system is already stressed, making you more vulnerable to an even greater yeast sensitivity. One way to reduce mold exposure is (at certain times of year when mold counts are high) to cut out the yeast and mold in your diet. This may decrease the degree of symptoms you experience.

It is important to remember that yeast overgrowth stresses the immune system, undermining your total health. When it comes to weight loss, a yeast overgrowth, in combination with mold sensitivity, may lead to a suppressed metabolism. This may deplete your body of the energy it takes to burn fat. Of course, there may well be other causes that we haven't yet identified. I think that the complete explanation of what *Candida* overgrowth does to the human body is still well in the future. (For a few common annoyances, see "Did You Know These Conditions Are Yeast Related?" on page 337.) But I do know from my medical practice that this is a problem that can cripple weight loss efforts.

What Can You Do?

If you think you might have excessive yeast in your system, your best bet is, in addition to controlling your carbohydrate intake, to cut out all yeast- and mold-containing foods and wait to see if your symptoms clear up. Give it four to six weeks. If your symptoms do not improve, your problem may not be yeast alone. If you improve in some of the areas I mentioned earlier, then you may have identified a yeast problem or conceivably you may have removed a food to which you're allergic (see the next chapter). If you do improve after four to six weeks, cautiously reintroduce some of these foods to see if your symptoms return. It is possible that you may always have to consume yeast and mold foods in moderation.

Lingering symptoms that look yeast related are a reason to refrain from eating yeast- and mold-containing foods a while longer. If you live in a hot, humid climate, be aware that your house may contain a considerable quantity of mold. I've had patients benefit from installing a hepa-filter air purifier in their bedrooms so that they can decrease their allergy load of dust and mold spores, at least when they're asleep. A preferable solution would be to install such filters throughout the house, if your budget allows. (See "Good Housekeeping" on the opposite page for more ways to control mold in your home.)

Probiotics

Probiotics, or beneficial bacteria, are essential in dealing with yeast. If *Candida albicans* has overgrown, then repopulating your insides with good bacteria that compete with *Candida* is certain to be helpful. I recommend that you find a probiotic compound that contains not only *acidophilus*—which is a direct inhibitor of yeast overgrowth—but also such other beneficial bacteria as *bifidobacterium* and *bulgaricus*. Preparations that do not need to be refrigerated are preferable. The best products are sold in dark glass or plastic light-screening containers. Make sure that the probiotics are not in a milk base. It's worthwhile paying a bit extra to get a really good product.

Other nutrients that can have a favorable effect on a yeast overgrowth include caprylic or undecenylic acid, oil of oregano and olive leaf extract. For a full discussion of these and other natural remedies, I suggest you refer to *Dr. Atkins' Vita-Nutrient Solution*.

My final bit of advice is that you take yeast seriously. Like any allergy or infectious overload, it puts a great strain on the immune system. If it undercuts your weight loss program, it will also impair your relationship with Atkins, and that is certainly one relationship I hope to see you maintain for a lifetime.

Did You Know These Conditions Are Yeast Related?

- Athlete's foot
- A white-coated tongue
- Jock itch
- Fungal nail infections
- Ringworm
- Vaginitis

Good Housekeeping

To control the mold in your environment as much as possible, consider doing the following:

- Keep humidity low.
- Use an air conditioner or dehumidifier.
- Allow adequate ventilation.
- Avoid using humidiflers.
- Clean walls and add mold inhibitor to paint.
- Limit the number of houseplants (they carry pollen).
- Avoid foam rubber and feather pillows.
- Decrease dust exposure by minimizing the number of books and magazines.
- Vacuum carpets regularly, or, better yet, keep wood floors bare.
- Install an exhaust fan in each bathroom, or if this is not possible, be sure to open the window regularly.
- Vent the clothes dryer outdoors.

26

---ⅲ---

Food Intolerances:
Why We Each Require a Unique Diet

In the previous chapter you learned that eating foods containing yeast may be standing in the way of successfully overcoming your weight problem. Could there be other specific foods that will make you miserable and also block your best efforts? If your lifetime eating plan is to be a complete success, you have to restrict these foods. I've witnessed such a scenario hundreds, if not thousands, of times. This cautionary note to all of you is based on a simple, self-evident truth: Everyone is different.

An Individual Approach

A good nutritional plan can't be bought off the rack; it must be custom-fitted, like a made-to-order suit. Following a healthy controlled carbohydrate approach will do a lot for your body. Finding out what foods you can and can't handle will give you an Atkins nutritional approach that is truly yours alone.

Happily, the most common sources of food intolerance are generally found in foods I recommend you either avoid entirely or approach very cautiously. The foods to which people most commonly prove intolerant are grains, such as corn, wheat, rye and oats; soy, milk, cheese, brewer's and baker's yeast and eggs. The only three you might be eating during the Atkins weight loss phases are eggs, cheese and soy in the form of tofu and other products.

But those foods are hardly the end of the story. There are many others that produce intolerances. Strictly speaking, you could react badly to any food you eat. A few of the other very common allergy-causing foods are those in the night-shade family: white potato, tomato, eggplant, paprika, bell and other peppers and tobacco. Add to that sulfites, coffee, chocolate and citrus fruits. Among the acceptable foods when you do Atkins, shellfish, beef, chicken, onions, mush-rooms, pepper and other spices, plus artificial sweeteners, can also provoke a response.

Alas, the Foods You Love

Perhaps the first and most basic principle of a food intol-erance is this: The foods you eat the most often and love the best will frequently be part of your problem. Many Asians are allergic to rice, many Italians to wheat and many Mexi-cans to corn. This is yet another reason why many carbohy-drate addicts experience the elimination or reduction of nagging physical ills, from headaches to diarrhea, when they start to do Atkins.

Complicating the matter of food intolerances is that a siz-able proportion of us become addicted to the very foods to which we are intolerant. You will often see the term "al-lergy/addiction" used in papers by specialists in environ-mental medicine. It works like this: The foods that make us ill also make us feel better for a short time after we eat them. This is surely a classic addiction pattern: The sugar addict, the drug addict, the alcoholic all feel better when they get their fix. But before long, they all feel worse.

For each and every addicted person, there's the difficult

process of withdrawal. If you're allergic to a food that has become the mainstay of your diet, then you will suffer unpleasant withdrawal symptoms when you quit. The worse these symptoms are, the happier I am as a doctor. That's because the greater your addiction, the greater your physical improvement will be once you leap over the withdrawal hurdle. So put up with feeling worse for a few days. After you give up the food "you can't live without," you're almost certainly going to feel better. The general rule is that after two to five days withdrawal symptoms cease.

What Causes Food Intolerances?

No one knows for sure, but I believe many food intolerances are related to the weakening of the immune system, which may be a secondary result of such problems as yeast overgrowth. When this weakness becomes chronic, you may develop an allergy. Allergies, in turn, challenge the immune system, which can in turn suppress the metabolism, slowing down weight loss.

It is rare to find a person with a yeast overgrowth who doesn't also have some food intolerances, and the reverse is also true. The symptom list for food intolerance mimics the items found on both the "Blood-Sugar Symptom Test" (see pages 150–151) and in "Yeast Symptoms" (see page 332). In general, if there are symptoms from those lists that won't go away in spite of diligently adhering to a controlled carbohydrate eating plan, you have good reason to look for food intolerances.

Food intolerances are implicated in scores of other health disorders.[1] One impressive medical study was done in 1983 by five physicians at the Hospital for Sick Children in London. The researchers took eighty-eight children, all of whom had been having migraine headaches at least once a week for the previous six months, and put them on a rotation diet that strictly excluded many varieties of food for weeks at a time.

To the doctors' admitted astonishment, ninty-three percent of the children became headache-free once their intolerances were discovered and the foods were taken out of their diet. One child had reacted to twenty-four foods and was symptom-free when all those foods were withdrawn. Cow's milk, eggs, wheat, chocolate and oranges were all foods to which more than twenty children responded adversely. Of equal importance was the fact that the change of diet corrected (in a number of the children) such other disorders as abdominal pains, behavioral problems, epileptic seizures, asthma and eczema.[2]

Food intolerance, like most allergies, indicates that the body is being stressed.[3] Sometimes the problem can be a chronic inflammation of the mucous membranes of the bowel. When this happens, food is absorbed into the body through the intestinal wall before it is completely broken down. The situation is often called Leaky Gut Syndrome. Your body does not recognize food in this imperfectly digested form and treats it as an intruder. Your symptoms will be the result of your body's aggressive response.

How to Deal With the Problem

There are two basic approaches to addressing this problem: First, you must identify the foods to which you are reactive and determine the degree to which they affect you; second, you need to coddle your body.

Finding the foods that affect you is a little time consuming but not otherwise difficult. Your initial approach should be to exclude all yeast and mold foods. For many people this will do the trick. After all, controlling your intake of carbohydrate has already banished a significant percentage of the usual culprits.

If you suspect you have other remaining intolerances, keep a food diary for three weeks. Record every food you eat, and when you feel an unfavorable reaction after eating one or more, note that fact. If you alter the combination of foods at your meals, you will be able to isolate the offenders. Once you've found them, stop eating them for four to six weeks. Then reintroduce them slowly. Try once a week at first. Then twice a week. You will often discover that you can continue to eat these foods as long as you don't eat them too often.

If the foods you're allergic to are foods you shouldn't be eating in the first place, there would be no loss in excluding them forever. But since you're on a controlled carbohydrate plan, and you aren't eating anything that isn't healthy, you don't want to take something out of your nutritional regimen forever, if you don't have to.

What if you were to find you are intolerant of broccoli or legumes? In my experience, most people can reintroduce such foods—especially if they've also started a program of intelligent coddling. We all need coddling. Life is a handful, and you and I are a day older than we were yesterday. I can assure you that food intolerances, like yeast conditions, stress the metabolism and often arise because many other things have stressed the body in the first place.

By doing Atkins, you are taking the first and most critical step toward minimizing that which stresses your body. Having stable blood sugar—perhaps for the first time in years—is going to give your metabolism a much needed shot in the arm. Dealing with a food intolerance, if you have one, will be another great advance. But I'd also like you to coddle yourself by searching out your other stressors and seeing if you can't work out a strategy for minimizing them.

These stressors could be psychological or work related, and you will know them better than I. They could also be such very difficult physical conditions as intestinal parasites, heavy-metal body load or chronic viral problems. I can't treat you long distance, and, with problems like those, you almost certainly can't treat yourself. You might want to read up on some of these conditions, and, if any seem to apply to you, find a physician who practices complementary medicine.

I wouldn't want to be alarmist, but I would say this: If you follow Atkins conscientiously and you don't feel better than you have in many years, you should want to know why. Were I your doctor, I would certainly make sure you're not eating foods to which you're actually allergic. Sometimes very simple changes can produce enormous results.

KEY POINTS

- A sizeable portion of us becomes addicted to the very foods to which we are intolerant.
- Food intolerances cause blood-sugar instability and can complicate weight loss.
- The symptom list for food intolerance mimics the list found on both the "Blood-Sugar Symptom Test" and the "Yeast Symptoms" sidebar in this book.

TIPS:

- Keep a food diary to determine what foods cause unpleasant symptoms.
- Some people may tolerate a cooked food they can't tolerate raw.
- Learn to read food labels carefully. Sometimes wheat is listed as "gluten" on food labels; egg can be called "albumin."

Lifetime Protection for Your Heart

The sad story I am about to tell should be as familiar as the back of your hand once you have read the rest of this book: An individual with metabolic vulnerability to weight gain eats the sugar-filled, nutrient-impoverished diet of the Western world. It doesn't make him feel great, but he assumes his various complaints are a natural part of getting older. Pounds begin to gather; then a few more, then a lot. Now he acquires the risk factors that set him apart from most people who don't have a weight problem. Yes, *those* risk factors. Let's hear them one last time:

- Insulin levels that are far too high.
- Blood pressure that is rising, ever rising.
- Triglyceride levels that have gone absolutely ballistic.
- Total cholesterol that's through the roof.
- HDL that's down in the cellar.
- Blood sugar that's gone straight up.

What's next? There's an excellent chance that he is heading for diabetes. He—or she—is far from happy now and grasps for one variation or another of the typical carbohydrate-saturated American diet. Along the way, he may even push his dietary fat down to where the government says it should be. Victory? Well, no. That achievement won't prevent an eventual visit to the cardiac ward of the local hospital. After all, dietary fat never was the primary source of the problem.

That snapshot of a life depicts the lifestyle of many people, but it need not be yours. You now have the tools to correct and control your vulnerabilities—the risk factors for heart disease. You'll know *why* these tools work once you've read this chapter. You're doing a heart health plan that is precisely tailored to the needs of a person who's susceptible to weight gain. Atkins is the deliverance from your susceptibility.

What Didn't Happen, and Then What Did

Ten years ago, I used to smile somewhat painfully at the blasts of anger aimed at me by my attackers. They said I didn't respect the low-fat gospel. "Eating a controlled carbohydrate, high-fat diet was dangerous," they said. "Cholesterol would elevate wildly. Heart attacks would sprout like mushrooms in the rain."

Then something strange happened: The last decade of the twentieth century transformed everything. Millions of people did Atkins. Physicians could not ignore the fact that not only did these bold nutritional adventurers lose weight and feel fine, but they nearly always also showed improvements in their blood-lipid chemistries, which—when it comes to predicting the future—are the holy grails of medicine.

No doubt many doctors raised as disciples of the low-fat creed looked at those results and wondered: *Why? How does following Atkins do it? Why doesn't those people's cholesterol go up? Why do they seem so healthy? What does the guru of controlled carbohydrate eating know that I don't?*

Many of them—because doctors are an inquiring bunch—have since started to learn what I already knew. It never was a secret formula hidden away in a locked laboratory. The "secret" has been published repeatedly right out in the open in many of the world's most respected medical journals. The research that has made controlled carbohydrate nutrition so popular today was trotting along steadily in the 1970s and 1980s; by the late 1990s it was moving at a fast canter, and it is positively galloping now.

So here it is, and you should know it.

The Cluster Effect

What we are learning—careful readers will not be surprised—is that the risk factors for heart disease cluster together. A very prominent cluster is found among the overweight. A little over a decade ago, Norman Kaplan, MD, of the University of Texas's Southwestern Medical Center, dubbed four risk factors the "Deadly Quartet." These four—upper-body obesity, glucose intolerance, high triglyceride levels and hypertension—were consequences of a single cause.[1] That cause was our old friend, hyperinsulinism.

Kaplan made a diagram to make this relationship clear.

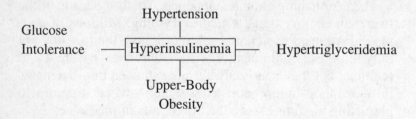

Kaplan had the good sense to notice the obvious. These conditions, he reasoned, occur in subjects with high insulin levels, and are likely to coexist in the same person. Thirty-nine million people in the United States are obese (twenty percent over ideal body weight)[2], and fifty million people are hypertensive.[3] Among the obese, hypertension is three times more common than among the non-obese. High triglyceride levels are twice as common among the obese than among the non-obese. The association is even stronger if one includes patients with upper-body obesity. The middle-aged man's paunch is related to metabolic factors that put him at risk for a heart attack.

If you still wonder how strong these associations are, listen to Albert Rocchini, MD, a medical scientist at the University of Minnesota. He writes: "It has been estimated that by the fifth decade of life, eighty-five percent of diabetic individuals are hypertensive and obese, eighty percent of obese subjects have abnormal glucose tolerance and are hypertensive, and sixty-seven percent of hypertensive subjects are both diabetic and obese."[4]

That's a pretty awe-inspiring—or more accurately—a terror-inducing cluster! Do you see yourself there? If you stand in one corner of the picture, the odds are good that—barring a nutritional change—you'll eventually occupy the whole image.

Kaplan's insight about the Deadly Quartet was probably dependent, as much modern thought about insulin is, on the work of Gerald Reaven, MD, of Stanford University. In his study of insulin, he has been pursuing the close connection between hyperinsulinism and cardiovascular risk factors with indefatigable zeal for over thirty years now. One piece of the puzzle that Reaven examined was that hypertension—which no serious medical theorist has ever questioned as a risk factor for both stroke and heart disease—is intimately related to hyperinsulinism. In 1989, in a major article titled "Hypertension as a Disease of Carbohydrate and Lipoprotein Metabolism," he wrote, "Patients with untreated hypertension have been shown to be resistant to insulin-stimulated glucose uptake and are both hyperinsulinemic and hypertriglyceridemic. . . ."[5] Let me translate into simpler language: If you have high blood pressure, you probably also have high insulin and triglyceride levels.

In 1988, Reaven noted a clustering of risk factors for coronary artery disease, all of which were associated with high insulin levels and increased insulin resistance.[6] These included hypertension, high triglyceride levels and decreased HDL cholesterol—the kind of cholesterol that has been found to be heart protective. Reaven has dubbed this collection of risk factors Syndrome X, and the name has stuck. Medical articles refer to the syndrome, and popular health books discuss it. It's a buzzword now, and since its implicit message is *be careful of excess carbohydrate intake*, I can only be happy about that.

Triglycerides and HDL

Meanwhile, responding in part to the urgent message of Syndrome X, medical research has moved beyond the limited predictive power of total cholesterol as an indicator of who will or will not get a heart attack. Many scientists now regard high triglycerides, high LDL (bad cholesterol) and low HDL (good cholesterol) as far more potent indicators. A series of papers coming out of Germany in the early 1990s indicated that men who had the combination of high triglycerides and low HDL were six times more likely to have heart attacks than men with the opposite propensities.[7]

A 1997 study led by Michael Gaziano, MD, of Harvard Medical School carried this relationship even further.[8] He investigated the heretofore ignored *ratio* of triglycerides to HDL and found it significant at all levels. A high ratio means a big number when triglycerides are divided by HDL level. People whose ratio was in the upper twenty-five percent were *sixteen times* more likely to have coronary trouble than were those in the lowest twenty-five percent. That predictive number is a striking finding for heart disease risk. William Castelli, MD, director of the famous Framingham study on heart disease, commented back in 1992, "The findings [from his study] swing the pendulum and show that high triglycerides can be a significant risk factor for some patients."[9]

A study published in *Circulation* by a research team in

Helsinki showed that those with high triglycerides plus an unfavorable LDL/HDL cholesterol ratio could lower their heart attack risk rate by seventy-one percent when these problems were corrected.[10]

An Insulin Assault

Now let's reverse this line of thought. High blood pressure, high triglycerides, low HDL and being overweight all turn out to be consistently associated with high insulin levels. If that's the case, then presumably high insulin itself should predict heart disease. Four significant studies done in Wales, Finland, France and Canada support this theory:

1. The Caerphilly, Wales, heart disease study, which observed 2,512 men aged 45 to 59, found a connection between fasting plasma insulin levels and heart disease that existed independently of other risk factors.[11]
2. In the Helsinki Policeman Study, 1,059 men aged 30 to 59 were tracked for five years. The data revealed that fatal (and nonfatal) heart attacks were most common in those who had the highest insulin levels.[12]
3. The Paris prospective study followed 7,246 men for an average of sixty-three months. Again coronary heart disease was proportionate to insulin levels, and the relationship was greater when the subjects were obese.[13]
4. A study done in Quebec was published in *The New England Journal of Medicine* in 1996. The researchers had collected blood samples from 2,103 men. Over five years, 114 of them had heart attacks. The insulin levels of these individuals were eighteen percent higher on average than those of the rest of the group.[14]

These large, statistically powerful epidemiological efforts really put insulin high on the list for concern when combined with the work done by Dr. Reaven. The total picture that he dubbed Syndrome X is becoming exceedingly clear. The abuse of highly refined and starchy carbohydrates in most regions of the modern world constitutes a long-term abuse of the body's insulin system. As that system begins to crumble, glucose intolerance and hyperinsulinism occur together with other damaging events. Arterial passageways are injured by insulin itself and by unhealthy cholesterol ratios. Arterial damage promotes high blood pressure, which will be even more aggravated in an overweight person. And let us not forget how being overweight, combined with blood-sugar and insulin imbalances, has resulted in an estimated twenty million diabetic Americans, plus an even greater number of pre-diabetic citizens.

For your heart health, it's vital to know about this combination of factors that cluster together to form Syndrome X. When you're doing Atkins, you're following the very nutritional approach that corrects this entire syndrome while nourishing yourself with healthy foods.

So heart disease isn't just about the other guy. No such luck. (And who would wish it on anyone?) If you've struggled with your weight, the message of this chapter is of crucial importance to *you*!

Better Late Than Never

My first forays into weight control began nearly forty years ago when I was a young cardiologist with a rapidly escalating weight problem and a strong desire to find a hunger-free way to deal with it. When I saw that my initial attempts worked, I was delighted. When I saw how much better I felt, I was happier still. But imagine my pleasure and astonishment when I began to comprehend the relationships between dietary carbohydrates and blood-sugar and insulin levels and the ability to eradicate the need for heart, high blood pressure and diabetes medications. In turn this led to my seeing how much healthier my patients were without the pharmaceuticals. This meant that I was working with a cutting-edge nutritional approach to helping overcome heart disease. This was unquestionably a defining moment in my life. What I now call the Atkins Nutritional Approach was born.

In the intervening decades, I have worked with thousands of heart patients, counseling them to abandon their junk food and eat the natural, healthy food that the Atkins plan emphasizes. And the results continue to support my thesis.

Occasionally, I need to convey the message twice. Fifteen years ago, Stanley Smith came to see me. At the age of 54, as he was helping a neighbor push his broken car into the garage, he had suddenly slumped to the pavement with chest pains. His wife knew a patient of mine who had achieved success doing Atkins, and the Smiths made an appointment with me soon after. Stan weighed 315 pounds and had extreme hyperinsulinism. After six months of doing Atkins, his weight was down to 225, his insulin had stabilized, his blood pressure medication was a thing of the past and, in his own words, "I felt 29 years old instead of 54."

Stan felt so good that in the next year or two he went back to his carb-laden ways. "I'd have a loaf of bread, half a gallon of ice cream and a quart of milk at one sitting," he recalls.

I didn't see Stan for more than a decade. In that time, his weight ratcheted back up to 310 and he returned to his blood pressure medication. Then about a year ago, on a flight from Florida to New York, he started having chest pain so severe that when the plane landed, he was rushed to a hospital. There he narrowly avoided a close encounter with the operating table. The next week I saw him in my office.

Talk about déjà vu. I put Stan back on the Atkins program he had abandoned ten years before and prescribed nutritional supplements. I also gave him adjunctive therapy including EECP (see "Twenty-First Century Diagnosis and Treatment" on pages 356–358). Naturally, I told him not to exert himself for a while. Stan tells the rest:

"Every week my wife drove me to my appointments with Dr. Atkins. For the first two weeks, I needed a wheelchair to get out of the car and to the elevator. By week three, I was able to push the wheelchair, using it to steady myself. Week four, I could shuffle up alone. By week five, I was able to drive in myself and walk from the parking garage. Over the next eight months I continued to see Dr. Atkins, and by then I was again leading a completely active, normal lifestyle.

"I'm still doing Atkins. I'm also painting the outside of my house, waxing my sedan and doing yard work. I go fishing and wear boots up to my knees to avoid the native stingrays. Those boots get heavy when they're wet, but carrying around the weight is no longer a problem. At age 69, I feel more robust and vigorous than I did when I was 50."

Stan got lucky. He could have died or suffered permanent, debilitating heart injury before he returned to the Atkins plan. He looks pretty good now; he has lost 60 pounds and is still losing 2 pounds a month, his lab work has improved astonishingly, and I am beginning to believe he will never go back to eating the way he ate before.

Go for the Whole Program, Friends!

What I've said in previous chapters almost makes my general position on your heart health self-explanatory. The vast majority of you will find that on a controlled carbohydrate regimen your recognized risk factors for present and future heart problems will steadily improve and will remain good as long as you follow this nutritional approach.

Your total cholesterol will probably go down—that's the most common result—but even if it doesn't or if it increases slightly, your ratio of HDL to LDL cholesterol is more likely to get better and your ratio of triglycerides to HDL is even more likely to do so. Those ratios are the real McCoy in terms of determining risk of a future coronary event. And if you were progressing toward diabetes—one of the great, grand gateways to heart disease—the improvements in your blood-sugar and insulin levels should astonish and delight your physician.

Half of all Americans still die of some form of heart disease.[15] I hope you will take the malign potential of this disease so seriously that you will eat the Atkins way for a lifetime—and follow the other components of nutritional supplementation and exercise. These two factors are not merely gaudy ribbons that I wave in front of you to impress you with the fact that the Atkins plan isn't only about weight loss.

I have stubbornly insisted throughout this book that you should exercise. It's good for your mood, good for your muscles, good for your energy level, especially good for your heart. Even if you've never exercised, it is not too late. (And you'll probably enjoy it once you start.)

The same advice applies to supplemental nutrients. Only the most hidebound physicians have failed to appreciate their value by now. I've written whole books promoting vitanutrients, so I'm sure you know I'm serious. Supplementation can have major positive effects on heart function. For supplements that address cardiovascular disease, see *Dr. Atkins' Vita-Nutrient Solution*.

The Atkins Nutritional Approach is like a three-legged stool, resting on a controlled carbohydrate way of eating, nutritional supplementation and exercise. Rely on just one or two of the legs, and the stool will not support you. But follow the whole plan faithfully, and you will be firmly positioned for ongoing cardiovascular health.

The Dangers of Trans Fats

Many Americans are still unaware that the most grossly harmful heart health trend of the last century was the gradual replacement of healthy natural fats and protein foods with foods such as margarine. They are constructed with hydrogenated and partially hydrogenated oils, which both contain fats never found in Nature. Called *trans fats*—meaning transformed from their natural state—they are manufactured by heating vegetable oils at a high temperature and bombarding them with hydrogen gas to form more stable oils. The process creates trans fats constructed of twisted, unnatural molecules that the body cannot process. The food industry sticks these hydrogenated and partially hydrogenated oils into virtually all baked goods and other junk food. The reasons are economic ones: Unlike butter, olive oil or other natural fats, trans fats have a shelf life from now to Doomsday.

Walter Willett, MD, chairman of the department of nutrition at the Harvard School of Public Health, was co-author of a 1993 report on the 85,095 women who were tracked in the Harvard Nurses Study. Women with a high intake of trans fats were one and a half times more likely to develop coronary heart disease than women with a low intake of these so-called "foods." Clearly this was not only due to the deleterious effects of eating junk food. For many people, the real shocker in this study was the statistic that women who ate the equivalent of four or more teaspoons of margarine per day had a sixty-six percent greater risk of heart disease than women who ate little or no margarine. But when it comes to butter, this vast study found no association between its consumption and the probability of contracting heart disease.[16]

Willett's report is shocking only if you have not had an eye on the research. Other scientists have demonstrated that while saturated fat (fats that are solid at room temperature, such as butter or the fat marbling a steak) has been reported to have both good and bad effects on cholesterol levels, the effects of trans-fatty acids are purely negative. Research also has shown that lipoprotein(a), one of the more damaging forms of chemical substances in cholesterol, consistently increases as a result of eating trans-fatty acids.[17]

This compelling research has had little effect on the packaged-food industry, but has, at least, persuaded some fast food chains to stop cooking with hydrogenated oils. And the FDA is considering mandating the listing of trans fats on the Nutrition Facts panel of food labels starting in 2002. Then, although foods would still contain these dangerous fats, you could choose to not purchase them. If enough consumers reject these foods, manufacturers would have to change their formulations.

In addition to boycotting junk foods, I strongly urge you to avoid cooking with margarine or vegetable shortening (that white, creamy stuff that comes in a can). Butter, olive oil and lard worked very well for our heart-healthy ancestors. Or if you find it difficult to resume eating saturated fat, use olive, canola or grape seed oil.

Food for Thought

If you've been saturated for years with old journalistic cliches about the terrors of fat and protein and the virtues of carbohydrate, try sinking your teeth into these crunchy little thought nuggets. Your physician might find them revealing as well.

- **1991:** A Canadian team substituted meat and dairy protein for carbohydrate in the diets of ten men and women with high cholesterol. The group lowered their total cholesterol by an average of six and a half percent, lowered their average triglycerides by twenty-three percent and raised their HDL cholesterol by an average of twelve percent.[18]
- **1996:** The INTERSALT, an international blood pressure study comparing 10,020 men and women in thirty-two countries, found that people with a dietary protein intake of thirty percent above the average had lower blood pressure than people with a lower intake of protein.[19]
- **1997:** In a twenty-year follow-up of 832 men tracked in the world-famous Framingham Heart Study, re-

searchers matched incidence of stroke (there were sixty-one in all) with dietary intake. The men with the highest intake of dietary fat had the fewest strokes; the men with the lowest had the most strokes.[20]

- **1998:** A Seattle team analyzed the data from seventeen different population-based studies that reported the relationship between triglycerides and heart disease. Men with higher triglycerides had a thirty-two percent increased risk of heart disease; women with higher levels had a seventy-six percent increased risk.[21]

- **1999:** The Harvard Nurses Study did a fourteen-year follow-up on 80,082 women, comparing incidence of heart disease. Findings show that the higher the intake of protein, the lower the risk of heart disease in this group of women who were 34 to 59 years old at the outset of the study.[22]

Twenty-First Century Diagnosis and Treatment

If you have any combination of risk factors, symptoms or family history that makes you wonder about your long-term prospects for heart disease, look for a physician with a really up-to-date approach. I recommend that he or she not only understand the conventional risk factors that we've talked about in this chapter, but also be familiar with other indicators of cardiac risk and test you for them. Note: These ranges are based on our forty years of clinical experience. The indicators include:

- **Total cholesterol:** Normal is considered 120 to 240 mg/dL; ideal is less than 200 mg/dL.
- **Low-density lipoprotein** (LDL) is the bad cholesterol. Normal levels range between 60 and 160 mg/dL; ideal is less than 130 mg/dL (the lower the better).
- **High-density lipoprotein** (HDL) is known as the

good cholesterol. Normal levels range between 35 and 80 mg/dL; ideal is more than 50 mg/dL (the higher the better).

- **Triglyceride** levels range normally between 30 and 160 mg/dL; ideal is less than 100 mg/dL (the lower the better).
- **HDL to total cholesterol ratio:** A measurement of your cardiovascular risk; average risk females: 4.4; average risk males: 4.9. (Ideal is to be below average. For both, the lower the better.)
- **Homocysteine** is a by-product of defective protein metabolism. An elevated level is a powerful marker for heart disease and stroke risk. High homocysteine levels also indicate a deficiency of folic acid, a B vitamin. (Homocysteine level can be reduced with the intake of vitamins B_6, B_{12}, and folic acid.) A normal level is 5 to 15 mmol/L; ideal is less than 8 mmol/L.
- **Lipoprotein(a)** is a high-risk component of LDL cholesterol. In the last ten years it has been recognized as a strong risk factor for heart disease and stroke. Elevated levels may indicate insufficient intake of vitamin C, which is needed to maintain healthy blood vessels. A normal level is below 20 mg/L; ideal is less than 15 mg/L.
- **C-reactive protein** is an antibody. It appears that some heart attack victims actually have an infectious component to their disease, which has little to do with following a sound dietary approach. The result is chronically inflamed blood vessels that are widely regarded as part of the atherosclerotic disease process. High levels of C-reactive protein have been found to increase the risk of heart disease by four and a half times.[23] The ideal is less than .55 mg/dL. Elevated levels would indicate you are at risk.

Therapy for heart disease goes far beyond bypass surgery and stents. I hope that your doctor will be open to the virtues of a less invasive but highly effective procedure called EECP.

Enhanced External Counter Pulsation (EECP). If you have diagnosed heart problems and a positive stress test, EECP is used to create collateral blood vessels supplying the heart muscle. Sometimes called a "natural bypass," EECP uses blood pressure cuffs applied to the patient's legs, which are repeatedly inflated and deflated, to force blood up from the legs to the heart. It has been government tested and funded, is currently being administered at four hundred sites in the United States and is reimbursed by health insurers. I strongly recommend it for our heart patients, so much so that the cardiology unit at The Atkins Center for Complementary Medicine provides about one hundred EECP treatments weekly.

The Lessons of History

Why did heart disease become a major problem when it did, and why is it so much more common in certain countries? Those questions have significant nutritional implications. Forty years ago, Ancel Keys, PhD, a prominent American nutritionist, argued that heart disease was common in countries that had high-fat diets. He drew a graph of seven nations to show that more fat meant more heart attacks.[24] This was an influential finding until a few years ago when George V. Mann, of Vanderbilt University, discovered that Keys had carefully selected those nations to make his case but suppressed the data in his preliminary report that showed exercise had a far more significant correlation with coronary heart disease risk than did any other factor.

A famous British nutritionist of the same period, Dr. John Yudkin, took a different view. He thought heart disease correlated with sugar consumption. It's difficult to isolate information on food habits in different nations.[25] Nearly all developed nations have high fat consumption *and* high sugar consumption. And nearly all underdeveloped nations have neither. Heart disease is high in the developed nations, but why?

One explanation proposed by T. L. Cleave, MD, in his book *Saccharine Disease: The Master Disease of Our Time*, argues that increases in the incidence of coronary artery disease could be traced to increases in refined carbohydrate intake.[26] He noted that diabetes, hypertension, ulcers, colitis and heart disease, to name a few, were all virtually nonexistent in primitive cultures until refined carbohydrates were introduced. He proposed his "Rule of Twenty Years," noting that it took that long after the introduction of refined carbohydrates before diabetes and heart disease began to appear.

Cleave's hypothesis does give one explanation of what brought about the heart disease epidemic in the industrialized world. Let's look at a couple of atypical western countries. In Iceland, heart disease (and diabetes) was almost unheard of until the 1930s, although the Icelanders ate a diet tremendously high in fat. In the early 1920s, however, refined carbohydrates and sugar arrived in the Icelandic diet, and true to Cleave's Rule of Twenty Years, the degenerative diseases arrived on schedule. Likewise, in the former Yugoslavia and in Poland, the development of high heart disease rates in the mid-twentieth century occurred in decades when the sugar rate was quadrupling and the animal-fat intake was falling.

I wouldn't regard these national trends as proof, but they certainly are suggestive. Suggestive also is the fact that in the Mediterranean countries fat consumption has been steadily increasing for the past thirty years and heart attack rates have been steadily falling.

The hypothesis that blames heart disease on high-fat diets is not on the ropes just yet, but it has taken some hard body blows, and is looking distinctly wobbly on its pins.

28

Spreading the Word

The great-granddaddy of the book you're holding in your hands right now became a bestseller way back in 1972. Between then and the original publication of *Dr. Atkins' New Diet Revolution* in 1992, controlled carbohydrate weight loss plans suffered a long, dry spell. Personally, that twenty-year stretch was deeply frustrating. I knew what this nutritional approach could do for overweight people as well as for people with blood-sugar imbalances. I had certainly witnessed permanent improvements in my patients' health and energy levels. Their successful weight loss efforts were equally real and long term. And the countless letters and phone calls I continue to receive from readers of my books confirm my clinical observations.

During those two decades—when low-fat diets were hawked as the only way to go, and high-carbohydrate foods such as pasta and bagels dominated the "health" landscape—the rate at which our population grew heavier and heavier accelerated. At the risk of sounding like a know-it-all, I have to tell you that this turn of events was no surprise to me. If you set out to become fat, there would be no better way to achieve it than with the diet of refined carbohydrates and starches so common in the United States.

Nowadays, the tide is flowing strongly in my direction. I only hope that it will continue long enough for the advantages of controlled carbohydrate eating to become apparent to tens of millions more people. Unfortunately, tides ebb and flow. There are still plenty of loyal followers of the low-fat doctrine who sincerely believe that their approach will ensure good health. And there are still plenty of food conglomerates committed to selling carb-laden junk food to Americans—and, increasingly, throughout the world.

What the Success of Atkins Will Mean

The best thing you can do for yourself and for the millions of others whose excess weight causes them both physical and psychological suffering is to tell them what has worked for you. Many people delude themselves about weight loss. They like to think they can lose those excess pounds by some magical burst of willpower, or they're waiting for the perfect drug to come along: Fen-Phen II without the deadly side effects. Your example can make them realize that instead of magic or drugs, the answer to lifetime weight control is simply a matter of a change in lifestyle.

The louder the voice of the controlled carbohydrate revolution, the better it will be for all of us. It's your voice that will help others understand that those boxes of junk food in the supermarket—and even in the health food store—proudly labeled "low fat" are to be avoided. It's your voice that will ensure that more and more restaurants, hotels and airlines offer controlled carbohydrate meal choices. It's your voice that will bring controlled carbohydrate products into your local supermarket so that you can enjoy ice cream made with controlled carb sweeteners, as well as tasty bread, muffins, bagels, chips and cookies—to name but a few. It is the people who have championed Atkins before you and raised their voices to create this demand that led to the development of such products which make doing Atkins easier than ever before. Now it's your turn to spread the word.

Calling All Revolutionaries

I dedicated my first book to the "diet revolutionaries" who would make a difference in the world. That term was then just a vague concept, but now it has real meaning. The world does indeed need diet revolutionaries, people who will organize into groups with meetings and membership rosters. While this book has focused on issues specific to your needs, you may want to get involved in the larger picture.

According to the most recent statistics from the Centers for Disease Control, childhood obesity has increased three-fold in the last twenty years.[1] Need I remind you that these are the same years in which carbohydrates have become a larger and larger component of the American diet and the period in which junk food has dominated the food industry? The point is that this is really more than just a matter of personal weight control and health objectives. It is a matter of concern for the health and longevity of our children and future generations.

I applaud the fact that so many Atkins followers have joined together in local groups and have participated in Internet chats and bulletin boards. Such activities not only enable people to help themselves, but also allow them to assist, motivate and inspire others to succeed in doing Atkins. In a more global way, those individuals who reach out to others by whatever means make the world understand that there are health choices far different from the ones that most people have been offered so far. If these words strike a responsive chord, you may wish to become a member of an existing group or help to form a new one.

If you are involved in groups that are determined to spread the word about the controlled carbohydrate lifestyle, I'd love for you to stay in touch. Keep me and my staff abreast of who you are, where you are based and what you are doing. See the end of this chapter for ways to get in touch with us. For those of you who are content merely to make your personal nutritional and weight loss experience as fulfilling and permanent as possible, the message is not very different: Keep in touch with us! Let us know of your progress, send us before-and-after pictures, tell us your story. My staff and I love to hear about experiences of men and women doing Atkins throughout the country and around the world.

There is no better way to stay in touch with all of our current activities and key nutritional and medical information updates than through our website (*www.atkinscenter.com*). As the number of people who visit our site has mushroomed well into the millions, we have recently upgraded it so that it offers the optimum in information and support to the growing contingent of Internet-savvy Atkins followers.

Visitors to our site will find a wealth of information about the Atkins Nutritional Approach, including:

- Atkins recipes and seasonal menus.
- A carb gram counter for printing out or for your Personal Digital Assistant (PDA).
- Tips from Atkins staff and others like you.
- Inspirational success stories.
- The latest scientific support of Atkins.
- Interaction with Atkins experts.
- Easy-to-find answers to your questions.
- Recent controlled carb news.
- A large selection of Atkins and other controlled carb products.
- An events calender of my upcoming media events and personal appearances.
- Updates on other Atkins events.
- Information on our increasingly popular "Atkins" cruises on Costa Cruise Lines NV.

On our website, you will also be able to sign up for a personalized area called "My Atkins," and participate in additional activities, including:

- A daily and weekly journal to track your progress and document your success.
- Customized controlled carb information and a "file cabinet" in which to save article clippings.
- Your own controlled carb recipe box.
- Shopping lists for Atkins recipes.
- The opportunity to inspire others by sharing your success story.
- Personal encouragement and reminders from Atkins.
- Simplified management of your product orders.
- Special discounts on Atkins products.

There are, of course, other ways in which you can make a difference in spreading the word about the value of a controlled carbohydrate approach to nutrition. Here are just a few ideas:

- Demonstrate with your purchasing power, demanding your local supermarkets and health food stores offer controlled carbohydrate alternatives.
- Let the restaurants you eat in know that you want more dishes that meet your needs—or take your business elsewhere.
- Lobby your elected officials at both the national and local level to pressure them into enacting appropriate food-labeling requirements.
- Contact your local school administration to pressure them to improve the nutritional quality of school lunches.
- Press for the removal of sugar-filled snacks and other junk food from school and office vending machines.
- Register with the National Weight Loss Registry at 1-800-606-NWLR so that a formal record of your weight loss success doing Atkins can be added to that database.

- Make your physician aware of your commitment to Atkins and share this book with him or her. Or if your doctor is unwilling to accept this approach to health and weight control, find another doctor who is.
- Support FAIM (Foundation for the Advancement of Innovative Medicine), an organization whose main purpose is to secure more health options—both procedures and nutrients—for you and the doctors who treat you. FAIM can be reached at the following address:
  FAIM
  P.O. Box 7016
  Albany, New York 12225-0016
- Contact the Dr. Robert C. Atkins Foundation to learn more about ongoing scientific research on controlled carbohydrate nutrition and to support its efforts in underwriting additional research through our website at *www.atkinscenter.com.*

These are just a few of the proactive steps you can take as an "Atkins revolutionary." We will continue to share ideas that can benefit from your involvement on our website and encourage you to do the same.

Here are the various ways to reach me:

1. Visit our website at *www.atkinscenter.com.*
2. Make an appointment for a telephone nutritional consultation or schedule an appointment to see us in person as a new patient (which includes a follow-up in person or via telephone) by calling 1-888-ATKINS-8.
3. Write or send photos to:
   Robert C. Atkins, MD
   Atkins Health and Medical Information Services
   150 East 50th Street
   New York, New York 10022

PART FIVE

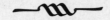

Food and Recipes

—⚭—

Food and Recipes to
Help You Do Atkins

It's important to get a healthy start on the day, and that means breakfast. There's plenty to choose from: omelettes, carbohydrate controlled cereals, smoothies, muffins, protein bars or quiches. The choice is yours and depends on which phase of Atkins you're doing and personal preference. I also encourage you to think "out of the breakfast box" and enjoy dinner leftovers, lunch salads and other protein-rich, controlled carb food in the mornings. At breakfast and throughout the day, variety is key, for both nutrition and taste.

For example, when making green salads, experiment with peppery greens such as arugula or watercress, crispy cabbages such as Savoy and Napa, or strong-tasting greens such as endive, escarole or dandelion. As you vary the greens, vary your salad dressings, too. Assertive greens stand up to strongly flavored dressings, such as blue cheese, where mild butter lettuces are best matched by soft tarragon vinaigrettes. Mixed green salads will depend on what is available in your local supermarket or greengrocer.

When it comes to the protein portion of your meal, keep entrées interesting by expanding your recipe repertoire and trying different condiments and spices. See the lists on pages 373–374 and 377-378 for some flavorful suggestions.

And be sure to make extra so that you have more on hand as fixings for future meals. Monday's dinner of roast pork can easily be turned into Wednesday's lunch of Chinese Moo-shoo pork (just mix in sautéed cabbage and sprouts, controlled carb hoisin sauce, and wrap the whole thing in a controlled carb tortilla). The variety principle applies to vegetables, too, especially since they will be your primary source of carbohydrate. Break away from the familiar broccoli, squash and cauliflower or you'll be bored in no time. Learn to love dark leafy greens: They are among the most nutritionally dense foods available, and when prepared well are delicious.

If you are not in the habit of eating soup, now is a good time to start. Hearty soups can be meals in themselves, and light soups or broths are great first courses: They will take the edge off your hunger and can prevent overeating. Eight soup recipes are included to add to your repertoire.

Finally, a word about sweets. Actually, two words: portion control. Some things are meant to be enjoyed in moderation, and controlled carbohydrate desserts, chocolate and sweets fall into that category. Even if an Atkins-acceptable cheesecake is only 5 grams of carbs per slice, that doesn't give you license to eat half a cake! If you need help controlling portions, freeze desserts and sweet treats in individual servings.

The Atkins Kitchen

Having the right foods in your pantry, freezer and fridge will help keep you on track as you learn to cook and eat the Atkins way. The following items will provide the basis for many a satisfying meal, so you'll never find yourself hungry and without any controlled carb options.

PANTRY

Savory Foods and Meal Builders

- Canned reduced-sodium beef, chicken and vegetable broths: These are the building blocks of soups, stews and gravies. Homemade is best, but feel free to rely on canned or dehydrated broths. In addition to cooking uses, a cup of broth before dinner or lunch helps fill you up.
- Boxed tomato sauce and chopped tomatoes: Check brands carefully! Some tomato sauces contain as little as 5 carbohydrate grams per half cup; others, made with sugar, can go as high as 10 grams.
- Tomato paste in tubes: Because its flavor is so concentrated, a little goes a long way. Tubes are more convenient than cans because you won't end up discarding unused portions that have gone bad.
- Sun-dried tomatoes in oil: A tablespoon or two adds depth of flavor to most vegetable dishes. Try mixing a teaspoon of chopped sun-dried tomatoes with mayonnaise and cream cheese to make a quick dip.
- Dried porcini mushrooms: Ounce for ounce, these morsels add more flavor to soups, stews and meat dishes than ingredients twice their weight. Don't throw away soaking water; strain and add to whatever dish you're preparing.
- Canned pumpkin: Loaded with beta-carotene, this ingredient contributes only 5 grams of carbohydrate per half cup.
- Wild rice: Cooked wild rice contains 16 digestible (remember, these are the only carbs that impact your blood-sugar levels) carbs per half cup. Use it in small amounts to add texture to soups or veggie side dishes.
- Cornmeal: Mixed with a controlled carbohydrate bake mix, cornmeal gives a pleasing crunch to fried foods.
- Marinated artichoke hearts: Eat as a snack or chop and add to salads.

- Roasted red peppers: Cut into strips and add to salads or chop finely and mix with mayonnaise or cream cheese for a dip or spread.
- Canned chilies: There's no quicker way to add zip to baked dishes or mild sauces.

Canned Protein

- Tuna: Tuna packed in oil has more flavor than tuna packed in water, but keep both on hand. For salads, tuna in water is milder and blends better with other ingredients. Tuna in oil (preferably olive oil) stands up well to cooked vegetables and stronger condiments, making it a better base for hot entrées.
- Salmon: Excellent in salads, and for making croquettes (see *www.atkinscenter.com* for recipe).
- Sardines: A terrific source of omega-3 fatty acids, they are inexpensive and versatile. If you find their flavor too assertive, try mackerel, which is less fishy-tasting than sardines and often moister than tuna packed in water.
- Black soybeans: Canned black soybeans contain only 4 grams of carbs per half cup, versus 8 to 15 for most other beans.
- White meat chicken: Handy in a pinch, especially when mixed with a flavorful mayonnaise and chopped green onions.

Baking Basics and Sweet Items

- Cocoa powder and unsweetened chocolate: Essential for homemade chocolate desserts and hot chocolate.
- Sugar substitute in granular form: For baking.
- Sugar substitute in packets: For sweetening beverages.
- Controlled carbohydrate sugar-free pancake syrup: Terrific not only to drizzle on waffles and pancakes, but to add a brown-sugar flavor to baked goods and glazes.
- Controlled carbohydrate bake mix: Made primarily from soy, this is an all-purpose substitute for wheat flour.

- Thicken Thin Not/Starch®: An excellent substitute for cornstarch, with a fraction of the carbs. A must-have item.
- Pure vanilla extract.
- Pure chocolate extract.
- Flavored citrus oils: Excellent substitutes for fruit juice flavor in cooking and baking.

Nuts, Seeds and Nut Butter Spreads

Nutritious, high in protein and healthy fats. Watch portions though: A small child's handful is about right for a snack.

- Macadamia nuts
- Almonds
- Walnuts
- Hazelnuts
- Pecans
- Sunflower seeds
- Pumpkin seeds

(Note: Store all nuts and seeds in the freezer—they'll stay fresher longer.)

- Macadamia or almond butter (unsweetened)
- Peanut butter (unsweetened)
- Sugar-free jams

Condiments

- Tabasco sauce
- Worcestershire sauce
- Reduced-sodium soy sauce
- Capers
- Mustard (countrystyle or Dijon)
- Sugar-free ketchup
- Sugar-free barbecue sauce
- Chipotle en adobo (smoked jalapeños in vinegar-tomato sauce): Hot, hot, hot—and tremendously flavorful.

- White horseradish: Use by itself or mix with mayo to make an instant sauce for beef.
- Pesto in a tube
- Canned or jarred anchovies: Essential for Caesar salads. In addition, a finely chopped half teaspoonful will add flavor to most sauces.

Oils and Vinegars

Vinegars vary in carbohydrates (1 to 3 grams per tablespoon), but since the amount you'll use is small, the difference is not that important. Avoid balsamic vinegar, which contains sugar. Aside from being a main ingredient in salad dressings, vinegar is also a great addition to many soups and even stir-fries (a splash added at the end of cooking will generally brighten up flavors).

- Safflower or peanut oil
- Olive oil
- Mayonnaise (regular, full-fat)
- White wine vinegar
- Red wine vinegar
- Tarragon vinegar

FREEZER

The following fruits and vegetables are all relatively low in carbohydrates:

- Chopped spinach
- Whole-leaf spinach
- Chopped kale
- Chopped collards
- Snow peas
- Green beans
- Artichoke hearts

- Asparagus spears
- Chopped broccoli
- Unsweetened strawberries
- Unsweetened blueberries
- Unsweetened raspberries
- Rhubarb

(Note: Buy frozen vegetables made without sauce and fruits not packed in syrup, which usually contains sugar.)

Plus:

- Frozen cooked shrimp
- Frozen crab meat (not artificial "crab product")

REFRIGERATOR

- **Cheese**: Try to keep several types in your refrigerator. Fresh cheeses include cottage cheese, ricotta, chèvre (soft goat cheese) and Italian mascarpone. They are terrific for breakfast or dessert with a sprinkling of chopped nuts and berries. Semi-soft cheeses such as Brie and Camembert are delicious with low-carb crackers and toasted protein bread. Firmer cheeses, such as Gruyère, Parmigiano-Reggiano, Dutch Gouda and cheddar can be eaten by themselves. Blue cheeses, such as French Roquefort, Italian Gorgonzola and American Maytag Blue pair well with salads and make wonderful sauces for vegetables. Buy cheese in small quantities and experiment until you find at least a half-dozen that you enjoy.
- **Cream/butter**: Add cream to your decaf coffee instead of milk for richer flavor and fewer carbs. Sweet butter is generally preferable to salted butter because it is purer in flavor. If you use butter for sautéing, mix it with a lit-

tle oil to increase the burn temperature. Or use ghee, which is clarified butter, instead. (The milk solids in butter that cause it to burn at low temperatures have been removed.)

- **Eggs**: Few foods are as versatile. Keep a half-dozen hard-boiled eggs on hand at all times. They are a perfect protein snack.
- **Protein**: Whether your protein preference is poultry, fish or red meat, try to make purchases as frequently as possible and prepare and cook the same day. Freezing is a convenient option, but shouldn't be a first choice. If you do freeze, be sure to wrap items carefully in freezer paper and defrost in the refrigerator. Most of us purchase whatever is on sale, but when your budget allows, experiment with more exotic quality proteins, such as buffalo, duck breasts and seasoned all-natural poultry sausages.
- **Cold cuts**: When possible, buy fresh from the deli counter (rather than prepackaged). Baked ham, smoked turkey, corned beef and sliced roast beef are great to have on hand for snacks and salad additions. Nitrate-free salami or pepperoni are good occasional treats, as is the more exotic Italian prosciutto de Parma.
- **Salad vegetables**: Buy only as much as you will consume in a five-day period. Wash and wrap greens as soon as you get home to preserve freshness and to ease salad preparation. Wash and spin-dry greens and pack in plastic bags with a sheet or two of paper towels in between to absorb excess moisture.
- **Vegetables/fruits**: Depending on the season, keep your vegetable bin filled with broccoli, green and yellow squash, cauliflower, eggplant, green beans, jicama, mushrooms, asparagus, bell peppers, green onions, leeks, spinach and broccoflower. When berry season rolls around, enjoy relatively low-carb strawberries, raspberries, blackberries and blueberries. Buy berries in

small quantities and use immediately—they don't keep well.

- **Tofu:** Firm tofu is great for stir-fries; and silken tofu is a high-protein, controlled carb substitute for bananas in smoothies. Pressed, seasoned tofu makes a quick entrée when sautéed with vegetables and can provide the protein in a luncheon salad.

Herbs and Spices

To assure freshness and flavor, buy spices in the smallest jars sold and, at home, sniff before using. Discard any spice that has a musty smell. To substitute dried herbs for fresh, the general rule is that one tablespoon fresh equals one teaspoon dried. Most spices contain less than 1 gram of carbohydrate per teaspoon; herbs, less than 1 gram of carbohydrate per two tablespoons. Make sure spice blends contain no sugar.

Suggested Spices
- Cajun spice blend
- Chili powder
- Chinese 5-spice powder (This mix of cinnamon, star anise, cloves, fennel seeds and pepper gives Chinese food its distinctive flavor.)
- Cinnamon
- Cumin
- Curry powder
- Garlic powder
- Marjoram (a more delicate version of oregano)
- Nutmeg
- Oregano
- Red pepper flakes
- Rosemary
- Sage
- Tarragon
- Thyme

Fresh Herbs

Fresh herbs liven up the flavor of most savory dishes.

- Basil
- Cilantro
- Chives
- Green onions
- Parsley: Flat-leaf, also known as Italian, is more flavorful than curly parsley.
- Ginger: A root, not an herb; buy as needed for recipes. Nothing beats the flavor and fragrance of freshly grated ginger.

Making the Change

Your meals will be built around protein, healthy fats and nutrient-dense carbohydrates, primarily in the form of vegetables. Most entrées fit easily into doing Atkins, with small modifications (see "Food Substitutions" below). As you approach your goal weight, your choice of foods will expand. When you reach Lifetime Maintenance, you will be able to eat most foods—with the exception of refined sugar, white flour and hydrogenated oils.

Food Substitutions

Instead of:	Substitute:
Refined flour	Equal parts controlled carb bake mix and finely ground nuts
Low-fat yogurt	Sour cream
Milk	Half 'n' half or heavy cream mixed with water
Yellow onions	Green onions (scallions) or leeks
Cornstarch	Thicken Thin Not/Starch®
Aspartame (Equal®, NutraSweet®)	Splenda®
Red salsa	Green salsa

Instead of:	Substitute:
Chips	Salted popped soy nuts or soy chips, pumpkin seeds\
Peaches (for cooking)	Rhubarb
Black or kidney beans	Black soybeans (canned)
Sliced bread	Controlled carb bread
Pasta	Spaghetti squash or controlled carb pasta
Margarine	Butter or ghee
Corn oil	Olive, safflower or peanut oil (cold-pressed)
Peanut butter	Sugar-free peanut butter
White rice	Wild rice
Potatoes	Cauliflower
Bananas (for smoothies)	Silken tofu

Pointers for Success

- Read labels carefully. Most commercial ketchups, barbecue sauces and other tomato-based sauces contain sugar or corn syrup and are high in carbohydrates.
- Shop in your local health food store, where you are likely to find products and brands not available in most supermarkets, including a wide range of sugar- and wheat-free baked goods.
- Make salad dressings at home. Not only are they tastier, but homemade dressings are sugar-free and contain all natural ingredients.
- Keep bottled lemon juice tucked away on a refrigerator shelf; lemons can be expensive and spoil quickly. A splash of bottled juice mixed with a packet of sugar substitute and some ice water makes instant lemonade.
- It is important to add variety to your diet through condiments, spices and new recipes.
- Butter and cream sauces should be occasional treats, not a daily part of your eating plan.

Sample Menus for the Four Phases of the Atkins Nutritional Approach

TYPICAL INDUCTION MENU

Breakfast:
Southwestern omelette with tomato, avocado and ham

Lunch:
Caesar Salad* with grilled chicken

Dinner:
Steak au Poivre*
Roasted asparagus
Mixed green salad with lemon vinaigrette
Gelatin dessert made with sucralose

Snack:
Celery stuffed with herb cream cheese

—⁓—

TYPICAL ONGOING WEIGHT LOSS MENU

Breakfast:
Two poached eggs over Fried Green Tomatoes*
Two strips of nitrate-free bacon

Lunch:
Grilled turkey burger with pepper Jack cheese and green salsa
Creamy Red Cabbage Slaw*

Dinner:
Cajun Pork Chops*
Sautéed Kale with Red Pepper*
Spicy Country Cornbread*

Snack:
Spiced pumpkin seeds

Recipe follows

TYPICAL PRE-MAINTENANCE MENU

Breakfast:
Belgian Waffles* with pancake syrup and strawberries

Lunch:
Almost Black Bean Soup*
Ham and cheese-filled tortilla

Dinner:
Roasted Salmon with Macadamia-Cilantro Crust*
Cauliflower-Leek Purée*
Arugula, radish and cucumber salad
Ginger Flan* with blueberries

Snack:
Two Chocolate Truffles*

—⁓—

TYPICAL LIFETIME MAINTENANCE MENU

Breakfast:
Two slices Cranberry-Orange Loaf*
Ricotta cheese omelette

Lunch:
Vegetable soup
Crab salad over mixed greens

Dinner:
Herbed-Roast Chicken with Lemon*
Wild rice with mushrooms
Bibb lettuce and watercress salad with French dressing
Molten Chocolate Cakes*

Snack:
Cantaloupe with lime juice

*Recipe follows

The Recipes

The recipes included here are all new to this edition of this book. Each one of them was carefully developed by our staff of nutritionists and reviewed by our food editor. Of course, we had them kitchen-tested and tasted.

Even so, we just didn't have enough space in this book to include all the outstanding recipes we have developed. Many more appear on our website at *www.atkinscenter.com*, as does an interactive area that allows you to submit your own recipe to us. Maybe we will find some that—with your permission—we will print in the next edition of this book!

Before you review the recipes that follow, let me remind you about the discussion in Chapter 8 about the carbs that count. Not all carbohydrates are created equal, and in fact there are certain types of carbs—specifically fiber—that don't affect blood-sugar levels. So when doing Atkins you can subtract the grams of fiber from the total carbohydrate count to get "the carbs that count when doing Atkins."

ENTRÉES (pages 414–455)

SEAFOOD (pages 414–422)
    Striped Bass with Fennel and Tomatoes
    Roasted Salmon with Macadamia-Cilantro Crust
    Maple Mustard-Glazed Salmon
    Atkins Crabcakes
    Shrimp and Feta Stew
    Asian Tuna Kabobs
    Pesto Scallops with Cherry Tomatoes
    Broiled Lobster with Garlic Oil
    Calamari with Basil and Lime

LAMB/VEAL (pages 423–428)
    Roast Leg of Lamb
    Lamb Chops with Mustard Sauce
    Veal Stew with Mushrooms and Smoked Provolone
    Veal Scallops with White Wine Caper Sauce
    Osso Buco

POULTRY (pages 429–438)
    Cheddar Chicken Roll-Ups
    Herbed-Roast Chicken with Lemon
    Sautéed Chicken Sausages with Red Peppers
    Duck Breasts with Blackberry-Wine Sauce
    Turkey Cutlets with Green Peppercorn Sauce
    Turkey Meatloaf with Pesto and Spinach
    Crispy Parmesan Chicken Legs
    Chicken Cacciatore
    Chicken Pot Pie

PORK (pages 439–444)
    Cajun Pork Chops
    Ginger Grilled Pork Tenderloin
    Kielbasa with Caraway Kraut
    Pork and Vegetable Ragout
    Shredded Pork Quesadillas

BEEF (pages 445–451)
Steak au Poivre
Italian Meatballs in Tomato Sauce
Two-Step Chili
Burgundy Beef Stew
Garlic-Rosemary Beef Rib Roast
Korean-Style Skirt Steak

VEGETARIAN (pages 452–455)
Stuffed Peppers
Eggplant Parmesan
Tofu Stir-Fry Over Baby Spinach

VEGETABLES (pages 456–468)

Artichoke and Cheese Squares
Fried Green Tomatoes
Sautéed Kale with Red Pepper
Broccoli with Toasted Pine Nuts and Garlic
Swiss Chard Gratin
Baked Spaghetti Squash with Garlic-Sage Cream
Sesame Snow Peas
Cauliflower-Leek Purée
Roasted Green Beans
Ratatouille Bake
Mixed Greens with Tomatoes and Ginger
Swedish Red Cabbage
Oven-Fried Turnips

SALADS AND DRESSINGS (pages 469–481)

Blue Cheese Dressing
Green Goddess Dressing
Ginger, Soy and Sesame Sauce
Classic Vinaigrette (and Variations)
Creamy Italian Dressing
Chicken Salad

Creamy Red Cabbage Slaw
Jicama Pico de Gallo
Radicchio, Gorgonzola and Bacon Salad
Cobb Salad
Greek Spinach Salad
Cauliflower "Potato" Salad
Caesar Salad
Asian Cucumber Salad
Crab and Avocado Salad

DESSERTS/SWEETS (pages 482–491)

Ginger Flan
Molten Chocolate Cakes
Chocolate Truffles
Italian Almond Cream
Banana Custard with Candied Pecans
Sunshine Cake
Chocolate Hazelnut Biscotti
Pumpkin Pie with Nut Crust
Coconut Macaroons

Breakfast, Brunch and Bread

Basque Eggs

The trick to this dish is to reduce the tomato mixture to a thick sauce that won't "break" and liquefy when added to the eggs. If you've never made scrambled eggs this way before, you're in for a treat. Steady, slow cooking turns them incredibly creamy.

Prep time: 30 minutes
Cook time: 12 minutes
6 servings

3 tablespoons olive oil
1 medium onion, sliced
6 garlic cloves, chopped
2 medium green or red bell peppers, roasted
2 plum tomatoes, chopped
¼ teaspoon cayenne pepper
salt and pepper
12 eggs
¾ stick (6 tablespoons) butter
⅓ cup thinly sliced fresh basil
6 ounces thinly sliced ham

1. Heat oil in large heavy skillet over medium heat. Sauté onion 5 minutes, until softened; add garlic and cook 1 minute more. Add roasted peppers, tomatoes and cayenne. Cover and cook 10 minutes, until vegetables are very soft, stirring occasionally. Uncover and simmer over medium heat until sauce is thick, about 10 minutes, stirring often. Season to taste with salt and pepper. (Mixture can be made up to 2 days ahead and reheated.)

2. In large bowl, beat eggs until blended. In large non-stick skillet, melt butter over low heat. Add eggs and basil. Cook, stirring constantly with rubber spatula, 12 minutes, until soft curds form and eggs are barely set. Add pepper mixture and ham; stir just until mixed.

Total carbohydrates per serving: 7 grams (count only 6 "digestible" carbs when doing Atkins); protein: 19 grams; fat: 30 grams; calories: 371

Belgian Waffles

Belgian-style waffles are thicker than standard waffles, but this recipe can be prepared in either type of waffle maker. Waffles can be made ahead and frozen individually for quick weekday breakfasts.

Prep and cook time: 10 minutes per batch
8 servings

1 cup Atkins™ Bake Mix
1 tablespoon baking powder
3 packets sugar substitute
1 teaspoon salt
¼ cup heavy cream
3 eggs
1 teaspoon vanilla extract
¼ cup ice water

1. Heat waffle iron. Whisk together bake mix, baking powder, sugar substitute and salt. Add cream, eggs, vanilla extract and ice water. Batter will be stiff; add a little more water if necessary, 1 tablespoon at a time, until batter spreads easily.
2. Place approximately 3 tablespoons of batter in center of waffle iron. Cook according to manufacturer's directions until crisp and dark golden brown. Repeat with remaining batter.

Total carbohydrates per serving: 4 grams (count only 3 "digestible" carbs when doing Atkins); protein: 3 grams; fat: 6 grams; calories: 112

Blueberry Clafoutis

Clafoutis is a French baked pudding dessert and is usually made with cherries. We've substituted lower-carb blueberries for the cherries. This would make a fine addition to a brunch menu.

Prep time: 10 minutes
Bake time: 45 minutes
6 servings

4 tablespoons butter
4 tablespoons Atkins™ Bake Mix, divided
3 packets sugar substitute
pinch salt
⅔ cup heavy cream
⅓ cup water
3 large eggs
½ teaspoon almond extract
1 cup fresh or frozen blueberries, patted dry

1. Heat oven to 350°F. Place butter in a 10-inch tart pan or 9-inch pie plate. Place in oven to melt. Remove from oven.

2. In medium bowl combine 3 tablespoons bake mix, sugar substitute and salt. In small bowl whisk cream, water, eggs and almond extract. Pour in melted butter, leaving enough to coat tart pan. Pour liquid mixture into dry ingredients; mix until smooth.
3. Toss blueberries with remaining 1 tablespoon bake mix; gently fold into batter. Pour into prepared pan. Bake 45 minutes or until golden and puffy. Serve immediately.

Total carbohydrates per serving: 6 grams (count only 5 "digestible" carbs when doing Atkins); protein: 4 grams; fat: 21 grams; calories: 234

California Breakfast Burritos

These tasty burritos are perfect for brunch. For variety, add ½ cup chopped cooked ham or smoked turkey to the filling.

Prep time: 20 minutes
Cook time: 5 minutes
4 servings

4 controlled carb flour tortillas
1 tablespoon peanut or canola oil
3 green onions, chopped
1 can (4 ounces) green chiles, drained, patted dry and chopped
1 small tomato, diced
½ teaspoon salt
¼ teaspoon black pepper
8 eggs, beaten
pinch cayenne pepper
2 tablespoons chopped cilantro
¼ cup green salsa
½ cup grated cheddar cheese

1. Heat oven to 325°F. Wrap tortillas in foil and heat in oven 5 to 10 minutes.
2. In a medium nonstick skillet, heat oil over medium-high heat. Add green onions, chiles, tomato, salt and pepper; sauté 3 minutes. Push mixture to side of pan.
3. Add eggs and cayenne to skillet. Cook 1 to 2 minutes, stirring occasionally with rubber spatula, until soft, creamy curds form. Stir vegetable mixture into eggs.
4. Divide mixture among warm tortillas, sprinkle with cilantro, a tablespoon of salsa and 2 tablespoons cheese. Roll up tortillas.

Total carbohydrates per serving: 16 grams (count only 6 "digestible" carbs when doing Atkins); protein: 21 grams; fat: 21 grams; calories: 317

Cranberry-Orange Loaf

Toasted, ground nuts give this loaf extra flavor. For variety, you may substitute 2 teaspoons cinnamon for the orange rind.

Prep time: 20 minutes
Bake time: 50 minutes
Yield: 20 slices

1 cup fresh or frozen cranberries, thawed
1¼ cups Atkins™ Bake Mix
½ cup walnuts, toasted and ground
16 packets sugar substitute
1 teaspoon baking soda
½ teaspoon salt
1 stick (8 tablespoons) butter, softened
2 tablespoons sour cream
2 eggs
1 tablespoon grated fresh orange rind

1 teaspoon vanilla extract
2 egg whites

1. Heat oven to 350°F. Grease a 9-inch-by-5-inch loaf pan; set aside. Coarsely chop cranberries; set aside. In a large bowl, whisk bake mix, walnuts, sugar substitute, baking soda and salt until combined.
2. In a medium bowl, with an electric mixer on medium, beat butter 3 minutes until fluffy. Beat in sour cream, eggs, orange rind and vanilla extract. Fold in cranberries.
3. Beat bake mix mixture into butter mixture. In a separate bowl, beat egg whites until stiff, but not dry. In three additions, fold egg whites into batter.
4. Spoon batter into prepared pan. Bake 50 to 55 minutes or until a toothpick inserted in center comes out clean. Cool on wire rack. Cut loaf into thin slices.

Total carbohydrates per serving: 4 grams (count only 2.5 "digestible" carbs when doing Atkins); protein: 2 grams; fat: 8 grams; calories: 106

Crustless Quiche

So tasty, you'll never miss the crust!

Prep and cook time: 20 minutes
Bake time: 1 hour 15 minutes
8 servings

4 ounces nitrate-free bacon
½ yellow onion, thinly sliced
6 eggs
¾ cup heavy cream
2 boxes (10 ounces each) frozen chopped broccoli or spinach, thawed and squeezed dry
½ pound Gruyère cheese, shredded

½ teaspoon salt
¼ teaspoon pepper

1. Heat oven to 350°F. Butter a 10-inch tart pan or 9-inch deep pie plate.
2. In a large skillet over medium heat, cook bacon until crisp. Drain on paper towels; coarsely chop.
3. Remove all but 1 tablespoon bacon drippings from skillet. Add onion and cook 5 minutes, until softened but not brown. In a large bowl, combine eggs, cream, broccoli, cheese, salt and pepper. Stir in bacon and onion.
4. Pour mixture into prepared pan. Bake 1 hour and 15 minutes (tenting with foil, if necessary, to prevent over-browning) or until a knife inserted in center comes out clean. Cool 5 minutes before cutting into wedges.

Total carbohydrates per serving: 6.5 grams (count only 4 "digestible" carbs when doing Atkins); protein: 17 grams; fat: 27 grams; calories: 329

Mushroom and Swiss Cheese Omelettes

White mushrooms are fine in this recipe, but more exotic varieties, such as morel, shiitake or cremini, would be even tastier.

Prep time: 15 minutes
Cook time: 10 minutes
2 servings

2 tablespoons butter, divided
4 ounces mushrooms, sliced
¼ cup finely chopped red onion
2 cloves garlic, chopped
½ teaspoon dried thyme
½ teaspoon grainy Dijon mustard
salt and pepper

6 eggs
¼ cup chopped fresh parsley
¾ cup shredded Swiss cheese

1. Melt 1 tablespoon butter in a small nonstick skillet over medium-high heat; sauté mushrooms, onion, garlic and thyme 4 minutes, until tender. Stir in mustard and season with salt and pepper; transfer to a bowl.
2. In medium bowl, whisk eggs, parsley and ¼ cup cheese until mixed. In skillet, melt ½ tablespoon butter over medium-high heat and add half the egg mixture. Tilt skillet or spread eggs to cover bottom. Cook until set, lifting omelette with rubber spatula to allow uncooked egg to flow underneath.
3. Top omelette with ¼ cup shredded cheese and half the mushroom mixture. Fold up filled portion over center of omelette and roll it out onto serving plate. Repeat with remaining butter, egg mixture, cheese and mushroom mixture.

Total carbohydrates per serving: 19 grams (count only 14.5 "digestible" carbs when doing Atkins); protein: 39 grams; fat: 42 grams; calories: 611

Pancakes With Ricotta-Apricot Filling

The cheesecake-inspired filling in the pancakes is not too sweet to serve for brunch. Once you've mastered making the pancakes, vary the flavor of the filling by trying different fruit spreads.

Prep time: 15 minutes
Cook time: 20 minutes
4 servings

3 eggs
3 tablespoons Atkins™ Bake Mix

¼ teaspoon salt
⅓ cup heavy cream
¾ cup ricotta cheese
¼ cup sugar-free apricot jam
1 packet sugar substitute
1½ tablespoons butter

1. In a medium bowl, whisk eggs, bake mix and salt until smooth. Gradually whisk in cream. Let stand 5 minutes.
2. Press ricotta through a fine sieve into a small bowl. Mix in jam and sugar substitute.
3. Melt butter in a small nonstick skillet over medium heat. Pour in 2 tablespoons batter and tilt skillet to coat bottom. Cook until golden on bottom; turn over. Cook 1 minute more. Transfer to a plate. Repeat with remaining batter.
4. Spread pancakes with ricotta mixture, roll up and serve.

Total carbohydrates per serving: 3 grams (count only 3 "digestible" carbs when doing Atkins); protein: 3 grams; fat: 5.5 grams; calories: 76

Spicy Country Cornbread

This quick cornbread can be ready in less than 30 minutes from the get-go. If you wish, stir half a cup of finely diced extra sharp cheddar cheese into the dry ingredients.

Prep time: 10 minutes
Bake time: 25 minutes
8 servings

4 tablespoons butter
1½ cups Atkins™ Bake Mix
½ cup yellow cornmeal
3 packets sugar substitute

2 teaspoons baking powder
1 teaspoon crushed red pepper flakes
½ cup heavy cream
½ cup water
2 eggs

1. Heat oven to 425°F. Place butter in an 8-inch square baking pan. Place in oven to melt. Remove from oven. In a large bowl, mix bake mix, cornmeal, sugar substitute, baking powder and red pepper flakes.
2. In a small bowl, mix cream, water and eggs. Add most of the butter, leaving enough to coat pan. Mix liquid mixture into dry ingredients. Blend just to combine. Transfer batter to prepared pan.
3. Bake 25 minutes, until golden brown. Cool 5 to 10 minutes in pan before cutting into squares.

Total carbohydrates per serving: 13.5 grams (count only 11 "digestible" carbs when doing Atkins); protein: 16 grams; fat: 15 grams; calories: 253

Strawberry Smoothie

Silken or soft tofu makes breakfast smoothies protein-rich and creamy, and it is very mild tasting. Vary the flavor of your smoothies by using different berries. This is for later phases of Atkins, because it is relatively high in carbs.

Prep time: 5 minutes
4 servings

1 cup soft tofu
2 cups frozen unsweetened strawberries, slightly thawed
3 tablespoons sugar-free strawberry syrup

3 packets sugar substitute
1 teaspoon vanilla extract
1 cup cold water

1. Place all ingredients in a blender.
2. Blend at high speed until very smooth. Serve immediately.

Total carbohydrates per serving: 12 grams (count only 10 "digestible" carbs when doing Atkins); protein: 4.5 grams; fat: 2 grams; calories: 80

Atkins Yorkshire Pudding

This is basically a giant popover and the perfect accompaniment to our Garlic-Rosemary Beef Rib Roast (see page 449). Wheat gluten is what makes bread chewy, and is available in health food stores.

Prep time: 5 minutes
Cook time: 35 minutes
9 servings

½ cup Atkins™ Bake Mix
¼ cup wheat gluten
3 eggs
1 cup whole milk
1 teaspoon salt
⅓ cup beef drippings (fat) or vegetable oil

1. Heat oven to 450°F. Whisk together bake mix, gluten, eggs, milk and salt.
2. Pour drippings or oil into an 8-inch square baking dish; place on center rack in oven for 10 minutes, until smoky hot. Add batter; bake 15 minutes. Lower temperature to

350°F; cook 20 minutes more, until lightly browned. Cut into squares before serving.

Total carbohydrates per serving: 5 grams (count only 4 "digestible" carbs when doing Atkins); protein: 5 grams; fat: 11 grams; calories: 149

Zucchini Nut Bread

Feel free to use this batter for muffins, too. Divide in 12 muffin tins and reduce baking time to 30 minutes. (Add 2 extra "digestible" carbs per serving, though, because the serving size will be larger.)

Prep time: 15 minutes
Bake time: 1 hour
Yield: 20 slices

1 scant cup Atkins™ Bake Mix
1 scant cup finely ground almonds
1½ cups granular sugar substitute
2 teaspoons cinnamon
1 teaspoon salt
1 teaspoon baking soda
½ teaspoon baking powder
1 cup vegetable oil
4 eggs
1 medium zucchini, coarsely grated
1 teaspoon vanilla extract

1. Heat oven to 350°F. Grease an 8-inch-by-4-inch loaf pan; set aside. In a large bowl whisk together bake mix, almonds, sugar substitute, cinnamon, salt, baking soda and baking powder. In a medium bowl, mix oil, eggs, zucchini and vanilla extract.

2. Pour zucchini mixture into bake mix mixture. Mix well. Pour batter into prepared pan. Bake 1 hour until golden brown and a cake tester inserted in center comes out clean. Cool on wire rack before cutting into thin slices.

Total carbohydrates per serving: 4 grams (count only 3 "digestible" carbs when doing Atkins); protein: 2.5 grams; fat: 14.5 grams; calories: 167

—∽—

Appetizers

Guacamole

For richer flavor, use pebbly skinned Haas avocados instead of the smooth skinned variety. Prepare just before serving; avocados oxidize (turn brown) after they've been cut.

Prep time: 15 minutes
Yield: 2 cups (8 servings)

3 green onions, white and 1" green part, chopped
1 jalapeño pepper, seeded and finely chopped
1 medium tomato, chopped
2 ripe avocados
1 tablespoon fresh lime juice
2 tablespoons chopped fresh cilantro
salt

1. Place onions, pepper and tomato in a medium bowl. Slice avocados in half lengthwise, remove pits and scoop pulp into bowl with a spoon. Mash mixture coarsely with a fork.
2. Mix in lime juice and cilantro. Add salt to taste.

Total carbohydrates per serving: 6 grams (count only 2 "digestible" carbs when doing Atkins); protein: 2 grams; fat: 11 grams; calories: 121

Chili Roasted Macadamia Nuts

You can buy raw macadamia nuts in the health food store. High in protein and fiber, macadamias are heart-healthy because they are packed with monounsaturated fats.

Prep time: 5 minutes
Bake time: 20 minutes
6 servings

2 cups raw shelled macadamia nuts
1 teaspoon canola oil
1½ teaspoons chili powder
1 teaspoon salt

1. Heat oven to 300°F. Toss nuts with oil, spread on a sheet pan and bake 25 minutes until golden.
2. Transfer to a bowl; immediately toss nuts with chili powder and salt. Allow to cool before serving.

Total carbohydrates per serving: 6 grams (count only 2.5 "digestible" carbs when doing Atkins); protein: 4 grams; fat: 35 grams; calories: 329

Roasted Garlic and Vegetable Dip

This flavor-packed dip will keep in the refrigerator up to three days, though we doubt it will last that long! Serve with blanched broccoli and cauliflower florets, celery sticks, radishes or jicama sticks.

Prep time: 5 minutes
Cook time: 30 minutes
Chill time: 2 hours
Yield: 2 cups

1 head garlic, halved crosswise
2 tablespoons olive oil

1 jarred roasted red pepper, patted dry
2 green onions, chopped
½ carrot, chopped
12 ounces cream cheese (one 8-ounce plus one 4-ounce
*   package)*
½ cup crumbled feta cheese
8 brine-cured black olives, pitted

1. Heat oven to 375°F. Brush garlic with olive oil. Wrap in foil and bake 40 minutes, until tender. Cool slightly.
2. Squeeze garlic cloves from skin. Place in food processor and pulse until coarsely chopped. Add pepper, onions, carrot, cream cheese, feta cheese and olives. Pulse until well blended and almost smooth. Transfer to a bowl and chill 2 hours for flavors to blend.

Total carbohydrates per 2-tablespoon serving: 2 grams (count only 2 "digestible" carbs when doing Atkins); protein: 2.5 grams; fat: 10.5 grams; calories: 110

Chicken and Beef Satés With Peanut Dipping Sauce

These curry-marinated morsels are traditionally grilled, but the broiler makes them an in-house specialty. You can, of course, use either all chicken or all beef instead of a combination.

Prep time and cook time: 25 minutes
8 servings

16 10" wooden or bamboo skewers

1 cup heavy cream
½ small onion, chopped
5 garlic cloves, chopped
4 teaspoons curry powder

1½ teaspoons ground cumin
½ teaspoon cayenne pepper
1½ teaspoons salt
1 boneless, skinless chicken breast (8 ounces), cut into
   ½" strips
1 rib-eye steak (8 ounces) trimmed, cut into ½" strips

Dipping Sauce:
⅓ cup sugar-free peanut butter
⅓ cup water
1 garlic clove
2 tablespoons fresh lime juice
2 tablespoons soy sauce
1 packet sugar substitute
dash cayenne pepper

1. Soak skewers in cold water for at least 20 minutes (this prevents burning). In a blender, combine cream, onion, garlic, curry powder, cumin, cayenne and salt; blend until smooth. Transfer to a bowl and add chicken and beef strips; toss to coat. Cover and marinate at room temperature 15 minutes.
2. Make dipping sauce: In a blender, combine ingredients and blend until smooth. Transfer to a small bowl. (Sauce can be prepared up to 2 days ahead, covered and refrigerated.)
3. Heat broiler. Thread chicken and beef strips on skewers without crowding. Place on an oiled rack in a broiler pan and broil until cooked through, turning once, about 5 minutes. Serve with dipping sauce.

Total carbohydrates per serving: 3 grams (count only 3 "digestible" carbs when doing Atkins); protein: 14 grams; fat: 8 grams; calories: 144

Italian Tuna Pâté

Simple and quick to make, this spread is perfect when unexpected guests drop by.

Prep time: 10 minutes
8 servings

1 can (6 ounces) tuna packed in olive oil, lightly drained
¼ cup tightly packed fresh parsley leaves
1 stick unsalted butter, softened
1 tablespoon lemon juice
salt and pepper

1. In a food processor, pulse tuna and parsley until parsley is finely chopped.
2. Add butter and lemon juice; process until smooth.
3. Season to taste with salt and freshly ground black pepper. Serve with blanched vegetables low in carbohydrate or controlled carb crackers.

Total carbohydrates per 2-tablespoon serving: 0 grams (count only 0 "digestible" carbs when doing Atkins); protein: 5 grams; fat: 16 grams; calories: 163

—w—

Soups

Almost Black Bean Soup

This quick and hearty main dish soup is high in fiber and iron. Black soybeans look and taste similar to black beans.

Prep and cook time: 25 minutes
4 servings

1 tablespoon vegetable oil
1 small onion, chopped
2 cloves minced garlic
1 can (16 ounces) black soybeans, drained
½ teaspoon dried thyme
¼ teaspoon dried sage
½ pound smoked ham or turkey, cut into ¼" cubes
1 can (14½ ounces) reduced-sodium beef broth, plus
* 1 can water*

1. Heat oil in a medium saucepot over medium heat. Cook onion 5 minutes, until softened. Add garlic and cook 30 seconds more. Remove saucepot from heat.
2. Add beans to saucepot. With a potato masher, coarsely

mash beans; return to stove. Stir in thyme, sage, smoked ham, broth and water. Bring to a boil. Reduce heat and simmer 20 minutes for flavors to blend, stirring occasionally.

Total carbohydrates per serving: 8 grams (count only 5 "digestible" carbs when doing Atkins); protein: 13 grams; fat: 6 grams; calories: 145

Beef Vegetable Soup

Double the recipe and freeze extra portions in small zipper bags for a quick and nutritious lunch or dinner. Antioxidant-rich escarole adds flavor and texture. The ingredients list is long, but preparation is simple.

Prep time: 25 minutes
Cook time: 35 minutes
8 servings

2 tablespoons butter
1 teaspoon dried thyme
8 ounces mushrooms, sliced
1 portobello mushroom, diced
1½ teaspoons salt, divided
¾ teaspoon black pepper, divided
½ cup red wine
2 tablespoons olive oil
1 small onion, diced
2 cloves garlic, chopped
1½ pounds beef stew meat, trimmed and cut into ½" dice
1 small carrot, diced
1 celery stalk, diced
1 cup canned diced tomatoes
2 cans (14½ ounces each) beef broth, plus 2 cans water
1 bunch escarole, ribs removed and leaves cut into ½" strips

1. In large nonstick skillet, melt butter over medium-high heat; add thyme and mushrooms; sprinkle with 1 teaspoon salt and ¼ teaspoon pepper. Cook 10 minutes or until almost dry. Add wine; cook 3 minutes until syrupy.
2. Meanwhile, toss meat with remaining ½ teaspoon salt and ½ teaspoon pepper. In large pot over medium-high heat, heat olive oil; add onion and garlic. Cook 3 to 5 minutes until onions are translucent, stirring occasionally. Raise heat to high; add meat. Cook 10 minutes until browned. Add carrots, celery, tomatoes, broth and water. Bring to boil, reduce heat, simmer 15 minutes; add escarole. Simmer 10 minutes until escarole is cooked.

Total carbohydrates per serving: 7 grams (count only 4 "digestible" carbs when doing Atkins); protein: 20 grams; fat: 13 grams; calories: 231

Manhattan Clam Chowder

Substituting zucchini for potatoes keeps the carb count down, while you get the benefits of lycopene-rich tomatoes.

Prep time: 15 minutes
Cook time: 25 minutes
6 servings

4 slices bacon, chopped
½ onion, chopped
2 celery stalks, chopped
2 cloves garlic pushed through a press
½ teaspoon dried thyme
1 can (14½ ounces) stewed tomatoes, chopped
1 medium zucchini, cut into ½" cubes
1 can (14½ ounces) vegetable broth
1 bottle (8 ounces) clam juice
2 cans (6½ ounces each) chopped clams, undrained

salt and pepper
2 tablespoons chopped fresh parsley

1. Sauté bacon in a large saucepot over medium heat until fat is released. Add onion, celery, garlic and thyme. Cook 8 minutes, stirring occasionally, until vegetables are softened.
2. Stir in tomatoes, zucchini, broth and clam juice. Cook 10 minutes, until zucchini is tender. Add clams with their juice. Cook 1 minute. Season to taste with salt and pepper. Sprinkle with parsley before serving.

Total carbohydrates per serving: 8 grams (count only 6 "digestible" carbs when doing Atkins); protein: 6 grams; fat: 5.5 grams; calories: 97

Escarole Soup With Turkey Meatballs

Italians traditionally use pork sausage in this soup, but we used turkey instead.

Prep time: 15 minutes
Cook time: 40 minutes
6 servings

2 tablespoons olive oil, divided
6 green onions, finely chopped, divided
3 garlic cloves, thinly sliced
1 bunch of escarole, ribs removed and leaves cut into
   ½" strips
2 cans (14½ ounces each) reduced-sodium chicken broth,
   plus 1 can water
½ teaspoon dried rosemary, divided
1½ pounds ground turkey
1 slice controlled carb bread, lightly toasted and ground
   into crumbs

1 egg
¾ teaspoon salt
½ teaspoon pepper
½ cup grated Parmesan cheese

1. Heat 1 tablespoon oil in a large soup pot over medium heat. Add two-thirds of the green onions and cook 3 minutes, until softened. Add garlic and cook 1 minute more. Stir in escarole, mix to coat in oil.
2. Add broth, water and ¼ teaspoon rosemary; bring to a boil. Reduce heat and simmer, partially covered, 10 minutes.
3. To make meatballs: Mix remaining green onions, turkey, bread crumbs, egg, salt, pepper and remaining ¼ teaspoon rosemary. Form into 1½-inch diameter balls. Heat remaining tablespoon of oil in a large skillet. Brown the meatballs on all sides, about 3 minutes. Add to soup. Cook soup 5 minutes more, until meatballs are cooked through. Ladle soup into bowls; sprinkle with Parmesan cheese.

Total carbohydrates per serving: 7 grams (count only 3 "digestible" carbs when doing Atkins); protein: 31 grams; fat: 20 grams; calories: 331

Cream of Spinach Soup

This is a soup version of that all-time favorite, creamed spinach. Substitute broccoli or cauliflower if you prefer.

Prep time: 5 minutes
Cook time: 20 minutes
6 servings

2 boxes (10 ounces each) frozen spinach, thawed
2 tablespoons butter

1 small onion, finely chopped
3 tablespoons Thicken Thin Not/Starch®
½ teaspoon ground nutmeg
½ teaspoon ground cumin
1 can (14½ ounces) reduced-sodium chicken broth plus
  1 can water
1 garlic clove, pushed through a press
1 cup heavy cream
salt and pepper

1. Squeeze excess moisture from spinach; blot with paper towels. Finely chop and set aside.
2. In a large saucepan, melt butter over medium heat. Add onion; cook 3 to 4 minutes, until softened. Stir in thickener, nutmeg and cumin; mix until smooth.
3. Add spinach, broth, water and garlic to saucepan. Mix well. Reduce heat to low and simmer 10 minutes.
4. Add cream and cook on low until heated through. Season to taste with salt and pepper.

Total carbohydrates per serving: 9 grams (count only 5 "digestible" carbs when doing Atkins); protein: 5 grams; fat: 19.5 grams; calories: 220

Egg Drop Soup

Few soups can be prepared as quickly—or hit the spot—quite like this one. Halve the recipe if you want just 2 servings.

Prep and cook time: 10 minutes
4 servings

2 cans (14½ ounces each) reduced-sodium chicken broth
2 thin slices fresh ginger (optional, but recommended)
2 eggs, beaten

2 green onions, chopped
½ teaspoon sesame oil

1. Bring broth and ginger to a boil in a small saucepan.
2. Hold a serving spoon upside down over the pan and slowly pour the eggs over the spoon so they drip in ribbons into the simmering soup.
3. Add green onions and sesame oil. Remove ginger; serve immediately.

Total carbohydrates per serving: 2 grams (count only 2 "digestible" carbs when doing Atkins); protein: 6.5 grams; fat: 4 grams; calories: 74

Cool As a Cucumber Soup

Soup made from scratch doesn't get much easier than this, Just blend, season and chill! Hothouse, or English, cucumbers have very small seeds, and are sweeter in taste and firmer in texture than regular cucumbers.

Prep time: 15 minutes
Chill time: 1 hour
4 servings

4 green onions, chopped
1 garlic clove, pushed through a press
1 medium hothouse cucumber, peeled, seeded and sliced
½ teaspoon dried tarragon
1 can (14½ ounces) reduced-sodium chicken broth
1 tablespoon fresh lemon juice
1 cup buttermilk
salt and pepper
¼ cup chopped fresh parsley

1. Combine all ingredients except parsley in a blender. Puree until smooth.

2. Add salt and pepper to taste. Chill 1 hour. Garnish with parsley before serving.

Total carbohydrates per serving: 7 grams (count only 6 "digestible" carbs when doing Atkins); protein: 5 grams; fat: 2 grams; calories: 57

Homemade Chicken Soup

Two professional techniques are used here: The chicken breast is added toward the end of cooking to keep it moist, and most of the vegetables are added for flavor and discarded before serving.

Prep time: 15 minutes
Cook time: 1 hour
6 servings

2 large ribs celery
2 carrots, peeled
2 onions
1 parsnip, peeled
3 sprigs parsley
1 whole stewing hen or chicken, about 5 pounds, cut into 8 pieces, breast meat reserved
10 black peppercorns
2 bay leaves
1 tablespoon kosher salt
2 quarts cold water

1. Finely chop 2 tablespoons each of celery, carrot, onion and parsnip and set aside; leave remaining large pieces of vegetable whole. Place whole vegetables, parsley, chicken (except reserved breast meat), peppercorns, bay leaves and salt in a large soup pot. Pour in water.

2. Bring to a rapid boil; skim off any foam that rises to the surface. Lower heat to a gentle simmer. Cook 1 hour. Discard all cooked solids. Strain soup into a smaller soup pot.
3. Halve chicken breasts horizontally. Bring soup back to boil. Add chicken and chopped vegetables; cover and remove from heat. Allow to sit 10 to 15 minutes, until chicken is cooked through and vegetables are tender.
4. Remove chicken breasts from stock, cut into strips and return to broth. Reheat soup and serve.

Total carbohydrates per serving: 1 gram (count only 1 "digestible" carb when doing Atkins); protein: 14 grams; fat: 1.5 grams; calories: 77

—∞—

Entrées—Seafood

Striped Bass With Fennel and Tomatoes

Fennel tastes like a cross between licorice and celery. Its slightly sweet flavor becomes very mild when cooked. If you can't find bass, substitute snapper fillets.

Prep time: 15 minutes
Bake time: 25 minutes
6 servings

1 small fennel bulb
2 tablespoons olive oil, divided
1 red pepper, cut into thin strips
1 medium onion, halved and thinly sliced
4 plum tomatoes, seeded and chopped
3 garlic cloves, pushed through a press
1 teaspoon salt, divided
¾ teaspoon dried thyme
½ teaspoon pepper
¼ cup dry white wine or water
6 skinned striped bass fillets (2½ pounds total)
1 tablespoon Pernod (optional)

1. Heat oven to 400°F. Cut fennel bulb in half lengthwise. Remove center core and cut bulb and 2 inches of stalk into thin slices. Save feathery tips for garnish.

2. In a 9-inch-by-13-inch baking dish, toss fennel slices with 1 tablespoon oil, red pepper, onion, tomatoes, garlic, ½ teaspoon salt, thyme and pepper until evenly coated. Bake 20 minutes, stirring occasionally during baking time.
3. Pour wine over vegetables. Arrange fish fillets in a single layer over vegetables, sprinkle with remaining salt and additional black pepper, if desired. Sprinkle fish with Pernod and remaining tablespoon of oil.
4. Bake 10 to 15 minutes more, until fish is cooked through.

Total carbohydrates per serving: 7 grams (count only 5 "digestible" carbs when doing Atkins); protein: 36 grams; fat: 9 grams; calories: 270

Roasted Salmon With Macadamia-Cilantro Crust

This delicious, easy entrée is a classic example of quality ingredients equaling more than the sum of their parts.

Prep time: 5 minutes
Roast time: 12 minutes
6 servings

¼ cup macadamia nuts
¼ cup fresh cilantro leaves
4 tablespoons butter, at room temperature, divided
1 teaspoon grated lemon rind
1 2½-pound salmon fillet
salt and pepper
1 tablespoon fresh lemon juice

1. Heat oven to 450°F. In a food processor, process macadamia nuts and cilantro until finely chopped; add 3 tablespoons butter and lemon rind; pulse until combined.

2. Grease a jellyroll pan with remaining tablespoon of butter. Place salmon in pan, flesh side up. Season with salt and pepper. Rub macadamia-cilantro butter over fish. Roast 12 to 15 minutes for medium-rare. Transfer to a serving platter. Drizzle with lemon juice.

Total carbohydrates per serving: 1 gram (count only 0 "digestible" carbs when doing Atkins); protein: 38 grams; fat: 32 grams; calories: 447

Maple Mustard-Glazed Salmon

A low-carb variation on the honey-mustard theme, using sugar-free maple syrup as a substitute for the honey.

Prep time: 5 minutes
Cook time: 10 minutes
4 servings

4 eight-ounce salmon steaks
salt and pepper
2 tablespoons sugar-free maple or pancake syrup
1 tablespoon countrystyle Dijon mustard
2 teaspoons reduced-sodium soy sauce

1. Heat broiler; line broiler pan with aluminum foil. Rinse and pat dry salmon steaks. Sprinkle with salt and pepper.
2. In a small bowl, combine syrup, mustard and soy sauce. Place salmon on broiler pan; brush with half the mixture. Broil 4 minutes. Turn salmon; brush with remaining mixture and broil 2 to 3 minutes more for medium doneness.

Total carbohydrates per serving: 1 gram (count only 0.5 "digestible" carbs when doing Atkins); protein: 49 grams; fat: 20 grams; calories: 387

Atkins Crabcakes

A neat kitchen trick to make a loose crab mixture hold together in a nice shape is to pack it into a measuring cup. Try these tender crabcakes with mayo, spiced with a dash of Old Bay seasoning.

Prep and cook time: 40 minutes
Chill time: 1 hour and 20 minutes
4 servings

3 tablespoons vegetable oil, divided
1 small red bell pepper, finely chopped
3 green onions, finely chopped
1 pound lump crabmeat, picked over
1 cup fresh breadcrumbs (made from 2 slices controlled carb bread), divided
¼ cup mayonnaise
3 tablespoons chopped fresh parsley
1 tablespoon Old Bay™ seasoning

1. Heat 1 tablespoon oil in a large nonstick skillet over medium heat. Cook pepper and onions 3 minutes, until slightly softened. Transfer vegetables to a large bowl. Add crab, 2 tablespoons breadcrumbs, mayonnaise, parsley and Old Bay. Mix with a fork until combined. Cover and refrigerate 20 minutes.
2. Sprinkle a layer of breadcrumbs on the bottom of a ⅓ cup metal measuring cup or a clean, empty tuna can. Fill measure with crab mixture and pack lightly using the bottom of a ¼ cup measuring cup. Sprinkle a layer of breadcrumbs on top and pack lightly with the measuring cup. Invert crabcake onto a plastic-wrap-lined baking sheet. Repeat with remaining breadcrumbs and crab mixture to make 8 crabcakes. Cover with plastic wrap and refrigerate at least 1 hour or up to 24 hours.

3. Heat oven to warm setting. Heat 1 tablespoon oil in large nonstick skillet over medium heat. Transfer four crabcakes to skillet using a wide metal spatula. Cook 5 minutes, until golden on bottom; flip with a spatula, and cook 5 minutes more. Transfer crabcakes to baking sheet and put in oven to keep warm; cook remaining crabcakes.

Total carbohydrates per serving: 7 grams (count only 3.5 "digestible" carbs when doing Atkins); protein: 27 grams; fat: 24 grams; calories: 340

Shrimp and Feta Stew

This recipe works with any firm-fleshed white fish, too. Just cut fish into 1-inch pieces. The cooking time should be about the same—fish turns opaque white when done.

Prep time: 20 minutes
Cook time: 15 minutes
4 servings

3 tablespoons olive oil
½ small onion, chopped
2 garlic cloves, pushed through a press
1 cup diced tomatoes, with juice, plus ½ cup water
½ cup dry white wine
½ teaspoon fresh oregano, chopped
½ teaspoon salt
1½ pounds large shrimp, peeled and deveined
4 ounces feta cheese, crumbled
2 tablespoons chopped parsley

1. Heat oil in a large nonstick skillet over medium heat. Sauté onion 3 minutes, until soft. Add garlic and cook 1 minute more. Add tomatoes with their juice, water,

wine, oregano and salt to skillet. Cook 10 minutes, stirring occasionally, until mixture thickens.

2. Add shrimp to skillet, cook 2 to 3 minutes until just cooked through. Stir in cheese and parsley. Serve immediately.

Total carbohydrates per serving: 5 grams (count only 4 "digestible" carbs when doing Atkins); protein: 26 grams; fat: 17.5 grams; calories: 302

Asian Tuna Kabobs

Cooked tuna should be crispy on the outside and rare to medium rare on the inside—like a steak. If you prefer your fish completely cooked through, substitute swordfish in this recipe and increase cooking time to 8 minutes.

Prep time: 25 minutes (including marinating)
Cook time: 6 minutes
4 servings

8 wooden skewers

2 pounds tuna steaks, cut into 24 equal-sized cubes
16 large mushrooms, quartered
1 red pepper, seeded and cut in 8 pieces
4 green onions, cut in 12 pieces

Marinade:
⅓ cup reduced-sodium soy sauce
⅓ cup dry sherry
2 tablespoons dark sesame oil
1 tablespoon fresh ginger, finely chopped
2 garlic cloves, pushed through a press
1 packet sugar substitute

1. On 8 skewers, alternately thread tuna cubes and vegetables. Combine marinade ingredients in a 9-inch-by-13-inch baking dish. Lay skewers in dish and marinate 15 minutes.
2. Heat broiler or prepare a medium grill. Broil or grill tuna and veggies 2 to 3 minutes per side, just to sear (tuna should be rare in center).

Total carbohydrates per serving: 7 grams (count only 5 "digestible" carbs when doing Atkins); protein: 56 grams; fat: 2 grams; calories: 298

Pesto Scallops With Cherry Tomatoes

Bright in color and flavor, this dish can be enjoyed all year long thanks to refrigerated pesto and year-round availability of cherry tomatoes.

Prep and cook time: 20 minutes
Chill time: 1 hour
2 servings

1 pound sea scallops (or medium shrimp, peeled)
¼ cup prepared pesto
2 tablespoons olive oil
2 tablespoons chopped parsley
1 teaspoon grated fresh lemon rind
8 cherry tomatoes, halved

1. Bring 4 cups of lightly salted water to a boil. Add scallops (or shrimp); remove from heat. After 8 minutes, remove scallops with slotted spoon.

2. In a large bowl, mix pesto, olive oil, parsley and lemon rind. Gently stir in scallops. Before serving, lightly mix in cherry tomato halves.

Total carbohydrates per serving: 11 grams (count only 9 "digestible" carbs when doing Atkins); protein: 43 grams; fat: 30 grams; calories: 489

Broiled Lobster With Garlic Oil

If you've only steamed lobsters before, give broiling a try. Broiling concentrates lobster's naturally sweet flavor. Have the lobsters split lengthwise for you in the fish store or supermarket and hurry home to prepare this dish!

Prep time: 10 minutes
Cook time: 15 minutes
4 servings

2 garlic cloves, finely chopped
¼ cup extra-virgin olive oil
1 tablespoon melted butter
4 fresh lobsters (about 1½ pounds each), split lengthwise
coarse (kosher) salt
1 lemon

1. Heat broiler; place rack at least 6" from heat source.
2. In a small saucepan heat garlic, olive oil and melted butter over low heat.
3. Brush lobsters liberally with garlic mixture, and sprinkle lightly with coarse salt.
4. Broil four minutes; baste with garlic mixture. Broil 3 minutes more. Serve with lemon wedges.

Total carbohydrates per serving: 4 grams (count only 4 "digestible" carbs when doing Atkins); protein: 128 grams; fat: 23 grams; calories: 766

Calamari With Basil and Lime

A quick marinade in fresh basil and lime imbues flavor and tenderizes the calamari (Italian for squid). A quick sauté finishes the dish.

Prep time: 20 minutes
Marinate time: 20 minutes
Cook time: 5 minutes
2 servings

1 pound cleaned squid, bodies cut into ½″ rings and
  tentacles halved
½ cup chopped fresh basil leaves
2 tablespoons olive oil
2 tablespoons fresh lime juice
1 garlic clove, pushed through a press
¼ teaspoon dried hot red pepper flakes
1 tablespoon peanut oil

1. Combine squid, basil, olive oil, lime juice, garlic and red pepper flakes in a bowl and mix well. Refrigerate at least 20 minutes or up to an hour.
2. Heat a heavy skillet over medium-high heat until a drop of water sizzles on the surface. Pour peanut oil into skillet, add squid, and cook, stirring frequently, about 2 minutes, until squid is opaque. Serve immediately.

Note: To turn this dish into a refreshing seafood salad, cool the finished dish in the refrigerator. Add ½ cup chopped celery, ½ cup chopped cucumber and ¼ cup chopped bell pepper. Toss with an additional tablespoon each of oil and lime juice. Season to taste with salt and pepper. Serves 3.

Total carbohydrates per serving: 9.5 grams (count only 9 "digestible" carbs when doing Atkins); protein: 36 grams; fat: 23.5 grams; calories: 397

Entrées—Lamb/Veal

Roast Leg of Lamb

Roast leg of lamb is both easy to make and impressive—and provides great leftovers. It's important to let the roast rest at room temperature for at least 10 minutes after removing it from the oven, before carving, to allow natural juices to flow back into the meat.

Prep time: 10 minutes
Cook time: 2 hours
8 servings

1 bone-in leg of lamb (about 8 pounds)
4 garlic cloves, cut into 5 slices each
¼ cup flat-leaf parsley leaves
1 tablespoon kosher salt
freshly ground black pepper

1. With the tip of a sharp knife, poke 20 holes in the leg of lamb about 1½ inches deep. Into each hole, stuff one slice of garlic and one parsley leaf. Rub the leg of

lamb all over with salt and pepper. (This step can be done up to one day in advance.)

2. Heat oven to 425°F. Place lamb in a roasting pan; roast 30 minutes. Reduce heat to 325°F, and baste the leg with any juices that have accumulated in the pan. Cook about 2 hours, until an instant-read thermometer registers 130°F (medium rare doneness) in the thickest part. Remove roast from oven and allow to rest at least 10 minutes.

3. Transfer roast to a cutting board. Carve in thin slices, parallel to the bone. If desired, make a natural gravy: Remove fat from pan drippings, add 1 cup of water to the pan, and simmer on the stovetop over a medium flame, scraping up browned bits with a wooden spoon. Cook until reduced to ¾ cup.

Total carbohydrates per serving: 1 gram (count only 1 "digestible" carb when doing Atkins); protein: 60 grams; fat: 16 grams; calories: 408

Lamb Chops With Mustard Sauce

This zesty sauce provides just the right flavor balance to the rich taste of lamb.

Prep and cook time: 20 minutes
4 servings

8 double-thick lamb rib chops
salt and pepper
¼ cup dry red wine
1 cup reduced-sodium beef broth, thickened with 1 table-
*   spoon Thicken Thin Not/Starch® thickener*
2 tablespoons Dijon mustard
2 teaspoons whole grain mustard (optional)
1 tablespoon butter

1. Season lamb chops well with black pepper. In a heavy 12-inch skillet over high heat, brown chops in two batches, moving them as little as possible in the pan. Transfer to a plate. Reduce heat to low.
2. Return all the chops back to the pan. Cook 5 minutes for medium doneness. Transfer to a plate. Pour red wine into pan; increase heat to high. Scrape up any browned bits with a wooden spoon. Cook wine until almost dry, 1 minute. Add broth-thickener combination. Bring to a boil, cook 1 minute, and remove from heat.
3. Stir in mustards and butter. Season to taste with salt.

Total carbohydrates per serving: 2 grams (count only 1 "digestible" carb when doing Atkins); protein: 54.5 grams; fat: 78 grams; calories: 949

Veal Stew With Mushrooms and Smoked Provolone

Like most stews, this tastes even better if prepared a day ahead.

Prep time: 20 minutes
Cook time: 1 hour
6 servings

2 pounds veal stew meat, cut in 1½" cubes
1 teaspoon salt
½ teaspoon pepper
2 tablespoons Atkins™ Bake Mix
3 tablespoons butter, divided
2 tablespoons olive oil, divided
2 cups sliced portobello mushrooms
3 celery stalks, diced
1 medium onion, chopped
4 garlic cloves, chopped

1 teaspoon paprika
1 can (14½ ounces) reduced-sodium chicken broth
¾ cup shredded smoked provolone or mozzarella
¼ cup chopped fresh parsley

1. Sprinkle veal with salt, pepper and bake mix. In a Dutch oven (or large nonstick skillet with a cover) melt 1 tablespoon butter and 1 tablespoon oil over medium heat. Sauté half the veal until lightly browned. Transfer to a platter; repeat with remaining veal.
2. Melt remaining tablespoon of butter in Dutch oven. Add mushrooms, celery, onion and garlic. Cook vegetables 5 minutes, stirring occasionally, until softened.
3. Add paprika, broth, and veal; bring to a simmer. Cover and cook over low heat 45 to 55 minutes, until veal is tender. Just before serving, stir in cheese and parsley.

Total carbohydrates per serving: 6 grams (count only 5 "digestible" carbs when doing Atkins); protein: 33 grams; fat: 30 grams; calories: 379

Veal Scallops With White Wine Caper Sauce

This recipe works equally well with thinly sliced turkey or chicken breasts.

Prep time: 10 minutes
Cook time: 10 minutes
2 to 3 servings

¼ cup Atkins™ Bake Mix
½ teaspoon salt
¼ teaspoon pepper
2 tablespoons olive oil
1 pound veal scallops, pounded ¼" thick

½ cup dry white wine
½ cup reduced-sodium chicken broth
½ cup diced stewed tomatoes
1 tablespoon nonpareil capers
1 tablespoon butter
1 tablespoon chopped fresh parsley

1. Mix bake mix, salt and pepper in a shallow plate. Heat half the oil in a large nonstick skillet over medium heat. Lightly coat scallops in mixture; tap off excess. Sauté half the scallops 2 to 3 minutes per side, until light golden brown. Repeat with remaining oil and scallops. Transfer to a platter and keep warm.
2. Add wine to skillet and cook 2 minutes, scraping up brown bits on bottom. Add broth, tomatoes and capers. Cook 5 minutes, stirring frequently, until mixture thickens. Swirl in butter and parsley. Spoon sauce over veal.

Total carbohydrates per serving: 8 grams (count only 6 "digestible" carbs when doing Atkins); protein: 68 grams; fat: 29 grams; calories: 618

Osso Buco

Osso Buco is a classic Italian braised dish. Made from veal shanks and flavored with onions, carrots, celery and a twist of lemon peel, it is wonderfully satisfying.

Prep time: 15 minutes
Cook time: 2 hours (largely unattended)
6 servings

2 tablespoons olive oil
4 pounds veal shank, cut across the bone in 2" slices
salt and pepper

1 small onion, chopped
1 small carrot, chopped
3 garlic cloves, chopped
1 cup diced tomatoes, with their juice
1 cup dry white wine
1 teaspoon dried oregano leaves
2 strips lemon peel, 2" by ½"
¼ cup roughly chopped flat-leaf parsley
1 tablespoon freshly grated Parmesan cheese

1. In a Dutch oven or large, heavy-bottomed pot, heat oil over medium heat. Pat shanks dry, sprinkle with salt and pepper. Brown two or three at a time. Transfer to a plate. Add onion, carrot, garlic and 1 teaspoon salt to Dutch oven and cook 5 minutes, until vegetables are soft. Add tomatoes, wine and oregano and lemon peel. Return veal to pot.
2. Bring to a boil; reduce heat to low. Simmer partially covered until veal is very tender, about 1½ hours. Transfer veal to a serving platter. Cook sauce uncovered, 10 minutes more, until slightly thickened; remove lemon peel. Add parsley. Pour sauce over shanks. Sprinkle with cheese and parsley before serving.

Total carbohydrates per serving: 4 grams (count only 3 "digestible" carbs when doing Atkins); protein: 59 grams; fat: 17 grams; calories: 447

—⚭—

Entrées—Poultry

Cheddar Chicken Roll-Ups

Store-bought cooked chicken makes this a quick week-night meal.

Prep time: 15 minutes
Bake time: 20 minutes
4 servings

2 cups shredded roasted chicken
1/3 cup green salsa
1/3 cup sour cream
4 green onions, divided
8 controlled carb flour tortillas
1 1/2 cups controlled carb tomato sauce (such as Rao's), divided
1 cup shredded cheddar cheese
1 cup shredded iceberg lettuce
2 to 3 tablespoons jarred nacho jalapeños
1/4 cup chopped fresh cilantro or parsley

1. Heat oven to 375°F. In a large bowl, mix chicken, salsa, sour cream and half the green onions. Spread 1/3 cup of

the filling on each tortilla. Roll up tortillas into cylinders.
2. Spread ¾ cup tomato sauce over bottom of a baking dish large enough to hold tortillas in a single layer. Arrange tortillas seam side down. Spread with remaining sauce and top with cheese. Bake 20 minutes, until filling is hot and cheese is melted. Place 2 tortillas on each plate and top with lettuce, jalapeños and cilantro.

Total carbohydrates per serving: 31 grams (count only 12 "digestible" carbs when doing Atkins); protein: 39 grams; fat: 23 grams; calories: 436

Herbed-Roast Chicken With Lemon

Simple, and simply delicious. Check chicken for doneness with an instant-read thermometer.

Prep time: 10 minutes
Cook time: about 1 hour
4 servings

1 chicken (about 3 pounds), rinsed and patted dry
1 teaspoon salt
¼ teaspoon black pepper
2 teaspoons chopped fresh herbs (thyme, parsley,
*   oregano, sage or a mixture) or 1 teaspoon dried*
1 large lemon, ½ sliced into rounds, ½ intact
2 tablespoons butter

1. Heat oven to 350°F. Rub chicken with salt, pepper and herbs inside and out. At cavity end, loosen skin from breast and stuff 2 slices of lemon and 1 tablespoon butter onto each side of breast. Place remaining lemon directly in chicken cavity. Transfer to a roasting pan.
2. Roast 1 hour, basting occasionally. Check chicken for doneness. An instant-read thermometer should regis-

ter 170°F in the thickest part of the thigh (not touching bone). Transfer chicken to a cutting board; wait 10
minutes before carving to allow juices to redistribute.
3. Pour pan juices into a measuring cup, let stand 5
minutes, and spoon off excess fat. Pour over chicken.

*Total carbohydrates per serving: 0 grams (count only 0
"digestible" carbs when doing Atkins); protein: 45 grams;
fat: 28 grams; calories: 441*

Sautéed Chicken Sausages With Red Peppers

Need a fast fix for a weeknight dinner? Here's one that can
be whipped up in a flash—you may already have most of the
ingredients on hand.

Prep and cook time: 30 minutes
4 servings

1½ tablespoons olive oil, divided
8 pre-cooked chicken sausages
½ red onion, thinly sliced
1 red bell pepper, cut lengthwise into ¼" strips
½ teaspoon dried thyme
3 garlic cloves, chopped
¼ cup coarsely chopped flat-leaf parsley
salt and pepper

1. Heat ½ tablespoon olive oil in a large skillet over
   medium-high heat. Add sausages and brown on all
   sides, about 5 minutes. Transfer to a plate.
2. Heat remaining tablespoon oil in skillet over medium-
   low heat. Add onion, pepper and thyme. Cook 8
   minutes, stirring occasionally, until vegetables are
   soft. Add garlic and cook 1 minute more.

3. Return sausages to skillet; cook on low 10 minutes for flavors to blend. Before serving, stir in parsley; season to taste with salt and pepper.

Total carbohydrates per serving: 5.5 grams (count only 4 "digestible" carbs when doing Atkins); protein: 22 grams; fat: 28 grams; calories: 335

Duck Breasts With Blackberry-Wine Sauce

Fruit and duck are a classic flavor combination. Here we use blackberries, but you can substitute raspberries.

Prep time: 5 minutes
Cook time: 30 minutes
4 servings

1 cup blackberries
1 cup red wine
2 packets sugar substitute
2 tablespoons sugar-free maple or pancake syrup
1 teaspoon dried thyme, divided
4 duck breast portions (about 8 ounces each)
2 tablespoons olive oil
½ teaspoon salt
½ teaspoon coarsely ground black pepper
½ teaspoon dried thyme
2 tablespoons chopped fresh parsley

1. In small saucepan, combine blackberries, wine, sugar substitute, pancake syrup and half the thyme. Bring to a boil over medium-high heat. Reduce heat and simmer 30 minutes, until reduced by one-third. Strain through a fine sieve into a clean small saucepan, pressing on the berries with the back of a spoon to extract all the juices. Set sauce aside.

2. While sauce simmers, prepare grill or preheat broiler. Rub duck breasts with oil and season with salt, pepper and remaining thyme. Grill or broil skin side down until skin is browned and crisp, 5 to 6 minutes. Turn duck over and cook 5 to 6 minutes more for medium-rare doneness. Transfer to warm platter. Cut breasts crosswise into thin slices; pour sauce over duck. Sprinkle with chopped parsley.

Total carbohydrates per serving: 7 grams (count only 5 "digestible" carbs when doing Atkins); protein: 30 grams; fat: 20 grams; calories: 368

Turkey Cutlets With Green Peppercorn Sauce

Green peppercorns have a floral, nutty taste with a hint of sweetness, and are much less pungent than black peppercorns. They come in jars and should be rinsed before use to eliminate excess salt.

Prep time: 10 minutes
Cook time: 20 minutes
4 servings

½ cup Atkins™ Bake Mix
½ teaspoon salt
¼ teaspoon pepper
2½ pounds turkey cutlets
2 tablespoons butter
1 tablespoon vegetable oil
⅔ cup reduced-sodium chicken broth
⅔ cup cream
2 tablespoons green peppercorns, rinsed and lightly crushed

1 packet sugar substitute
salt and pepper

1. Heat oven to warm setting. Combine bake mix, salt and pepper on a shallow plate. Lightly coat cutlets in mixture; tap off excess.
2. Heat butter and oil in a large nonstick skillet over medium heat. Cook cutlets 2 to 3 minutes per side until light golden brown and just cooked through. Transfer to a platter; place in oven to keep warm.
3. Add chicken broth and cream to skillet. Cook, stirring occasionally, 10 minutes, until liquid is reduced to 1 cup. Stir in peppercorns and sugar substitute. Cook 3 minutes more. Season to taste with salt and pepper. Spoon sauce over cutlets.

Total carbohydrates per serving: 4 grams (count only 3 "digestible" carbs when doing Atkins); protein: 76 grams; fat: 19 grams; calories: 544

Turkey Meatloaf With Pesto and Spinach

For a delicious twist on traditional meatloaf, try this turkey version. Prepared pesto and oregano add lots of flavor.

Prep time: 15 minutes
Bake time: 45 minutes
4 servings

1 pound ground turkey
1 (10 ounce) package frozen spinach, thawed
1 slice controlled carb bread, grated into crumbs
1 egg, beaten
3 tablespoons prepared pesto
¼ cup cream
1 garlic clove, pushed through a press

1 teaspoon dried oregano
½ teaspoon salt
¼ teaspoon pepper

1. Heat oven to 375°F. In a large bowl, combine turkey and spinach until well blended. Mix in breadcrumbs, egg, pesto, cream, garlic, oregano, salt and pepper.
2. Transfer mixture to a 9-inch-by-5-inch loaf pan. Bake 45 to 50 minutes, or until an instant read thermometer inserted in center registers 160°F. Cool 5 minutes before cutting into slices.

Total carbohydrates per serving: 8 grams (count only 3.5 "digestible" carbs when doing Atkins); protein: 30 grams; fat: 23 grams; calories: 354

Crispy Parmesan Chicken Legs

Real fried chicken is a bit of work: but worth it! Parmesan cheese adds extra flavor.

Prep time: 10 minutes
Standing time: 15 minutes
Bake time: 30 minutes
6 servings

½ cup grated fresh Parmesan cheese, divided
¼ cup Atkins™ Bake Mix
½ teaspoon black pepper
3 slices controlled carb bread, toasted
½ teaspoon oregano
½ teaspoon salt
2 eggs
3 pounds chicken legs, cut into drumstick and thigh pieces
vegetable oil for frying

1. Mix ¼ cup Parmesan cheese, bake mix and pepper in a shallow plate. In a food processor, pulse toasted bread until fine crumbs form (or use a box grater); add remaining ¼ cup cheese, oregano and salt; pulse to combine. Transfer to plate and stir. Beat eggs in a bowl.
2. Dip chicken pieces into eggs. Tap off excess. Lightly coat pieces in breadcrumb mixture and place on a wire rack to dry 15 minutes.
3. Heat oven to warm setting. Heat ½ inch of oil to 325°F in a large skillet over medium heat. Fry half the chicken, covered, 10 minutes, until rich golden brown. Turn over pieces and cook uncovered 10 to 12 minutes more, until other side is browned and chicken is cooked through. Transfer chicken to oven to keep warm while frying remaining chicken.

Total carbohydrates per serving: 5 grams (count only 2 "digestible" carbs when doing Atkins); protein: 39 grams; fat: 30 grams; calories: 459

Chicken Cacciatore

Serve over a portion of steamed spaghetti squash tossed with chopped fresh basil.

Prep time: 25 minutes
Cook time: 35 minutes
4 servings

3 tablespoons extra-virgin olive oil
1 chicken (3 to 3½ pounds), cut into 8 pieces
1 small onion, thinly sliced
2 garlic cloves, chopped
2 teaspoons dried rosemary
½ cup dry white wine or reduced-sodium chicken broth
¾ teaspoon salt

¹⁄₄ teaspoon crushed red pepper flakes
1¹⁄₂ cups canned plum tomatoes, drained and coarsely chopped

1. In large skillet, heat oil over medium-high heat. Brown chicken in 2 batches, about 8 minutes. Transfer to a plate.
2. Add onion, garlic and rosemary to pan; cook 4 minutes, until onion is softened. Add wine and bring to a boil, stirring to loosen any browned bits. Add salt and pepper flakes.
3. Add chicken, skin side up, and accumulated juices to skillet. Boil until almost all the wine has evaporated, about 2 minutes. Add tomatoes. Cover, reduce heat to low and simmer 30 minutes, until chicken is cooked through.
4. Transfer chicken to a serving platter. Boil sauce 2 minutes to thicken; spoon over chicken.

Total carbohydrates per serving: 7 grams (count only 5 "digestible" carbs when doing Atkins); protein: 50 grams; fat: 34 grams; calories: 560

Chicken Pot Pie

Creamy chicken and vegetables nestled under a crisp pie crust will make this a family favorite. You can make both the filling and crust up to 2 days ahead, but assemble just before baking.

Prep and cook time: 50 minutes
Bake time: 18 minutes
6 servings

1 recipe Atkins Pie Crust rolled out to a 10" circle (see recipe on page 438)
1¹⁄₂ pounds chicken breast fillets, cut into 1¹⁄₂" pieces
1 can (14¹⁄₂ ounces) reduced-sodium chicken broth plus 1 cup water

1 small onion, chopped
1 carrot, thinly sliced
2 celery stalks, thinly sliced
½ teaspoon crushed fennel seeds
½ cup cream
2 tablespoons Thicken Thin Not/Starch®
2 tablespoons chopped fresh parsley
salt and pepper

1. Heat oven to 375°F. Place chicken, broth, water, onion, carrot, celery and fennel seeds in a medium saucepot. Bring to a simmer over low heat and cook 20 minutes, until chicken is cooked through and vegetables are tender. Strain stock into a small saucepan; mix in cream and bring to a boil. Stir in Thicken Thin Not/Starch®; cook 2 minutes until mixture thickens. Pour sauce over chicken and vegetables; stir to coat. Add parsley. Season to taste with salt and pepper.
2. Spoon mixture into a 9-inch deep-dish pie plate. Lay dough over filling; press onto edges of pie plate. Bake 18 minutes, until crust is golden and baked through.

Total carbohydrates per serving: 9.5 grams (count only 5.5 "digestible" carbs when doing Atkins); protein: 29 grams; fat: 29 grams; calories: 446

Atkins Pie Crust:

¾ cup plus 2 tablespoons Atkins™ Bake Mix
4 tablespoons butter, softened
3 ounces cream cheese, softened
1 tablespoon sour cream

1. In medium bowl with an electric mixer on medium speed, beat bake mix, butter, cream cheese and sour cream just to combine.
2. Shape into a disc; wrap in plastic. Chill 20 minutes before rolling out between pieces of waxed paper.

Entrées—Pork

Cajun Pork Chops

A spicy dry rub adds zest to pork chops. You can also purchase a commercial Cajun mix if you don't feel like making
your own. Don't overcook the pork—it should still be juicy
in the center.

Prep and cook time: 20 minutes
4 servings

1 tablespoon paprika
½ teaspoon ground cumin
½ teaspoon salt
½ teaspoon sage
½ teaspoon freshly ground pepper
½ teaspoon garlic powder
¼ teaspoon cayenne pepper (or to taste)
4 boneless center-cut pork chops, ½" thick
½ tablespoon butter
½ tablespoon oil

1. Combine paprika, cumin, salt, sage, pepper, garlic powder and cayenne in a bowl. Coat chops with seasoning mixture on both sides.
2. Heat butter and oil over high heat in a large skillet until very hot. Place chops in skillet, reduce heat to medium and cook 7 to 8 minutes, turning once halfway through cooking time.

Total carbohydrates per serving: 2 grams (count only 1 "digestible" carb when doing Atkins); protein: 53 grams; fat: 15 grams; calories: 364

Ginger Grilled Pork Tenderloin

When purchasing fresh ginger, look for a plump, unwrinkled piece. It is not necessary to peel the ginger before grating—just rinse and pat dry.

Prep time: 10 minutes
Marinate time: 2 hours
Cook time: 15 to 20 minutes
4 servings

2 whole pork tenderloins (1½ pounds total)
2 cups dry white wine or reduced-sodium chicken broth
3 tablespoons grated fresh ginger
2 tablespoons reduced-sodium soy sauce
2 tablespoons sesame oil
1 packet sugar substitute
3 garlic cloves, pushed through a press
4 green onions, thinly sliced

1. Combine pork, wine, ginger, soy sauce, sesame oil, sugar substitute and garlic in a resealable plastic storage bag. Refrigerate 2 hours or overnight.

2. Remove tenderloins from marinade; discard marinade. Heat gas grill to medium and grill tenderloins 15 to 20 minutes in covered grill, turning occasionally, until an instant-read thermometer registers 150° to 155°F. Slice pork, garnish with green onion and serve immediately.

Total carbohydrates per serving: 4 grams (count only 3 "digestible" carbs when doing Atkins); protein: 37 grams; fat: 13 grams; calories: 362

Kielbasa With Caraway Kraut

This classic combo makes a hearty and satisfying main course, especially suited to cold weather.

Prep time: 5 minutes
Cook time: 55 minutes
6 servings

1 tablespoon vegetable oil
1 small onion, thinly sliced
1 package (1 pound) refrigerated sauerkraut, with juice
1 cup reduced-sodium chicken broth
1 tablespoon Dijon mustard
1 bay leaf
½ teaspoon caraway seeds
½ teaspoon black peppercorns, lightly crushed with a knife
1½ pounds kielbasa sausage, cut into ½" slices

1. Heat oil in large saucepan over medium-high heat. Sauté onion 5 minutes until soft. Add sauerkraut, broth, mustard, bay leaf, caraway seeds and peppercorns; mix well.

2. Cover pan; reduce heat to low. Simmer mixture 30 minutes. Add sausage, mix well and simmer 20 minutes more. Remove bay leaf before serving.

Total carbohydrates per serving: 7 grams (count only 4 "digestible" carbs when doing Atkins); protein: 17.5 grams; fat: 33 grams; calories: 397

Pork and Vegetable Ragout

Here's a stew with long-simmering flavor—in a flash! The secret? Tender pork chops cut down on cooking time.

Prep time: 15 minutes
Cook time: 20 minutes
4 servings

3 tablespoons Atkins™ Bake Mix
½ teaspoon salt
½ teaspoon pepper
4 boneless pork chops (about 1½ pounds total), cut into
   ¾" cubes
2 tablespoons olive oil, divided
½ small onion, chopped
2 celery stalks, thinly sliced
½ medium green bell pepper, chopped
2 garlic cloves, finely chopped
1 medium zucchini, halved lengthwise and sliced
   ½" thick
1 cup diced tomatoes
1 teaspoon dried basil
½ teaspoon dried oregano

1. Combine bake mix, salt and pepper in a plastic bag. Add pork pieces and shake to coat. Set aside.

2. Heat 1 tablespoon oil in Dutch oven (or large heavy pot) over medium heat. Add onion, celery and green pepper and cook 5 minutes, until vegetables are softened. Add garlic; cook 1 minute more. Transfer to a bowl.
3. Wipe out Dutch oven; heat remaining tablespoon of oil. Brown pork on all sides. Stir in zucchini, tomatoes, basil, oregano and onion mixture.
4. Bring to a boil. Reduce heat, cover and simmer 10 minutes, stirring occasionally, until pork is tender.

Total carbohydrates per serving: 8 grams (count only 5 "digestible" carbs when doing Atkins); protein: 41 grams; fat: 16 grams; calories: 356

Shredded Pork Quesadillas

This recipe works equally well with chicken or beef. If you enjoy spicy heat, use pepper Jack cheese instead of Monterey.

Prep and cook time: 15 minutes
Bake time: 5 minutes
4 servings

2 tablespoons vegetable oil, divided
½ small onion, chopped
1 pound cooked pork roast, cut into very thin strips
1 cup grated Monterey Jack cheese
¼ cup green salsa
1 jalapeño pepper (optional), seeded and finely chopped
¼ cup chopped cilantro
½ teaspoon pepper
¼ teaspoon salt
8 controlled carb flour tortillas

1. Heat oven to 450°F. Heat 1 tablespoon oil in large skillet over medium-high heat. Cook onion 5 minutes,

until softened. Transfer to a bowl and add pork, cheese, salsa, jalapeño, cilantro, pepper and salt. Mix well.

2. Brush one side of each tortilla with remaining oil. Spoon one-eighth of pork mixture over half of non-oiled side. Fold in half over filling.

3. Arrange on a baking sheet. Bake 5 minutes, until crisp and golden. Serve with additional salsa.

Total carbohydrates per serving: 26 grams (count only 7 "digestible" carbs when doing Atkins); protein: 40 grams; fat: 32 grams; calories: 505

Entrées—Beef

Steak au Poivre

This classic French dish combines peppercorns, Cognac and cream in a simple and elegant sauce.

Prep and cook time: 25 minutes
2 servings

2 tablespoons crushed black peppercorns*
2 boneless sirloin shell steaks (each about 1" thick)
2 tablespoons olive oil
½ cup heavy cream
1 tablespoon unsweetened ketchup
1 tablespoon Cognac
½ teaspoon salt

1. Spread peppercorns on a work surface and press onto both sides of steaks in an even layer. Heat oil in a large, heavy skillet over medium-high heat until very

*To crush peppercorns, place in a plastic bag and pound them with a rolling pin or the flat side of a knife.

hot. Cook steaks 5 minutes per side for medium-rare. Remove steaks from skillet and keep warm.

2. Add cream, ketchup, Cognac and salt to skillet. Bring to a boil, stirring to loosen any browned bits from bottom of skillet. Lower heat and simmer sauce for 2 minutes until slightly thickened. Pour sauce over steaks and serve immediately.

Total carbohydrates per serving: 7 grams (count only 2 "digestible" carbs when doing Atkins); protein: 62 grams; fat: 55.5 grams; calories: 798

Italian Meatballs in Tomato Sauce

Try these very tender meatballs over baked spaghetti squash or controlled carb pasta.

Prep time: 20 minutes
Cook time: 20 minutes
4 servings

2 slices controlled carb bread, crusts removed, torn into small pieces
¼ cup cream
1½ pounds ground beef chuck
¼ cup freshly grated Parmesan cheese
2 tablespoons finely chopped fresh parsley
1 egg yolk
1 garlic clove, pushed through a press
¾ teaspoon salt, divided
½ teaspoon black pepper
2 tablespoons olive oil
1 (8-ounce) jar controlled carb marinara sauce
1 tablespoon minced fresh basil leaves or 1 teaspoon dried

1. In a large bowl soak bread in cream until soft. Add ground chuck, Parmesan cheese, parsley, egg yolk,

garlic, salt and pepper. Mix well. Form mixture into 1½-inch meatballs.

2. Heat olive oil in large skillet over medium heat. Add meatballs and brown on all sides, about 10 minutes. Transfer meatballs to a plate lined with paper towels to drain. Wipe out skillet.

3. Add sauce and basil to skillet. Bring to a simmer over medium heat. Add meatballs and cook on low 5 minutes until heated through.

Total carbohydrates per serving: 9 grams (count only 6 "digestible" carbs when doing Atkins); protein: 43 grams; fat: 38 grams; calories: 544

Two-Step Chili

Thanks to canned tomatoes and salsa (which provides some of the heat), this delicious twist on chili couldn't be easier. Ask the butcher to cube the beef for you to cut prep time.

Prep and cook time: 2 hours (largely unattended)
6 servings

2 tablespoons vegetable oil
3 pounds boneless beef chuck, cut into 1" pieces
1 can (14½ ounces) diced tomatoes
1 cup reduced-sodium beef broth
2 garlic cloves, pushed through a press
½ cup medium-heat chunky salsa
2 tablespoons chili powder
1 teaspoon dried oregano leaves
sour cream (optional)
thinly sliced green onions (optional)

1. Heat oil in a Dutch oven or large pot over medium heat until hot. Brown beef in batches. Return beef and accumulated juices to Dutch oven.

2. Stir in tomatoes, broth, garlic, salsa, chili powder and oregano. Bring to a boil; reduce heat to low. Cover tightly and simmer 1½ to 1¾ hours, until beef is tender. Serve with sour cream and green onions, if desired.

Total carbohydrates per serving: 8 grams (count only 5.5 "digestible" carbs when doing Atkins); protein: 45 grams; fat: 43 grams; calories: 599

Burgundy Beef Stew

Reducing the wine before adding the beef allows for almost all the alcohol to burn off, producing a very rich sauce.

Prep and cook time: 2 hours (largely unattended)
6 servings

½ cup Atkins™ Bake Mix
3 pounds beef chuck or round, cut into 1½" cubes
¼ pound sliced bacon
1 tablespoon olive oil
1 medium onion, chopped
1 carrot, chopped
1 celery stalk, chopped
2 garlic cloves, pushed through a press
2 cups dry red wine
1 can (14½ ounces) reduced-sodium beef broth plus
   1 can water
1 bay leaf
½ teaspoon dried thyme
1 tablespoon butter
½ pound button mushrooms

1. Spread bake mix on a plate; lightly coat beef pieces, tap off excess. In a large Dutch oven or large pot over medium heat, cook bacon until crisp. Remove bacon, crumble and set aside.

2. Add oil to bacon fat in Dutch oven. Brown beef in batches. Transfer to a platter. Add onion, carrot and celery to Dutch oven; cook 8 minutes, until softened. Add garlic and cook 1 minute more. Pour in wine; increase heat to high. Boil until wine is reduced to 1 cup, about 5 minutes.

3. Return beef and accumulated juices to Dutch oven. Pour in beef broth and water; add bay leaf and thyme. Reduce heat to low; cover partially and simmer 1½ hours, until beef is tender.

4. Melt butter in a large skillet over medium heat. Sauté mushrooms until golden brown, about 5 minutes. Add mushrooms to stew along with reserved bacon. Remove bay leaf.

Total carbohydrates per serving: 9 grams (count only 7 "digestible" carbs when doing Atkins); protein: 52 grams; fat: 38 grams; calories: 662

Garlic-Rosemary Beef Rib Roast

This classic rib roast requires little adornment—but do try it with our Yorkshire Pudding! The beef will continue to cook as it sits before being sliced, so be careful to remove it from the oven when the thermometer registers about 10 degrees less than desired temperature for doneness.

Prep and cook time: 2 hours, 25 minutes to 3 hours
(largely unattended)
8 servings

2 teaspoons dried rosemary leaves, crushed
1 teaspoon dried thyme
4 garlic cloves, pushed through a press
¾ teaspoon salt
½ teaspoon freshly ground pepper
6- to 7-pound beef rib roast, well trimmed

1. Heat oven to 350°F. Combine rosemary, thyme, garlic, salt and pepper in a bowl; rub onto surface of beef. Arrange roast, fat side up, in a shallow roasting pan. Insert meat thermometer in thickest part of beef, not touching bone. Roast 2½ hours for medium-rare (145°F) or 2¾ hours for medium (160°F). Let stand 15 minutes before cutting into slices.

2. Pour off fat from roasting pan (if making Yorkshire Pudding, use fat). Add ¾ cup of water to roasting pan. Place pan over two stovetop burners over medium heat. Scrape up browned bits with a wooden spoon; cook 2 to 3 minutes. Strain and serve with beef.

Total carbohydrates per serving: 0.5 grams (count only 0 "digestible" carbs when doing Atkins); protein: 58 grams; fat: 75 grams: calories: 922

Korean-Style Skirt Steak

Skirt steak isn't just for fajitas. Try this Asian style recipe for a delicious change of pace.

> Prep time: 5 minutes
> Marinate time: 1 hour
> Cook time: 8 minutes
> 4 servings

1½ pounds beef skirt steak
2 green onions, finely chopped
4 garlic cloves, pushed through a press
3 tablespoons reduced-sodium soy sauce
1 tablespoon sesame oil
1 tablespoon rice wine vinegar or white wine vinegar
1 packet sugar substitute

1. Place all ingredients in a resealable plastic bag; turn to coat. Refrigerate 1 hour, turning meat once or twice.

2. Preheat grill or broiler. Remove meat from marinade; discard marinade. Grill or broil steak 4 to 5 minutes per side for medium-rare doneness.Thinly slice.

Total carbohydrates per serving: 0.5 grams (count only 0.5 "digestible" carbs when doing Atkins); protein: 35 grams; fat: 14 grams; calories: 274

—ɯ—

Entrées—Vegetarian

Stuffed Peppers

These flavorful stuffed peppers are delicious, colorful, and packed with fiber and vitamins.

Prep time: 40 minutes
Cook time: 40 minutes
8 servings

Tomato Sauce:
1 tablespoon olive oil
3 green onions, finely chopped
2 garlic cloves, chopped
3 ripe tomatoes, peeled, seeded and chopped, or 1½ cups
*   canned chopped tomatoes, drained*
salt

Peppers:
*8 assorted red, green and yellow peppers, roasted and peeled**

1 pound smoked mozzarella or Swiss Gruyère cheese, cut into ¼ " by 2½" sticks

½ cup frozen chopped kale or collard greens, thawed

1 tablespoon dried basil

salt and freshly ground black pepper

½ cup freshly grated Parmesan cheese

1. Heat oil in a heavy medium skillet over medium heat. Add green onions and cook, stirring occasionally, until translucent, about 5 minutes. Add garlic and cook 1 minute more. Add tomatoes; reduce heat and simmer 10 minutes, stirring occasionally, until sauce thickens. Season to taste with salt and remove from heat.
2. Heat oven to 375°F; grease a 2-quart shallow baking dish. Make a 2-inch slit along side of each pepper. Rinse out seeds and gently pull out white pulp with your fingers. Pat dry.
3. Insert cheese strips and kale into peppers. Sprinkle with basil, salt and pepper. Arrange peppers in a single layer, filled side up. Pour sauce on top. Sprinkle evenly with Parmesan. Bake 40 to 45 minutes, until lightly browned.

Total carbohydrates per serving: 10 grams (count only 8 "digestible" carbs when doing Atkins); protein: 15 grams; fat: 16 grams; calories: 241

To roast peppers, broil them 4 inches from heat source, turning occasionally until skin blackens and blisters. Place in a container or bowl covered with plastic wrap, and cool for 5 minutes. Peel off skins.

Eggplant Parmesan

In this easy-to-make update of the classic version, un-breaded eggplant is broiled, not fried, and then baked. Less work; less mess—and just as delicious.

Prep time: 45 minutes
Bake time: 30 minutes
6 servings

2 medium eggplants, about 1½ pounds total
salt and pepper
3 tablespoons olive oil
1½ cups controlled carb tomato sauce
1 cup thinly sliced mushrooms
10 large basil leaves, torn in pieces
8 ounces mozzarella cheese, thinly sliced
½ cup Parmesan cheese

1. Slice eggplants into ⅓-inch-thick rounds. Sprinkle with salt and let stand for 30 minutes for bitter juices to drain. Rinse and pat dry.
2. Heat broiler. Arrange eggplant slices in a single layer. Brush each side with oil. Broil 5 to 6 inches from heat source 2 to 3 minutes per side until browned.
3. Heat oven to 375°F; lightly oil a 9-inch-by-13-inch baking dish; set aside. Combine tomato sauce, mushrooms and half the basil in a saucepan and bring to a boil. Cook 3 minutes. Season to taste with salt and pepper.
4. Spread one half of the sauce on bottom of baking dish. Top with eggplant slices, mozzarella slices and remaining basil. Spread remaining sauce over layers. Sprinkle surface evenly with Parmesan cheese. Bake 30 minutes until bubbling.

Total carbohydrates per serving: 15 grams (count only 10 "digestible" carbs when doing Atkins); protein: 12 grams; fat: 16 grams; calories: 239

Tofu Stir-Fry Over Baby Spinach

Light yet filling, this entrée can be ready in less than a half-hour. Be sure to buy firm tofu—it keeps its shape in stir-fries.

Prep and cook time: 25 minutes
4 servings

1 pound firm tofu, cut into 1" cubes
1 tablespoon canola oil
4 green onions, cut in ¼" slices
1 tablespoon fresh ginger, finely chopped
1 teaspoon Chinese 5-spice powder
8 cherry tomatoes, halved
4 garlic cloves, finely chopped
½ teaspoon salt
2 (6 ounce) bags pre-washed baby spinach

1. Gently press tofu cubes between layers of paper towels to absorb excess moisture.
2. Heat oil in large nonstick skillet over medium heat. Add green onions; cook 4 minutes, until wilted. Increase heat to medium-high. Add ginger, 5-spice powder and tofu cubes. Cook 3 to 4 minutes, until tofu starts to brown. Add tomatoes, garlic and salt. Cook 1 minute more.
3. Divide spinach among four plates. Top with hot tofu mixture. Serve immediately.

Total carbohydrates per serving: 10 grams (count only 7 "digestible" carbs when doing Atkins); protein: 12 grams; fat: 9 grams; calories: 153

Vegetables

Artichoke and Cheese Squares

This easy side dish can be made up to 3 days ahead, and goes well with pork, chicken or fish.

Prep time: 10 minutes
Bake time: 30 minutes
8 servings

1 12-ounce jar marinated artichoke hearts, drained,
   liquid reserved
1 small onion, finely chopped
2 garlic cloves, pushed through a press
4 whole eggs, beaten
2 tablespoons Atkins™ Bake Mix
½ teaspoon salt
¼ teaspoon pepper
¼ teaspoon oregano
¼ teaspoon Tabasco sauce
8 ounces shredded Monterey Jack cheese
2 tablespoons chopped parsley

1. Heat oven to 325°F. Chop artichoke hearts and set aside. Heat the reserved marinade liquid in a medium skillet, and cook the onion and garlic in it until softened, about five minutes.
2. In a mixing bowl, combine eggs, bake mix, salt, pepper, oregano and Tabasco. Mix in cheese, parsley, artichokes, onions and garlic.
3. Spoon mixture into a shallow 1½-quart baking dish. Bake 30 minutes, until set. Cool 10 minutes before cutting into squares.

Total carbohydrates per serving: 6 grams (count only 4.5 "digestible" carbs when doing Atkins); protein: 12 grams; fat: 14 grams; calories: 200

Fried Green Tomatoes

A Southern tradition, these tasty tomatoes are great as a side dish and/or for breakfast topped with a slice of cheddar cheese and a poached egg.

Prep time: 5 minutes
Cook time: 10 minutes per batch
6 servings

4 medium green (unripe) tomatoes
⅓ cup stone-ground cornmeal
⅓ cup Atkins™ Bake Mix
½ teapoon salt
¼ teaspoon pepper
3 tablespoons canola oil

1. Cut tomatoes crosswise into ½-inch-thick slices. In a plate, combine cornmeal, bake mix, salt and pepper. Press tomato slices in cornmeal mixture to lightly coat.

2. Heat oil in a large nonstick skillet over medium-high heat. Fry tomatoes in batches, 8 to 10 minutes, turning once, until golden brown. Drain on a wire rack, or pat with paper towels to remove excess oil.

Total carbohydrates per serving: 11 grams (count only 9 "digestible" carbs when doing Atkins); protein: 2 grams; fat: 8 grams; calories: 128

Sautéed Kale With Red Pepper

Kale is an excellent source of vitamins A and C and folic acid.

Prep and cook time: 25 minutes
6 servings

1 large head kale
3 tablespoons olive oil
½ small red onion
1 diced roasted red pepper
2 garlic cloves, pushed through a press
3 tablespoons red wine vinegar
1 packet sugar substitute
salt and pepper

1. Bring a large pot of lightly salted water to a boil. Remove and discard stems from kale leaves. Rinse leaves thoroughly under cold water. Cook 4 to 5 minutes, until just tender. Drain in a colander; press down to express liquid. Coarsely chop kale.*
2. Heat oil in a large skillet over medium heat. Add onion and red pepper; cook 3 minutes or until onion softens. Add garlic to pan; cook 30 seconds more. Stir in kale;

*Kale may be prepared up to 3 days ahead up to this point. Cover with plastic and refrigerate.

cook 3 minutes, stirring frequently. Transfer mixture to a large bowl.

3. Add vinegar and sugar substitute to pan; cook 1 minute. Pour sauce over kale; toss to coat. Season to taste with salt and pepper.

Total carbohydrates per serving: 9 grams (count only 7 "digestible" carbs when doing Atkins); protein: 2 grams; fat: 7 grams; calories: 102

Broccoli With Toasted Pine Nuts and Garlic

This classic Italian side dish can be made with regular broccoli florets, tender broccolini or slightly bitter broccoli rabe. Don't omit the pine nuts—they add a delicate crunch and creamy flavor.

Prep time: 10 minutes
Cook time: 10 minutes
4 servings

1 head broccoli cut into florets (about 3 cups)
2 tablespoons extra-virgin olive oil
3 garlic cloves, finely chopped
¼ cup Italian pine nuts, toasted slightly in a dry pan until golden
salt and pepper
crushed red pepper flakes (optional)
lemon wedges

1. Cook broccoli in a large pot of lightly salted water until crisp-tender, about 6 minutes. Drain and pat dry.
2. In a large skillet, heat oil over medium heat. Add garlic and cook 30 seconds until lightly golden (do not allow

garlic to brown). Add pine nuts and broccoli. Add salt, pepper and red pepper to taste. Cook, stirring occasionally, until warmed through. Serve with lemon wedges.

Total carbohydrates per serving: 5 grams (count only 3 "digestible" carbs when doing Atkins); protein: 4 grams; fat: 11 grams; calories: 126

Swiss Chard Gratin

Delicious prepared with fresh chard, in a pinch this dish can also be made with two 10-ounce boxes of frozen spinach.

Prep and cook time: 15 minutes
Bake time: 45 minutes
6 servings

butter for greasing casserole dish
2 pounds Swiss chard, washed and cut into 2" pieces*
¼ cup Atkins™ Bake Mix
½ cup heavy cream mixed with ½ cup water
¼ cup sour cream
3 eggs
2 tablespoons mixed chopped fresh herbs (parsley,
  cilantro, chives, tarragon, dill, etc.)
½ teaspoon salt
¼ teaspoon freshly ground pepper

1. Heat oven to 375°F. Butter a shallow casserole or gratin dish.

---

* Swiss chard leaves and stems are often cooked as two different vegetables: the leaves like spinach and the stems like celery. However, if the chard is young and the stems are soft and narrow, leaves and stems can be cooked together.

2. Cook chard in lightly salted boiling water for 5 minutes; drain and squeeze dry. (May be prepared up to 1 day ahead). Spread in prepared dish in an even layer.
3. In a large bowl, whisk together bake mix, cream and water, sour cream, eggs, herbs, salt and pepper. Pour mixture over chard.
4. Bake 45 minutes, until set and lightly browned.

Total carbohydrates per serving: 8 grams (count only 5 "digestible" carbs when doing Atkins); protein: 7 grams; fat: 13 grams; calories: 175

Baked Spaghetti Squash With Garlic-Sage Cream

A few simple ingredients—sage, garlic and Parmesan cheese—transform a mild-tasting vegetable into a memorable side dish.

Prep time: 10 minutes
Bake time: 45 minutes
6 servings

1 large (about 2½ pounds) spaghetti squash
¾ cup heavy cream
1 garlic clove, pushed through a press
3 finely chopped fresh sage leaves or ½ teaspoon dried sage
salt and pepper
¼ cup Parmesan cheese

1. Heat oven to 400°F. Prick squash in several places. Bake 45 minutes until tender. Allow to cool slightly, cut in half and scoop out seeds. Pull out squash strands from each side with a fork. Transfer to a warmed bowl.
2. While squash is baking, heat cream, garlic and sage in a small saucepan over medium heat. Cook 10 minutes,

until cream is thick enough to coat the back of a spoon. Pour sauce over squash; toss lightly until combined. Add salt and pepper to taste. Sprinkle with Parmesan cheese and serve immediately.

Total carbohydrates per serving: 12 grams (count only 2 "digestible" carbs when doing Atkins); protein: 3.5 grams; fat: 13 grams; calories: 168

Sesame Snow Peas

Snow peas have the lowest carb count of all peas—only 5 grams of "digestible" carbs per 5 ounces—and they are high in fiber, too. Very brief cooking keeps them bright green and crunchy.

Prep and cook time: 10 minutes
4 servings

½ pound snow peas, trimmed and strings discarded
1 teaspoon sesame oil
1 green onion, sliced thinly on the diagonal
2 teaspoons sesame seeds, toasted lightly
salt and pepper

1. Cut snow peas on diagonal into long thin slices. Set up a large bowl of ice and cold water.
2. Blanch snow peas 30 seconds in a large pot of boiling, lightly salted water. Drain in a colander. Immediately transfer to ice water to stop cooking. Drain well.
3. In a bowl toss snow peas with oil, green onion and sesame seeds. Season to taste with salt and pepper.

Total carbohydrates per serving: 4 grams (count only 3 "digestible" carbs when doing Atkins); protein: 2 grams; fat: 2 grams; calories: 42

Cauliflower-Leek Purée

Leeks are relatively low in carbs (for a member of the onion family) and have a fresh, grassy onion flavor that balances the sweetness of cauliflower. The single leek used here transforms cauliflower purée into something resembling garlic mashed potatoes.

Prep time: 15 minutes
Cook time: 15 minutes
6 servings

1 head cauliflower, separated into florets
1 leek, white and 1" green, well washed, cut into ½" slices
3 tablespoons butter
3 tablespoons cream
⅛ teaspoon nutmeg (optional)
salt and pepper

1. Cook cauliflower and leek in lightly salted boiling water until very tender, about 15 minutes. Drain; return vegetables to pot and toss over high heat to thoroughly remove excess moisture.
2. Place half the vegetables in food processor with half the butter and cream and salt. Process until smooth. Repeat with remaining vegetables, butter and cream. Mix in nutmeg; season to taste with salt and pepper.

Total carbohydrates per serving: 7 grams (count only 5 "digestible" carbs when doing Atkins); protein: 2 grams; fat: 9 grams; calories: 110

Roasted Green Beans

Say goodbye to boring green beans—these are so good you'll be snitching them with your fingers. Try mixing green and wax beans.

Prep time: 10 minutes
Cook time: 30 minutes
8 servings

3 pounds thin green beans
1½ tablespoons olive oil
salt to taste

1. Heat oven to 375°F. In a large bowl, combine green beans, oil and salt. Toss to coat.
2. Spread out beans in a single layer on 2 jellyroll pans or shallow baking pans.
3. Roast beans until lightly browned and crisp-tender, 30 minutes, shaking pans occasionally.

Total carbohydrates per serving: 13 grams (count only 8 "digestible" carbs when doing Atkins); protein: 3 grams; fat: 3 grams; calories: 80

Ratatouille Bake

This is an herbed French vegetable mélange that became well known in the United States in the 1970s. Great as a side dish, it also makes a super omelette filling and a topping for low-carb pasta.

Prep time: 30 minutes
Bake time: 45 minutes
6 servings

1 small eggplant (about 1¼ pounds), cut into 1" pieces
⅓ cup olive oil
4 garlic cloves, pushed through a press
1 teaspoon salt
½ teaspoon dried rosemary
½ teaspoon dried thyme
¼ teaspoon black pepper
1 medium zucchini, cut into 1" pieces
1 yellow squash, cut into 1" pieces
1 small red pepper, cut into ½" pieces
1 small tomato, cut into ½" pieces
1 small onion, thinly sliced

1. Sprinkle eggplant with salt; place in a colander and let bitter juices drain 20 minutes. Rinse eggplant and pat dry.
2. Heat oven to 425°F. In a 10-inch-by-15-inch baking dish, mix oil, garlic, salt, rosemary, thyme and pepper. Add vegetables, toss to coat evenly with oil mixture.
3. Cover dish with foil and bake 15 minutes. Uncover and cook 30 minutes more, mixing occasionally, until vegetables are tender and browned.

Total carbohydrates per serving: 11 grams (count only 7 "digestible" carbs when doing Atkins); protein: 2 grams; fat: 12 grams; calories: 154

Mixed Greens With Tomatoes and Ginger

An array of sweet, tangy, peppery and bitter greens mixes textures and flavors. Serve hot or at room temperature.

Prep time: 15 minutes
Cook time: 15 minutes
6 servings

3 tablespoons butter
½ small onion, finely chopped
1 garlic clove, pushed through a press
2 medium tomatoes, seeded and finely chopped
1 tablespoon grated fresh ginger
2 pounds mixed fresh greens such as arugula, chard,
    collard, dandelion, mustard, sorrel and turnip,
    trimmed, coarsely chopped (blanch collard, mustard
    and turnip greens after chopping)
salt and pepper

1. Melt butter in a large saucepan over medium heat. Add onion; cook 5 minutes until softened. Add garlic and cook 30 seconds more. Add tomatoes and ginger and cook 5 minutes, stirring occasionally.
2. Stir in greens. Mix well, cover and cook 5 minutes, until wilted. Season with salt and pepper to taste.

Total carbohydrates per serving: 11 grams (count only 6.5 "digestible" carbs when doing Atkins); protein: 4 grams; fat: 7 grams; calories: 108

Swedish Red Cabbage

Sweet and sour red cabbage pairs beautifully with wild game, goose, duck and roasted red meats. This dish can be made up to 3 days ahead.

Prep time: 15 minutes
Cook time: 45 minutes
8 servings

½ stick butter
2 tart apples (such as Granny Smith), peeled, cored and roughly chopped
1 small onion, thinly sliced
2 pounds red cabbage, shredded
2 packets sugar substitute
2 tablespoons cider vinegar
1 teaspoon salt
¼ teaspoon ground cloves
¼ teaspoon ground allspice
⅓ cup dry red wine
salt and pepper

1. Melt butter in a large, heavy Dutch oven or heavy pot over medium heat. Add apples and onion. Cook 10 minutes until very tender. Stir in cabbage and cook 8 minutes, stirring frequently, until slightly wilted. Mix in sugar substitute, cider vinegar, salt, cloves and allspice.
2. Cover and cook 10 minutes, stirring occasionally. Uncover, add wine. Cook 10 to 15 minutes more, until vegetables are soft. Season to taste with salt and pepper.

Total carbohydrates per serving: 12 grams (count only 9 "digestible" carbs when doing Atkins); protein: 2 grams; fat: 6 grams; calories: 109

Oven-Fried Turnips

While they'll never be mistaken for French fries, these root veggies taste great and are perfect for dipping into controlled carb ketchup.

Prep time: 15 minutes
Bake time: 30 minutes
6 servings

4 turnips, trimmed and peeled (about 1¼ pounds)
2 tablespoons olive oil
1 teaspoon kosher salt
½ teaspoon chili powder

1. Heat oven to 425°F. Cut turnips into 2-inch-by-½-inch sticks. Place on a foil-lined jellyroll pan. Drizzle with oil and sprinkle with salt and chili powder. Toss with your hands to coat. Spread out in a single layer.
2. Roast fries 30 minutes, turning halfway through cooking time for even browning. Serve immediately.

Total carbohydrates per serving: 4.5 grams (count only 2 "digestible" carbs when doing Atkins); protein: 1 gram; fat: 5 grams; calories: 59

Salads and Dressings

Blue Cheese Dressing

Just a few ingredients and so much better than the bottled kind!

Prep time: 5 minutes
Yield: 1 cup

4 ounces blue cheese (i.e., Stilton, Gorgonzola, Danish blue, Roquefort, Maytag)
¼ cup mayonnaise
¼ cup sour cream
1 tablespoon white wine vinegar
1 teaspoon Dijon mustard
⅓ cup olive oil
salt and pepper

1. In a medium bowl, mash cheese. Mix in mayonnaise, sour cream, vinegar and mustard until well combined (mixture doesn't have to be smooth).

2. Whisk in olive oil until blended. Season to taste with salt and freshly ground black pepper.

Total carbohydrates per 2-tablespoon serving: 2 grams (count only 2 "digestible" carbs when doing Atkins); protein: 3 grams; fat: 20 grams; calories: 200

Green Goddess Dressing

The anchovy paste is optional, but it is the secret ingredient.

Prep time: 10 minutes
Yield: 1 cup

½ cup mayonnaise
½ cup sour cream
1 tablespoon white wine vinegar
¼ cup chopped parsley
2 tablespoons chopped fresh chives or green onions
1 tablespoon chopped fresh tarragon
1 teaspoon anchovy paste (optional)
salt and pepper

1. Process all ingredients except salt and pepper in a blender or food processor. Add 2 tablespoons of water and blend until smooth. Add salt and pepper to taste.

Total carbohydrates per 2-tablespoon serving: 1 gram (count only 1 "digestible" carb when doing Atkins); protein: 1 gram; fat: 14 grams; calories: 132

Ginger, Soy and Sesame Sauce

This Asian sauce has myriad uses: as a sauce for grilled meats or poultry, dressing for salads, even as a marinade.

Prep time: 5 minutes
Yield: ¾ cup

¼ cup reduced-sodium soy sauce
¼ cup reduced-sodium chicken broth
2 tablespoons sesame oil
2 tablespoons rice wine vinegar or cider vinegar
1 packet sugar substitute
1 teaspoon grated fresh ginger
1 garlic clove, pushed through a press

1. In a small bowl, whisk together all ingredients.

Total carbohydrates per tablespoon: 1.5 grams (count only 1 "digestible" carb when doing Atkins); protein: 1 gram; fat: 2 grams; calories: 29

Classic Vinaigrette (and Variations)

Vinaigrette isn't just for salads—drizzle it on cooked vegetables such as asparagus, cauliflower or green beans. It also makes a great marinade for chicken, pork or fish. The carb count on the variations will vary by a negligible ½ gram per serving.

Prep time: 5 minutes
Yield: 1 cup

¼ cup red or white wine vinegar
1 teaspoon Dijon mustard
¼ teaspoon salt

⅛ teaspoon freshly ground pepper
¾ cup extra-virgin olive oil

1. In a small bowl, whisk together vinegar, mustard, salt and pepper. Whisk in the olive oil in a slow, steady stream until completely incorporated.

Variations:

Herb Vinaigrette: Add 3 tablespoons of finely chopped fresh herbs, such as parsley, basil, cilantro, dill or chervil.

Lemon Vinaigrette: Substitute lemon juice for the vinegar; add 1 teaspoon grated lemon rind and 1 tablespoon finely chopped shallot or green onion.

Mustard Vinaigrette: Increase mustard to 2 teaspoons; add 1 garlic clove pushed through a press, 2 tablespoons sour cream, 1 tablespoon chopped fresh parsley and ¼ packet sugar substitute.

Total carbohydrates per 2 tablespoons basic vinaigrette: 1 gram (count only 1 "digestible" carb when doing Atkins); protein: 0 grams; fat: 20 grams; calories: 182

Creamy Italian Dressing

Wonderful over hearty greens, this dressing also makes a savory sauce for cooked vegetables.

Prep time: 5 minutes
Chill time: 30 minutes
Yield: 1 cup

½ cup mayonnaise
¼ cup heavy cream
1 tablespoon white wine vinegar

1 garlic clove
½ teaspoon dried oregano
½ teaspoon dried basil
salt and pepper

1. Mix all ingredients. Add salt and pepper to taste. Chill in refrigerator 30 minutes for flavors to blend.

Total carbohydrates per 2-tablespoon serving: 1 gram (count only 1 "digestible" carb when doing Atkins); protein: 0 grams; fat: 14 grams; calories: 127

Chicken Salad

Capers and dill pickles make this chicken salad zestier than the usual version.

Prep time: 10 minutes
6 servings

2 large chicken breasts (about 1¼ pounds), cooked
2 dill pickles, chopped
3 hard boiled eggs, chopped
3 green onions, chopped
⅓ cup mayonnaise
⅓ cup sour cream
2 tablespoons drained capers
2 tablespoons fresh dill, chopped
½ teaspoon freshly ground pepper
½ cup pecan halves

1. Cut chicken into strips. Mix pickles, eggs, green onions, mayonnaise, sour cream, capers, dill and pepper in a large bowl.

2. Add chicken to bowl; toss well to thoroughly combine ingredients. Sprinkle with pecans before serving.

Total carbohydrates per serving: 4 grams (count only 2.5 "digestible" carbs when doing Atkins); protein: 24 grams; fat: 27.5 grams; calories: 356

Creamy Red Cabbage Slaw

This colorful slaw is a nice change of pace from green cabbage. To turn this into a light lunch, add 4 ounces of sliced baked ham to each serving.

Prep time: 15 minutes
6 servings

1 pound red cabbage, cored, quartered and thinly sliced
1 small red onion, very thinly sliced
⅓ cup sour cream
⅓ cup mayonnaise
1 tablespoon chopped fresh tarragon (or 1 teaspoon dried)
1 tablespoon balsamic vinegar
¼ packet sugar substitute
salt and pepper

1. In large bowl, combine cabbage and onion. In small bowl, mix sour cream, mayonnaise, tarragon, vinegar and sugar substitute. Add salt and pepper to taste.
2. Add dressing to cabbage mixture and toss to coat. Cover and refrigerate at least 1 hour for flavors to blend. (May be made up to 1 day ahead.) Serve chilled or at room temperature.

Total carbohydrates per serving: 6 grams (count only 4 "digestible" carbs when doing Atkins); protein: 2 grams; fat: 12.5 grams; calories: 139

Jicama Pico de Gallo

A jicama (HEE-kah-mah) looks like a round, overgrown potato. But this low-carb veggie has a crunchy texture and a flavor reminiscent of apples.

Prep time: 35 minutes (including marinating)
6 servings

1 small jicama (about the size of a baseball), peeled and diced into ¼" cubes
1 or 2 jalapeño peppers, finely chopped
3 green onions, chopped
½ cup canned tomatillos, chopped
½ teaspoon salt
2 tablespoons lime juice
¼ cup chopped fresh cilantro
½ packet sugar substitute

1. Mix all ingredients in a bowl. Let flavors blend at least 15 minutes before serving.

Total carbohydrates per serving: 7 grams (count only 4 "digestible" carbs when doing Atkins); protein: 1 gram; fat: 0 grams; calories: 32

Radicchio, Gorgonzola and Bacon Salad

This hearty, beautiful salad is almost a meal in itself. Slightly bitter radicchio pairs well with smoky bacon and tangy blue cheese.

Prep and cook time: 10 minutes
4 servings

6 nitrate-free bacon slices
3 tablespoons extra-virgin olive oil

1 tablespoon fresh lemon juice
salt and pepper
1 small head Boston or bibb lettuce, torn into bite-sized pieces
1 head radicchio (about ½ pound), thinly sliced
½ cup Gorgonzola cheese (about 2 ounces), crumbled
2 tablespoons flat-leaf parsley leaves

1. Cook bacon until crisp. Drain on paper towels, crumble and set aside.
2. In a large bowl whisk olive oil and lemon juice. Add salt and pepper to taste. Add Boston lettuce, radicchio, cheese and parsley. Toss gently to coat. Divide evenly among 4 plates; sprinkle with bacon.

Total carbohydrates per serving: 4 grams (count only 3 "digestible" carbs when doing Atkins); protein: 8 grams; fat: 19.5 grams; calories: 218

Cobb Salad

Improvise on this basic recipe by adding any low-carb veggies you have on hand. Chopped mushrooms, diced zucchini or sliced celery would all be great additions.

Prep time: 25 minutes
4 servings

3 cups chopped Romaine lettuce (about ⅓ head)
3 cups chopped iceberg lettuce (about ⅓ head)
1 pound cooked chicken or turkey breast, in one piece, diced
8 slices bacon, cooked and crumbled
1 tomato, seeded and diced
4 green onions, chopped
¼ cup red wine vinegar
1 teaspoon Dijon mustard
½ packet sugar substitute
½ cup olive oil

¾ cup (about 6 ounces) crumbled Roquefort cheese
1 hard-boiled egg, very finely chopped
1 large avocado, peeled and sliced

1. In a large bowl, mix lettuces, chicken, bacon, tomato and green onions.
2. In a small bowl, whisk vinegar, mustard and sugar substitute until combined. Slowly whisk in olive oil. Pour ¾ of the dressing over salad and mix well. Divide salad on 4 plates.
3. Sprinkle cheese and chopped egg over salads. Arrange avocado slices on top; drizzle with remaining dressing.

Total carbohydrates per serving: 12 grams (count only 6 "digestible" carbs when doing Atkins); protein: 47 grams; fat: 57 grams; calories: 739

Greek Spinach Salad

Nuggets of salty white feta nestle in iron-rich spinach leaves covered with a garlicky vinaigrette. If you can't find tender baby spinach, coarsely chop regular spinach.

Prep time: 15 minutes
4 servings

3 tablespoons red wine vinegar
1 garlic clove, pushed through a press
¼ cup olive oil
1 package (10 ounces) baby spinach, pre-washed
½ red onion, thinly sliced
8 ounces feta cheese, crumbled
½ jar (4 ounces) roasted red peppers, drained, cut into strips
¼ cup coarsely chopped walnuts

1. In a large salad bowl, combine vinegar and garlic. Add oil in a thin, steady stream, whisking constantly until smooth.

2. Add spinach and onion to dressing and toss to coat. Gently mix in feta and pepper strips. Divide salad on plates; sprinkle with walnuts.

Total carbohydrates per serving: 10 grams (count only 7 "digestible" carbs when doing Atkins); protein: 12 grams; fat: 31 grams; calories: 351

Cauliflower "Potato" Salad

Our low-carb version of this classic summer salad will complete your barbecue or picnic. For variety, add sliced, hard-boiled eggs. This dressing also works for coleslaw.

Prep and cook time: 25 minutes
Chill time: 30 minutes
6 servings

1 medium head cauliflower, broken into small florets
¼ cup mayonnaise
2 tablespoons lemon juice
2 packets sugar substitute
½ teaspoon dried mustard
3 green onions, chopped
1 very finely chopped jalapeño pepper or 2 tablespoons
   chopped green bell pepper (optional)
salt and pepper

1. Cook cauliflower in a large pot of boiling salted water 10 minutes, until very tender. Drain and rinse under cold water; pat dry.
2. In a large mixing bowl, mix mayonnaise, lemon juice, sugar substitute and mustard. Add cauliflower, green onions and pepper, if using. Mix well until vegetables are evenly coated with dressing. Add salt and pepper to taste. Chill 30 minutes for flavors to blend.

Total carbohydrates per serving: 4 grams (count only 2 "digestible" carbs when doing Atkins); protein: 2 grams; fat: 8 grams; calories: 85

Caesar Salad

As the story goes, the Caesar salad was invented by Caesar Ritz to commemorate the opening of his grand hotel. It has become America's favorite salad. Don't omit the anchovies in the dressing: they don't taste fishy and add lots of flavor.

Prep time: 15 minutes
4 servings

2 garlic cloves, pushed through a press
¼ cup mayonnaise
3 canned anchovy fillets, rinsed
1 tablespoon lemon juice
1 teaspoon Worcestershire sauce
2 tablespoons olive oil
2 tablespoons plus ¼ cup Parmesan cheese
1 medium head Romaine lettuce, cut into bite-sized pieces
Garlic Croutons (see recipe, below)

1. In a food processor, process garlic, mayonnaise, anchovy fillets, lemon juice and Worcestershire sauce until smooth. Add olive oil and 2 tablespoons cheese; blend just to combine.
2. Toss lettuce with dressing until evenly coated. Divide on plates; top with garlic croutons and remaining Parmesan cheese.

Total carbohydrates per serving: 7 grams (count only 4 "digestible" carbs when doing Atkins); protein: 3 grams; fat: 24 grams; calories: 264

Garlic Croutons:

Cut 2 slices controlled carb bread into ½ inch squares. Toss with 2 teaspoons olive oil and ¼ teaspoon salt. Toast on a baking sheet in a 350°F oven for 6 to 8 minutes until golden brown. Toss with 1 teaspoon Parmesan cheese, if desired.

To turn Caesar Salad into a hearty main course, add any of the following per serving:

1 grilled or sautéed chicken breast half, cut into strips
6 ounces grilled shrimp
2 hard-boiled eggs, quartered
6 ounces grilled or pan-fried steak, thinly sliced
1 6-ounce can of tuna in water or oil, drained

Asian Cucumber Salad

This light, refreshing salad is a perfect accompaniment to grilled or roasted meats.

Prep time: 5 minutes
4 servings

1 English cucumber, peeled and thinly sliced
3 green onions, thinly sliced
1 tablespoon rice wine vinegar
2 teaspoons soy sauce
1 teaspoon sesame oil
¼ packet sugar substitute

1. Combine all ingredients in a large bowl; toss until combined. Serve immediately.

Total carbohydrates per serving: 3 grams (count only 2.5 "digestible" carbs when doing Atkins); protein: 1 gram; fat: 1 gram; calories: 25

Crab and Avocado Salad

Sweet crabmeat and creamy avocado make a light yet filling salad. A mildly spicy dressing brings flavors together. Fresh cooked crabmeat is best, but canned works well, too.

Prep time: 20 minutes
4 servings

3 tablespoons mayonnaise
2 tablespoons lime juice
1 teaspoon cumin
½ teaspoon paprika
1 pound lump crabmeat, cooked
2 celery stalks, thinly sliced
salt and pepper
1 medium Haas avocado, peeled, pitted and cubed
2 bunches watercress, washed, stems removed

1. In a large bowl, mix mayonnaise, lime juice, cumin and paprika. Add crabmeat and celery. Mix well; add salt and pepper to taste. Gently stir in avocado cubes.
2. Divide watercress on 4 plates; top with salad.

Total carbohydrates per serving: 6 grams (count only 2 "digestible" carbs when doing Atkins); protein: 26 grams; fat: 18 grams; calories: 281

Desserts/Sweets

Ginger Flan

If you aren't partial to the flavor of ginger, omit it and increase the vanilla extract to 1 tablespoon.

Prep time: 10 minutes
Bake time: 30 minutes
Chill time: 3 hours
6 servings

3 egg yolks
2 eggs
1½ cups heavy cream
1 cup water
8 packets sugar substitute
1 teaspoon vanilla extract
1 tablespoon chopped fresh ginger

1. Heat oven to 350°F. Place a roasting pan on center rack in oven and fill almost halfway with boiling water.
2. In a blender, combine yolks, eggs, cream, water, sugar substitute, vanilla and ginger, process until very smooth. Pour through a sieve into a shallow 1-quart baking dish.

3. Carefully place dish in roasting pan (water should come halfway up sides). Bake 30 to 35 minutes until a knife inserted in center comes out clean. Transfer to wire rack; cool to room temperature.
4. Spray a piece of plastic wrap with cooking spray; lay directly over flan. Chill 3 hours in refrigerator before serving.

Total carbohydrates per serving: 4 grams (count only 4 "digestible" carbs when doing Atkins); protein: 5 grams; fat: 26 grams; calories: 269

Molten Chocolate Cakes

These chocolatey delights are supposed to be soft in the center—so don't overbake them.

Prep time: 5 minutes
Bake time: 8 to 9 minutes
4 servings

7 tablespoons butter
Atkins™ Bake Mix for dusting
2 ounces unsweetened chocolate, coarsely chopped
1 tablespoon Atkins™ Bake Mix
2 eggs, at room temperature
2 egg yolks, at room temperature
8 packets sugar substitute
1 teaspoon vanilla extract

1. Heat oven to 375°F. Generously grease four 6-ounce custard cups with 1 tablespoon butter and dust with bake mix. Place cups on a baking sheet.
2. Melt remaining 6 tablespoons butter and chocolate in a double boiler. Remove from heat; cool. Stir in 1 tablespoon bake mix. Transfer to a large bowl.

3. With an electric mixer on high, beat eggs, egg yolks, sugar substitute and vanilla until almost firm peaks form, about 4 minutes.

4. In three additions, fold egg mixture into chocolate mixture. Divide batter in cups.

5. Bake 8 to 9 minutes until toothpick inserted near edge comes out clean and inserted in center comes out coated with batter. Cool 3 minutes. Run knife around edge, turn upside down to release onto serving plates. Serve immediately.

Total carbohydrates per serving: 7 grams (count only 5 "digestible" carbs when doing Atkins); protein: 6 grams; fat: 30 grams; calories: 313

Chocolate Truffles

These are just about the easiest confections to make. If you like, place a walnut or pecan half atop each truffle.

Prep time: 20 minutes
Cook time: 5 minutes
Chill time: 2 hours
Yield: 48

1 cup heavy cream
8 ounces unsweetened chocolate, chopped
1¾ cups granular sugar substitute
2 tablespoons unsalted butter
1 tablespoon vanilla extract
unsweetened cocoa powder (for dusting)

1. In a large saucepan bring cream to a boil. Add chocolate and stir until melted. Remove from heat; add sugar substitute, butter and vanilla extract. Mix until smooth. Transfer to a large bowl. Refrigerate until cool and stiff, about 2 hours.

2. Sift cocoa powder onto a piece of waxed paper. Use a small melon ball scoop to form chocolate balls (or use 2 spoons). Roll in cocoa powder. Place truffles in foil candy holders if desired.

Total carbohydrates per truffle: 2 grams (count only 2 "digestible" carbs when doing Atkins); protein: 1 gram; fat: 5 grams; calories: 50

Italian Almond Cream

For a dessert that looks as good as it tastes, serve this with fresh sliced berries.

Prep time: 8 minutes
Cook time: 8 minutes
Chill time: 3 hours
6 servings

1 envelope gelatin
2 cups heavy cream
8 packets sugar substitute
½ teaspoon almond extract

1. Lightly spray six 6-ounce custard cups with cooking spray. In small bowl, sprinkle gelatin over 3 tablespoons cold water; let sit 5 minutes until softened. Meanwhile, in medium saucepan, combine cream, ½ cup water, sweetener and almond extract. Bring to a boil over medium heat. Remove from heat, add gelatin mixture; stir until melted.
2. Pour mixture into prepared cups. Cover surface with plastic wrap to prevent skin from forming. Refrigerate at least 3 hours. Turn out onto serving plates.

Total carbohydrates per serving: 3 grams (count only 3 "digestible" carbs when doing Atkins); protein: 3 grams; fat: 29 grams; calories: 280

Banana Custard With Candied Pecans

Banana flavor without high-carb bananas! Banana extract is available in most health food stores.

Prep time: 10 minutes
Bake time: 30 minutes
Chill time: 3 hours
6 servings

Custard:
5 egg yolks
6 packets sugar substitute
⅛ teaspoon salt
2 cups heavy cream
⅓ cup water
1½ teaspoons banana extract
½ teaspoon vanilla extract

Candied Pecans:
16 packets sugar substitute
6 tablespoons pecans, coarsely chopped

1. Heat oven to 300°F. Place six 6-ounce custard cups in baking pan; set aside. Bring 6 cups of water to a boil.
2. In a medium bowl, whisk yolks, sugar substitute and salt. In medium saucepan over medium-high heat, bring cream and water to a boil; remove from heat.
3. Slowly pour cream into yolk mixture, whisking constantly. Stir in extracts. Pour custard into cups. Place baking pan on oven rack and pour in enough boiling water to come halfway up sides of cups.
4. Bake 30 minutes until custards are just set in the middle. Immediately transfer cups to wire rack. Cool to room temperature, then chill in refrigerator 3 hours. (Before refrigerating, spray 6 small squares of plastic wrap with cooking spray and lay directly over custards to prevent skins from forming.)

5. For candied nuts: Spray a baking sheet with cooking spray; set aside. In small skillet heat sugar substitute and 2 tablespoons water over medium high heat about 5 minutes until sugar substitute turns a caramel color. Add nuts; swirl to coat. Remove from heat. Pour nuts onto prepared baking sheet; spread into a single layer with a spatula coated with cooking spray. Let cool before removing.

6. Sprinkle pecans over custards just before serving.

Total carbohydrates per serving: 7 grams (count only 7 "digestible" carbs when doing Atkins); protein: 5 grams; fat: 39 grams; calories: 393

Sunshine Cake

As close to a chiffon cake as low-carb baking can get. For maximum volume, make sure the egg whites are at room temperature before whipping them.

Prep time: 15 minutes
Bake time: 55 minutes
10 servings

1¾ cups Atkins™ Bake Mix
1 cup granular sugar substitute
¼ teaspoon salt
1 tablespoon grated orange rind
9 egg yolks
¾ cup cold water
½ cup vegetable oil
2 teaspoons vanilla extract
12 egg whites, at room temperature
½ teaspoon cream of tartar

1. Heat oven to 325°F. In a large bowl whisk bake mix, sugar substitute, salt and orange rind. In another bowl,

combine yolks, water, oil and vanilla extract. Slowly add liquid to dry mixture; fold in with a rubber spatula to combine. Mix well.

2. With an electric mixer on high, beat whites and cream of tartar until stiff, about 4 minutes.

3. In three additions fold whites into batter. Pour batter into an ungreased 10-inch tube pan. Bake 55 minutes until toothpick inserted in center comes out clean. Cool upside down. (If tube pan does not have legs, invert onto the neck of a heavy bottle.)

4. To unmold, run knife around center and outside of cake.

Total carbohydrates per serving: 8 grams (count only 5.5 "digestible" carbs when doing Atkins); protein: 8 grams; fat: 17 grams; calories: 260

Chocolate Hazelnut Biscotti

Perfect for dunking into decaf coffee or tea, these biscotti are a little more tender than most because they contain sour cream. To keep them crunchy, store in a metal container.

Prep time: 25 minutes
Bake time: 40 minutes
Yield: 40 cookies

1¼ cups Atkins™ Bake Mix
16 packets sugar substitute
½ cup unsweetened cocoa powder
1 teaspoon baking soda
1 teaspoon baking powder
½ teaspoon salt
¼ cup sour cream
4 eggs, lightly beaten
2 teaspoons vanilla extract
1½ sticks butter, at room temperature

2 teaspoons decaffeinated espresso powder
1½ cup toasted, chopped hazelnuts

1. Heat oven to 350°F. Whisk together bake mix, sugar substitute, cocoa powder, baking soda, baking powder and salt. In medium bowl mix sour cream, eggs and vanilla extract.
2. In a large bowl, with an electric mixer on medium speed, beat butter 3 minutes until creamy. Beat in espresso powder. Alternately add bake mix mixture and sour cream mixture to butter. Stir in hazelnuts.
3. Divide dough in half. On a baking sheet, form each dough half into a log measuring about 11 inches by 2½ inches (moisten hands if necessary to keep dough from sticking).
4. Bake logs 25 minutes, until almost firm. Transfer sheet to wire rack to cool 10 minutes. Reduce oven temperature to 325°F.
5. Carefully cut logs crosswise with a serrated knife, into ½-inch-wide slices. Arrange slices on baking sheet. Bake 15 minutes until firm and crisp. Cool slices on sheet before storing.

Total carbohydrates per biscotti: 2 grams (count only 2 "digestible" carbs when doing Atkins); protein: 3 grams; fat: 6 grams; calories: 75

Pumpkin Pie With Nut Crust

This recipe features a hint of orange flavor in the filling.

Prep and cook time: 15 minutes
Bake time: 10 minutes
Chill time: 3 hours
8 servings

6 ounces (1½ cups) pecan or walnut halves, chopped
18 packets sugar substitute

2 tablespoons butter, softened, plus more for preparing pan
1 packet gelatin
¼ cup water
1 teaspoon pumpkin pie spice
1 can (15 ounces) pumpkin purée
2 teaspoons grated orange rind
1½ cups heavy cream
2 teaspoons vanilla extract

1. Heat oven to 400°F. Butter a 9-inch springform pan. In medium bowl, combine pecans, 6 packets sugar substitute and butter. Mix well; press onto bottom and 1 inch up sides of prepared pan. Bake 10 minutes, until golden brown. Cool on wire rack.

2. In small bowl sprinkle gelatin over water; let sit 5 minutes until gelatin softens. Meanwhile, in a small skillet over medium heat, toast pumpkin pie spice 1 to 2 minutes until fragrant, stirring frequently. Reduce heat to low, stir in gelatin mixture and cook 1 to 2 minutes until gelatin melts. Remove from heat; cool to room temperature.

3. Place pumpkin purée in a large bowl and mash with a fork to loosen; mix in orange rind. In another large bowl, with an electric mixer on high, beat cream, remaining 12 packets sugar substitute and vanilla until soft peaks form. With a rubber spatula, slowly fold in cooled gelatin mixture. In three additions, gently fold whipped cream mixture into pumpkin purée. Pour filling into cooled pie shell; smooth top. Refrigerate at least 3 hours before serving.

Total carbohydrates per serving: 11 grams (count only 7.5 "digestible" carbs when doing Atkins); protein: 4 grams; fat: 35 grams; calories: 360

Coconut Macaroons

Halfway between a cookie and a candy, these are fun to make with kids. Purchase unsweetened coconut in a health food store.

Prep time: 15 minutes
Bake time: 12 minutes
Yield: 30 macaroons

Atkins™ Bake Mix (for dusting)
4 egg whites, at room temperature
1½ cups sugar substitute
½ teaspoon coconut extract
3 cups grated unsweetened coconut (about 8 ounces)

1. Heat oven to 325°F. Grease 2 baking sheets and dust with bake mix.
2. With an electric mixer, whip egg whites on low until medium peaks form; gradually beat in sugar substitute and coconut extract; continue beating until stiff peaks form.
3. Fold in coconut. Drop mixture by tablespoons onto prepared baking sheets. Shape into little mounds with wet fingertips.
4. Bake 12 minutes; cool on sheets 1 minute; then carefully transfer to wire racks to cool completely.

Total carbohydrates per macaroon: 3 grams (count only 2 "digestible" carbs when doing Atkins); protein: 1 gram; fat: 5 grams; calories: 59

Carbohydrate Gram Counter

| Portion | Food Item | Carbohydrate (in grams) | |
		Total Carbs	"Digestible" Carbs*
ALCOHOL			
12 fl oz	Beer	13.2	12.5
1 fl oz	Brandy, 86 proof	0.0	0.0
4 fl oz	Red wine	2.0	2.0
1 fl oz	Rum, 80 proof	0.0	0.0
1 fl oz	Tequila, 80 proof	0.0	0.0
1 fl oz	Vodka, 80 proof	0.0	0.0
4 fl oz	White wine, medium	0.9	0.9
BAKING PRODUCTS			
2 tbsp	All purpose white flour	11.9	11.5
¼ cup	Atkins™ Bake Mix	6.0	3.0
1 oz	Baking chocolate, unsweetened	8.0	3.7
2 tbsp	Chocolate chips, semisweet	13.3	12.0
½ tsp	Cinnamon	0.9	0.3
½ tsp	Cocoa powder, unsweetened	0.5	0.2
2 tbsp	Coconut, dried, unsweetened	2.4	0.8
2 tbsp	Coconut milk, canned	0.8	0.5
1 tsp	Sugar, brown	4.5	4.5

Count only these carbs when doing Atkins.

Portion	Food Item	Carbohydrate (in grams)	
		Total Carbs	"Digestible" Carbs*
1 tsp	Sugar, white	4.2	4.2
1 tsp	Thicken Thin Not/Starch®	1.5	0.0

BEANS

½ cup	Baby lima beans	21.2	14.2
½ cup	Black beans	20.4	12.9
½ cup	Red kidney beans	19.8	11.6
½ cup	Chickpea/Garbanzo beans	22.5	16.2
½ cup	Great Northern beans	18.7	12.5
2 tbsp	Hummus	6.2	4.6
½ cup	Lentils	19.9	14.2
½ cup	Navy beans	23.9	18.1
½ cup	Pinto beans	18.0	11.0
½ cup	Soybeans	9.9	6.2

BEEF AND VEAL

6 oz	All types, unless listed	0.0	0.0
1 oz	Beef jerky	3.1	2.6
6 oz	Calf liver	10.4	10.4
6 oz	Roast beef, deli	2.3	2.3

BREADS, ROLLS AND CRACKERS

1	Bagel, 2½ oz	38.0	36.3
1	Biscuit, 2 oz	27.6	26.6
1	Blueberry muffin, 2 oz	27.4	25.9
1	Bran muffin, 2 oz	23.8	19.8
1	Breadstick, sesame, small	2.2	2.1
1 piece	Cornbread, 2½" × 2½" × 1½"	22.7	20.7
1	Corn muffin, 2 oz	29.0	27.1
5	Crackers, butter-type	51.4	49.8
5	Crackers, rye wafers	44.2	31.6
1	Croissant	27.0	27.0
1	English muffin	26.0	24.5
1 slice	Italian bread	15.0	14.2
1	Pita pocket bread, 6½" diameter	33.4	32.1

Count only these carbs when doing Atkins.

Portion	Food Item	Carbohydrate (in grams)	
		Total Carbs	"Digestible" Carbs*
1 slice	Raisin bread	13.6	12.5
1 slice	Rye bread	15.5	13.6
1	Tortilla, corn	12.1	10.8
1	Tortilla, flour, 8" diameter	25.3	25.3
1 slice	White bread	14.9	14.2
1	White roll, hard	30.0	28.7
1 slice	Whole grain bread	11.8	10.7

CEREALS

Portion	Food Item	Total Carbs	"Digestible" Carbs*
1 cup	Corn Flakes	24.2	23.4
½ cup	Cream of Rice cereal, cooked	13.9	13.8
½ cup	Cream of Wheat, cooked	15.8	14.3
½ cup	Oatmeal, cooked	12.6	10.6
1 cup	Puffed Wheat cereal	11.1	10.5
1 cup	Raisin Bran	47.1	38.9
1 cup	Rice Krispies	22.8	22.5

CHEESES

Portion	Food Item	Total Carbs	"Digestible" Carbs*
1 piece	American cheese, ⅔ oz slice	0.3	0.3
2 tbsp	Blue cheese, crumbled	0.4	0.4
2 tbsp	Cheddar cheese, shredded	0.2	0.2
2 tbsp	Cream cheese	0.8	0.8
½ cup	Creamed cottage cheese, small curd	2.8	2.8
2 tbsp	Feta cheese, crumbled	0.8	0.8
2 tbsp	Fontina cheese, shredded	0.2	0.2
2 tbsp	Goat cheese, soft type	0.3	0.3
1 oz	Mascarpone cheese	0.6	0.6
2 tbsp	Monterey Jack cheese, shredded	0.1	0.1
2 tbsp	Mozzarella cheese, whole milk, shredded	0.3	0.3
2 tbsp	Muenster cheese, shredded	0.2	0.2
2 tbsp	Parmesan cheese, shredded	0.3	0.3
1 oz	Provolone cheese, diced	0.6	0.6
¼ cup	Ricotta cheese, whole milk	1.9	1.9
2 tbsp	Swiss cheese, shredded	0.5	0.5

Count only these carbs when doing Atkins.

Portion	Food Item	Carbohydrate (in grams)	
		Total Carbs	**"Digestible" Carbs***
CONDIMENTS			
1 tbsp	Balsamic vinegar	2.3	2.3
1 tbsp	Capers	0.4	0.1
1 tsp	Chili powder	1.4	0.5
1 tbsp	Cider vinegar	0.9	0.9
2 tbsp	Cranberry sauce	13.5	13.1
1 tsp	Dijon mustard	0.6	0.5
1 clove	Garlic	1.0	0.9
1 tbsp	Ginger, root slices	0.9	0.8
1 tsp	Honey	5.8	5.8
1 tsp	Horseradish, prepared	0.6	0.4
1 tsp	Jam	4.6	4.5
1 tsp	Jam, sugar-free	0.3	0.3
1 tbsp	Ketchup	4.2	4.0
1 tbsp	Maple syrup	13.4	13.4
5	Olives, black	1.4	0.7
5	Olives, green	2.5	2.5
1 tbsp	Pesto sauce	1.0	0.6
1 tbsp	Pickle relish	5.4	5.2
1 tbsp	Red wine vinegar	0.0	0.0
1 tbsp	Rice vinegar, seasoned	3.0	3.0
1 tbsp	Salsa, red	0.8	0.7
1 tbsp	Soy sauce	1.0	1.0
1 tbsp	Tahini	3.2	2.5
1 tbsp	White wine vinegar	1.5	1.5
1 tsp	Worcestershire sauce	0.9	0.9
DESSERTS AND PASTRIES			
1 slice	Cake, angel food, 1/12 cake	29.4	29.2
1 slice	Cake, chocolate layer, 3 oz	38.0	36.0
1 slice	Cake, pound, 1 oz	13.8	13.7
1 oz	Chocolate, dark	17.9	16.2
1	Cookie, chocolate chip, ½ oz	10.3	10.0
1	Cookie, oatmeal, ½ oz	12.4	11.9
1	Cookie, sugar, ½ oz	10.2	10.1
1	Doughnut, glazed	26.6	25.9

Count only these carbs when doing Atkins.

Portion	Food Item	Carbohydrate (in grams)	
		Total Carbs	"Digestible" Carbs*
½ cup	Ice cream, chocolate	18.6	17.8
½ cup	Ice cream, vanilla	15.6	15.6
1 slice	Pie, apple, ⅛ of 9" pie	57.5	55.3
1 slice	Pie, lemon meringue, ⅙ of 8" pie	53.3	52.0
1 slice	Pie, pecan, ⅛ of 9" pie	63.7	57.6
1 slice	Pie, pumpkin, ⅛ of 9" pie	40.9	36.7

EGGS

1	Whole	0.6	0.6

FATS, OILS AND DRESSINGS

1 tsp	Corn Oil	0.0	0.0
1 tsp	Mayonnaise	0.1	0.1
1 tsp	Olive Oil	0.0	0.0
2 tbsp	Salad dressing, Blue Cheese	2.3	2.3
2 tbsp	Salad dressing, Caesar	0.6	0.5
2 tbsp	Salad dressing, Italian	3.0	3.0
2 tbsp	Salad dressing, Ranch	1.4	1.4
2 tbsp	Salad dressing, Thousand Island	4.8	4.8
1 tsp	Sesame oil	0.0	0.0

FRUIT AND FRUIT JUICES

1	Apple, medium	21.0	17.3
¼ cup	Applesauce	6.9	6.2
1	Apricot, fresh	3.9	3.1
¼ cup	Apricots, dried	24.9	21.3
1	Avocado	14.9	4.8
1	Banana, small	23.7	21.2
¼ cup	Blackberries	4.6	2.7
¼ cup	Blueberries	5.1	4.1
¼ cup	Cantaloupe	3.3	3.0
¼ cup	Cherries	4.8	4.2
¼ cup	Cranberries, raw	3.0	2.0
1	Fig, fresh	9.6	7.9
¼ cup	Grapes	7.1	6.7

Count only these carbs when doing Atkins.

Portion	Food Item	Carbohydrate (in grams)	
		Total Carbs	**"Digestible" Carbs***
¼ cup	Honeydew Melon	3.9	3.6
½ cup	Juice, apple	14.5	14.4
½ cup	Juice, grapefruit	11.1	10.9
1 tbsp	Juice, lemon	1.3	1.3
½ cup	Juice, orange	13.4	13.2
½ cup	Juice, tomato	5.1	4.7
1	Kiwifruit	11.3	8.7
¼ cup	Mango	7.0	6.3
1	Nectarine	16.0	13.8
1	Orange	16.3	12.9
¼ cup	Papaya	3.4	2.8
1	Peach, medium	10.9	8.9
1	Pear, medium	25.1	21.1
¼ cup	Pineapple	4.8	4.3
1	Plum	8.6	7.6
¼ cup	Raspberries	3.6	1.5
¼ cup	Strawberries	2.7	1.8
1	Tangerine	7.8	6.2
¼ cup	Watermelon	2.8	2.6

GRAINS

Portion	Food Item	Total Carbs	"Digestible" Carbs*
½ cup	Barley, pearled, cooked	22.2	19.2
½ cup	Bulgur wheat, cooked	16.9	12.8
2 tbsp	Cornmeal	11.7	10.6
½ cup	Couscous, cooked	18.2	17.1
½ cup	Hominy, cooked	11.8	9.7
½ cup	Rice, brown, cooked	22.4	20.6
½ cup	Rice, white, cooked	22.3	21.9
½ cup	Rice, wild, cooked	17.5	16.0
2 tbsp	Wheat germ, toasted	7.0	5.2

GRAVIES AND SAUCES

Portion	Food Item	Total Carbs	"Digestible" Carbs*
2 tbsp	Barbecue Sauce	4.0	3.6
¼ cup	Gravy, canned (chicken, beef, turkey, etc)	3.2	3.0

Count only these carbs when doing Atkins.

Portion	Food Item	Carbohydrate (in grams)	
		Total Carbs	"Digestible" Carbs*
2 tbsp	Hollandaise Sauce	0.3	0.3
¼ cup	Spaghetti/Marinara Sauce	5.1	4.1
¼ cup	Sweet & Sour Sauce	15.1	15.1
2 tbsp	Tartar Sauce	1.2	1.1
2 tbsp	Teriyaki Sauce	5.7	5.7
¼ cup	Tomato Sauce	4.4	3.5

HERBS

Portion	Food Item	Total Carbs	"Digestible" Carbs*
1 tbsp	All types	0.1	0.1

LAMB

Portion	Food Item	Total Carbs	"Digestible" Carbs*
6 oz	All types	0.0	0.0

LUNCH MEATS

Portion	Food Item	Total Carbs	"Digestible" Carbs*
3 oz	Beef bologna	0.7	0.7
3 oz	Beef salami	2.4	2.4
3 oz	Deli ham	1.5	1.5
3 oz	Pork bologna	0.6	0.6
3 oz	Turkey breast	0.0	0.0

MILK, CREAM AND BUTTER

Portion	Food Item	Total Carbs	"Digestible" Carbs*
1 tsp	Butter	0.0	0.0
1 cup	Buttermilk, 1% lowfat	13.0	13.0
2 tbsp	Half 'n' Half cream	1.0	1.0
2 tbsp	Heavy whipping cream	0.8	0.8
1 oz	Milk, chocolate	16.8	15.8
1 cup	Milk, 2%	11.7	11.7
1 cup	Milk, whole	11.4	11.4
2 tbsp	Sour cream	1.2	1.2
1 cup	Yogurt, whole milk, plain	11.4	11.4

MISCELLANEOUS

Portion	Food Item	Total Carbs	"Digestible" Carbs*
2 tbsp	Chicken liver pâté, canned	1.7	1.7
1	Controlled carb tortilla	12.0	3.0

Count only these carbs when doing Atkins.

Portion	Food Item	Carbohydrate (in grams)	
		Total Carbs	"Digestible" Carbs*
NUTS AND SEEDS			
2 tbsp	Almond butter	6.8	5.6
2 tbsp	Almonds, whole	3.6	1.4
2 tbsp	Hazelnuts, whole	2.8	1.2
2 tbsp	Macadamia nuts	2.3	0.9
2 tbsp	Peanut butter, natural, no sugar added	6.9	4.8
2 tbsp	Peanuts	3.4	1.8
2 tbsp	Pecans, chopped	2.1	0.6
2 tbsp	Pine nuts	2.4	1.7
2 tbsp	Pistachio nuts	4.7	3.1
2 tbsp	Pumpkin seeds	3.1	2.4
2 tbsp	Sunflower seeds	3.4	1.5
2 tbsp	Walnuts, halves	1.7	0.9
PANCAKES, WAFFLES AND FRENCH TOAST			
1 slice	French toast, frozen	18.9	18.3
1	Pancake, homemade, 6" diameter	21.8	20.7
1	Waffle, homemade, 7" diameter	24.7	23.6
PASTA			
½ cup	Noodles, egg, cooked	19.9	19.0
½ cup	Pasta/noodles, cooked	19.8	18.6
½ cup	Pasta, spinach, cooked	18.3	15.9
½ cup	Pasta, whole wheat, cooked	18.6	16.6
PORK			
3 slices	Bacon	0.1	0.1
3 slices	Canadian bacon	0.9	0.9
6 oz	Ham, boneless	0.0	0.0
2 oz	Kielbasa	0.8	0.8
6 oz	Pork chop, center cut	0.0	0.0
2 oz	Pork Frankfurter	1.4	1.4
6 oz	Pork, ground	0.0	0.0

Count only these carbs when doing Atkins.

Portion	Food Item	Carbohydrate (in grams)	
		Total Carbs	"Digestible" Carbs*
6 oz	Pork loin, boneless	0.0	0.0
6 oz	Pork loin chops	0.0	0.0
2 links	Pork sausage	2.0	2.0
6 oz	Pork spareribs	0.0	0.0
6 oz	Pork tenderloin	0.0	0.0
6 oz	Prosciutto	0.9	0.9

POULTRY

6 oz	All types, unless listed	0.0	0.0
2 oz	Chicken/turkey sausage	0.3	0.3

SEAFOOD

6 oz	All types, unless listed	0.0	0.0
1 oz	Anchovies in oil and drained	0.0	0.0
6 oz	Clams, canned	8.7	8.7
6 oz	Mussels	8.4	8.4
6 oz	Oysters	12.5	12.5
6 oz	Scallops	3.9	3.9
6 oz	Squid	7.0	7.0
6 oz	Lobster, whole	2.2	2.2

SNACKS

10 piece	Potato chips	10.6	9.7
10 piece	Pretzels	47.5	45.6
½ oz	Soy nuts	4.5	2.0
10 piece	Tortilla chips	11.3	10.2

SOUPS

1 cup	Beef broth	1.0	1.0
1 cup	Black bean soup	19.8	15.4
1 cup	Chicken broth	1.5	1.5
1 cup	Chicken noodle soup	9.4	8.6
1 cup	Cream of tomato soup	22.3	19.6
1 cup	Minestrone soup	11.2	10.3
1 cup	New England clam chowder	16.6	15.1
1 cup	Onion soup	8.2	7.2
1 cup	Vegetable soup	19.0	17.8

Count only these carbs when doing Atkins.

Portion	Food Item	Carbohydrate (in grams)	
		Total Carbs	"Digestible" Carbs*
TOFU			
4 oz	Tofu, firm	4.9	2.2
4 oz	Tofu, silken	3.3	3.2
8 fl oz	Soy milk	4.4	1.2
VEGETABLES			
1	Artichoke	13.4	6.9
6	Asparagus spears	3.8	2.4
½ cup	Beans, green	4.9	2.9
½ cup	Broccoli	3.9	1.7
6	Brussels sprouts	10.9	7.6
½ cup	Cabbage, green	1.9	1.1
1	Carrot, medium	7.3	5.1
6	Cauliflower florets	4.4	1.5
1	Celery stalk	1.5	0.8
1	Chili pepper	0.0	0.0
4 oz	Collards	7.3	3.2
½ cup	Corn	16.0	14.1
½	Cucumber, small	2.5	1.8
½ cup	Daikon	1.8	1.1
½ cup	Eggplant	3.3	2.0
½ cup	Endive	1.8	0.4
½ cup	Escarole	0.8	0.1
½ cup	Fennel	3.2	1.8
1 cup	Greens, mixed	1.6	0.4
½ cup	Jicama	5.7	2.5
½ cup	Kale	3.7	2.4
1	Leek	12.6	11.0
1 cup	Lettuce, butterhead	1.3	0.7
1 cup	Lettuce, romaine	1.3	0.4
½ cup	Mushrooms, portobello	1.4	1.0
4 oz	Okra	7.5	5.0
1	Onion	9.5	7.5
¼ cup	Onions, green	1.8	1.2
½ cup	Peas, green	9.9	6.5
½ cup	Peppers, green	4.8	3.4

Count only these carbs when doing Atkins.

Portion	Food Item	Carbohydrate (in grams)	
		Total Carbs	"Digestible" Carbs*
½ cup	Peppers, red	4.8	3.3
1	Potato, sweet	22.4	19.2
½ cup	Potato, white	15.4	13.9
½ cup	Pumpkin	9.9	6.3
½ cup	Radicchio	0.9	0.7
6	Radishes	1.0	0.5
½ cup	Rhubarb	2.8	1.7
1 cup	Spinach, raw	1.1	0.2
½ cup	Squash, butternut	10.8	7.9
½ cup	Squash, spaghetti	5.0	3.9
½ cup	Swiss chard	0.7	0.4
½ cup	Tomatoes, canned	5.2	4.0
1	Tomato, small	4.2	3.2
½ cup	Turnips	3.8	2.3
½ cup	Watercress	0.2	0.0
½ cup	Squash, summer	2.5	1.4
1	Squash, zucchini	5.7	3.3

*Count only these carbs when doing Atkins.

References

Chapter 1

1. Willett, W. "Got Fat? Exploring Nutrition Myths: A News Digest from the Center for Health Communication of the Harvard School of Public Health," *World Health News Boston*, March 29, 2000.

2. Liu, S., et al. "A Prospective Study of Dietary Glycemic Load, Carbohydrate Intake, and Risk of Coronary Heart Disease in U.S. Women," *American Journal of Clinical Nutrition*, 71, 2000, pp. 1455–1461.

3. Westman, E., et al. "Effect of a Very Low Carbohydrate Diet and Nutritional Supplements on Serum Lipids in Mildly Overweight Individuals," abstract presentation at Southern Regional Society of General Internal Medicine, February 18, 2000.

4. Volek, J.S., et al. "Fasting Lipoprotein and Postprandial Triacylglycerol Responses to a Low-Carbohydrate Diet Supplemented with n-3 Fatty Acids," *Journal of the American College of Nutrition*, 19(3), 2000, pp. 383–391.

5. Nobels, F., et al. "Weight Reduction with a High Protein, Low Carbohydrate, Caloric Restricted Diet: Effects on Blood Pressure, Glucose and Insulin Levels," *Netherlands Journal of Medicine*, 35(5–6), 1989, pp. 295–302.

6. Abbasi, F., et al. "High Carbohydrate Diets, Triglyceride Rich Lipoproteins, and Coronary Heart Disease Risk," *American Journal of Cardiology*, 85, 2000, pp. 45–48.

7. Assman, G., et al. "The Emergence of Triglycerides as a Significant Independent Risk Factor in Coronary Artery Disease," *European Heart Journal*, 19(M), 1998, pp. M8–M14.

8. Manninen, V., et al. "Joint Effects of Serum Triglyceride and LDL Cholesterol and HDL Cholesterol Concentrations on Coronary Heart Disease Risk in the Helsinki Heart Study: Implications for Treatment," *Circulation*, 85, 1992, pp. 37–47.

9. Erkkila, A. T., et al. "Dietary Associates of Serum Total, LDL, and HDL Cholesterol and Triglycerides in Patients with Coronary Heart Disease," *Preventive Medicine*, 28(6), 1999, pp. 558–565.

10. Morris, K., et al. "Glycemic Index, Cardiovascular Disease, and Obesity," *Nutrition Reviews*, 57(9), 1999, pp. 273–276.

11. Miller, M., et al. "Normal Triglyceride Levels and Coronary Artery Disease Events: The Baltimore Coronary Observational Long-Term Study," *The American College of Cardiology*, 31(6), 1998, pp. 1252–1257.

12. Hu, F. B., et al. "Dietary Protein and Risk of Ischemic Heart Disease in Women," *American Journal of Clinical Nutrition*, 70, 1999, pp. 221–227.

13. Jeppesen, J., et al. "Triglyceride Concentration and Ischemic Heart Disease: An Eight-Year Follow-Up in the Copenhagen Male Study," *Circulation*, 97(11), 1998, pp. 1029–1036.

14. Stavenow, L., and Kjellstrom, T. "Influence of Serum Triglyceride Levels on the Risk for Myocardial Infarction in 12,510 Middle Aged Males: Interaction with Serum Cholesterol," *Atherosclerosis*, 147, 1999, pp. 243–247.

15. Miller, M. "Is Hypertriglyceridaemia an Independent Risk Factor for Coronary Heart Disease? The Epidemiological Evidence," *European Heart Journal*, 19, Supplement H, 1998, pp. H18–H22.

16. Reaven, G. M., et al. "Hypertension Is a Disease of Carbohydrate and Lipoprotein Metabolism," *American Journal of Medicine*, 87(supplement 6A), 1989, pp. 2S–6S.

17. McPhillips, J. B., et al. "Cardiovascular Disease Risk Factors Prior to the Diagnosis of Impaired Glucose Tolerance and Non-Insulin-Dependent Diabetes Mellitus in a Community of Older Adults," *American Journal of Epidemiology*, 131(3), 1990, pp. 443–453.

18. Wu, J. T. "Review of Diabetes: Identification of Markers for Early Detection, Glycemic Control, and Monitoring Clinical Complications," *Journal of Clinical Laboratory Analysis*, 7(5), 1993, pp. 293–300.

19. Gutierrez, M., et al. "Utility of a Short-Term 25% Carbohydrate Diet on Improving Glycemic Control in Type 2 Diabetes Mellitus," *Journal of the American College of Nutrition*, 17(6), 1998, pp. 595–600.

20. Buyken, A. E., et al. "Glycemic Index in the Diet of European Outpatients with Type 1 Diabetes: Relations to Glycated Hemoglobin and Serum Lipids," *American Journal of Clinical Nutrition*, 73(3), 2001, pp. 574–581.

21. Mayer-Davis, E.J., et al. "Insulin Secretion, Obesity, and Potential Behavioral Influences: Results from the Insulin Resistance Atherosclerosis Study (IRAS)," *Diabetes/Metabolism Research and Reviews*, 17(2), 2001, pp.137–145.

22. Fujita, Y., et al. "Basal and Post-Protein Insulin and Glucagon Levels During a High and Low Carbohydrate Intake and Their Relationships to Plasma Triglycerides," *Diabetes*, 24(60), 1975, pp.552–558.

23. Garg, A., et al. "Comparison of Effects of High and Low Carbohydrate Diets on Plasma Lipoproteins and Insulin Sensitivity in Patients with Mild NIDDM," *Diabetes*, 41(10), 1992, pp.1278–1285.

24. Salmeron, J., et al. "Dietary Fat Intake and Risk of Type 2 Diabetes in Women," *American Journal of Clinical Nutrition*, 73(6), 2001, pp.1001–1002.

25. Salmeron, J., et al. "Dietary Fiber, Glycemic Load, and Risk of NIDDM in Men," *Diabetes Care*, 20(4), 1997, pp.545–550.

26. National Center for Health Statistics, Centers of Disease Control. "Prevalence of Overweight and Obesity Among Adults: United States, 1999," *http://cdc.gov/nchs/products/pubs/pubd/hestats/obese/obse99.htm.* Accessed September 5, 2001.

27. Guyton, A.C. "Lipid Metabolism," *Textbook of Medical Physiology* (8th edition), 1991, chapter 68, pp.756–760.

28. Sondike, S., et al. "The Ketogenic Diet Increases Weight Loss but not Cardiovascular Risk: A Randomized Controlled Trial," *Journal of Adolescent Health*, 26, 2000, p.91.

29. Kasper, II., et al. "Response of Body Weight to a Low Carbohydrate, High Fat Diet in Normal Obese Subjects," *American Journal of Clinical Nutrition*, 26, 1973, pp.197–204.

30. Enns, C.W., et al. "Trends in Food and Nutrient Intakes by Adults: NFCS 1977–78, CSFII 1989–91 and CSFII 1994–95," *Family Economics and Nutrition Review*, 10(4), 1997, pp.2–15.

Chapter 2

1. Kekwick, A., and Pawan, L.S. "Calorie Intake in Relation to Body Weight Changes in the Obese," *Lancet*, 1956, pp.155–161.

2. Rabast, U., et al. "Dietetic Treatment of Obesity with Low and High-Carbohydrate Diets: Comparative Studies and Clinical Results," *International Journal of Obesity*, 3(3), 1979, pp.201–211.

3. Rabast, U., et al. "Loss of Weight, Sodium and Water in Obese Persons Consuming a High- or Low-Carbohydrate Diet," *Annals of Nutrition and Metabolism*, 25(6), 1981, pp.341–349.

4. Yang, M. U., and Van Itallie, T. B. "Composition of Weight Loss During Short-Term Weight Reduction. Metabolic Responses of Obese Subjects to Starvation and Low-Calorie Ketogenic and Nonketogenic Diets," *Journal of Clinical Investigation*, 58(3), 1976, pp. 722–730.

5. Young, C., et al. "Effect on Body Composition and Other Parameters in Obese Young Men of Carbohydrate Level of Reduction Diet," *American Journal of Clinical Nutrition*, 24, 1971, pp. 290–296.

6. Kasper, H., et al. "Response of Body Weight to a Low Carbohydrate, High Fat Diet in Normal Obese Subjects," *American Journal of Clinical Nutrition*, 26, 1973, pp. 197–204.

7. See reference #5.

8. Skov, A. R., et al. "Randomized Trial on Protein vs. Carbohydrate in *Ad Libitum* Fat Reduced Diet for the Treatment of Obesity," *International Journal of Obesity*, 23, 1999, pp. 528–536.

9. Willi, S. M., et al. "The Effects of a High-Protein, Low-Fat Ketogenic Diet on Adolescents with Morbid Obesity: Body Composition, Blood Chemistries, and Sleep Abnormalities," *Pediatrics*, 101(1), 1998, pp. 61–67.

10. Sharman, M.J., et al. "Fasting and Postprandial Lipoprotein Responses to a Ketogenic Diet," abstract presentation at American College of Sports Medicine, June 2001.

11. Garrow, J.S., and Summerbell, C.D. "Meta-Analysis: Effect of Exercise, with or Without Dieting, on Body Composition of Overweight Subjects," *European Journal of Clinical Nutrition*, 49(1), 1995, pp. 1–10.

12. See reference #2.

13. Lean, M.E., et al. "Weight Loss with High and Low Carbohydrate 1200 Kcal Diets in Free Living Women," *European Journal of Clinical Nutrition*, 51(4), 1997, pp. 243–248.

14. Benoit, F.L., et al. "Changes in Body Composition During Weight Reduction in Obesity: Balance Studies Comparing Effects of Fasting and a Ketogenic Diet," *Annals of Internal Medicine*, 63, 1965, pp. 604–612.

15. Sondike, S., et al. "The Ketogenic Diet Increases Weight Loss but not Cardiovascular Risk: A Randomized Controlled Trial," *Journal of Adolescent Health*, 26, 2000, p. 91.

16. Westman, E., et al. "Effect of a Very Low Carbohydrate Diet and Nutritional Supplements on Serum Lipids in Mildly Overweight Individuals," Abstract presentation at Southern Regional Society for General Internal Medicine, February 18, 2000.

17. Volek, J.S., et al. "Fasting Lipoprotein and Postprandial Triacylglycerol Responses to a Low-Carbohydrate Diet Supplemented with n-3 Fatty Acids," *Journal of the American College of Nutrition*, 19 (3), 2000, pp. 383–391.

18. Nobels, F., et al. "Weight Reduction with a High Protein, Low Carbohydrate, Caloric Restricted Diet: Effects on Blood Pressure, Glucose and Insulin Levels," *Netherlands Journal of Medicine*, 35(5–6), 1989, pp. 295–302.

19. Abbasi, F., et al. "High Carbohydrate Diets, Triglyceride Rich Lipoproteins, and Coronary Heart Disease Risk," *American Journal of Cardiology*, 85, 2000, pp. 45–48.

20. Assman, G., et al. "The Emergence of Triglycerides as a Significant Independent Risk Factor in Coronary Artery Disease," *European Heart Journal*, 19(M), 1998, pp. M8–M14.

21. Manninen, V., et al. "Joint Effects of Serum Triglyceride and LDL Cholesterol and HDL Cholesterol Concentrations on Coronary Heart Disease Risk in the Helsinki Heart Study: Implications for Treatment," *Circulation*, 85, 1992, pp. 37–47.

22. Erkkila, A. T., et al. "Dietary Associates of Serum Total, LDL, and HDL Cholesterol and Triglycerides in Patients with Coronary Heart Disease," *Preventive Medicine*, 28(6), 1999, pp. 558–565.

23. Morris, K., et al. "Glycemic Index, Cardiovascular Disease, and Obesity," *Nutrition Reviews*, 57(9), 1999, pp. 273–276.

24. Miller, M., et al. "Normal Triglyceride Levels and Coronary Artery Disease Events: The Baltimore Coronary Observational Long-Term Study," *Journal of the American College of Cardiology*, 31(6), 1998, pp. 1252–1257.

25. Hu, F. B., et al. "Dietary Protein and Risk of Ischemic Heart Disease in Women," *American Journal of Clinical Nutrition*, 70, (1999), pp. 221–227.

26. Jeppesen, J., et al. "Triglyceride Concentration and Ischemic Heart Disease: An Eight-Year Follow-Up in the Copenhagen Male Study," *Circulation*, 97(11), 1998, pp. 1029–1036.

27. Stavenow, L., and Kjellstrom, T. "Influence of Serum Triglyceride Levels on the Risk for Myocardial Infarction in 12,510 Middle Aged Males: Interaction with Serum Cholesterol," *Atherosclerosis*, 147, 1999, pp. 243–247.

28. Miller, M. "Is Hypertriglyceridaemia an Independent Risk Factor for Coronary Heart Disease? The Epidemiological Evidence," *European Heart Journal*, 19, 1998, Supplement H, pp. H18–H22.

29. Reaven, G. M., et al. "Hypertension Is a Disease of Carbohydrate and Lipoprotein Metabolism," *American Journal of Medicine*, 87 (supplement 6A), 1989, pp. 2S–6S.

30. McPhillips, J. B., et al. "Cardiovascular Disease Risk Factors Prior to the Diagnosis of Impaired Glucose Tolerance and Non-Insulin-Depen-

dent Diabetes Mellitus in a Community of Older Adults," *American Journal of Epidemiology*, 131(3), 1990, pp. 443–453.

31. Wu, J.T. "Review of Diabetes: Identification of Markers for Early Detection, Glycemic Control, and Monitoring Clinical Complications," *Journal of Clinical Laboratory Analysis*, 7(5), 1993, pp. 293–300.

32. Gutierrez, M., et al. "Utility of a Short-Term 25% Carbohydrate Diet on Improving Glycemic Control in Type 2 Diabetes Mellitus," *Journal of the American College of Nutrition*, 17(6), 1998, pp. 595–600.

33. Buyken, A.E., et al. "Glycemic Index in the Diet of European Outpatients with Type 1 Diabetes: Relations to Glycated Hemoglobin and Serum Lipids," *American Journal of Clinical Nutrition*, 73(3), 2001, pp. 574–581.

34. Mayer-Davis, E.J., et al. "Insulin Secretion, Obesity, and Potential Behavioral Influences: Results from the Insulin Resistance Atherosclerosis Study (IRAS)," *Diabetes/Metabolism Research and Reviews*, 17 (2), 2001, pp. 137–145.

35. Fujita, Y., et al. "Basal and Post-Protein Insulin and Glucagon Levels During a High and Low Carbohydrate Intake and Their Relationships to Plasma Triglycerides," *Diabetes*, 24(60), 1975, pp. 552–558.

36. Garg, A., et al. "Comparison of Effects of High and Low Carbohydrate Diets on Plasma Lipoproteins and Insulin Sensitivity in Patients with Mild NIDDM," *Diabetes*, 41(10), 1992, pp. 1278–1285.

37. Salmeron, J., et al. "Dietary Fat Intake and Risk of Type 2 Diabetes in Women," *American Journal of Clinical Nutrition*, 73(6), 2001, pp. 1001–1002.

38. Salmeron, J., et al. "Dietary Fiber, Glycemic Load, and Risk of NIDDM in Men," *Diabetes Care*, 20(4), 1997, pp. 545–550.

39. Baba, N.H., et al. "High Protein vs. High Carbohydrate Hypoenergetic Diet for the Treatment of Obese Hyperinsulinemic Subjects," *International Journal of Obesity*, 11, 1999, pp. 1202–1206.

40. Wolfe, B.M. "Potential Role of Raising Dietary Protein Intake for Reducing Risk of Atherosclerosis," *Canadian Journal of Cardiology*, 11(Supplement G), 1995, pp. 127G–131G.

41. Wolfe, B.M., and Giovannetti, P.M. "Short-Term Effects of Substituting Protein for Carbohydrate in the Diets of Moderately Hypercholesterolemic Human Subjects," *Metabolism*, 40(4), 1991, pp. 338–343.

42. Gumbiner, B., et al. "Effects of Diet Composition and Ketosis on Glycemia During Very-Low-Energy-Diet Therapy in Obese Patients with Non-Insulin-Dependent Diabetes Mellitus," *American Journal of Clinical Nutrition*, 63, 1996, pp. 110–115.

43. Parks, E., and Hellerstein, M. "Carbohydrate-Induced Hypertriacylglycerolemia: Historical Perspective and Review of Biological Mechanisms," *American Journal of Clinical Nutrition*, 7, 2000, pp. 412–433.

44. Daly, M.E., et al. "Dietary Carbohydrates and Insulin Sensitivity: A Review of the Evidence and Clinical Implications," *American Journal of Clinical Nutrition*, 66, 1997, pp. 1072–1085.

45. See reference #35.

46. Friedlander, Y., et al. "LDL Particle Size and Risk Factors of Insulin Resistance Syndrome," *Atherosclerosis*, 148, 2000, pp. 141–149.

47. See reference #20.

48. Carantoni, M., et al. "Relationship Between Insulin Resistance and Partially Oxidized LDL Particles in Healthy Nondiabetic Volunteers," *Arteriosclerosis Thrombosis and Vascular Biology*, 18, 1998, pp. 762–767.

49. Lamarche, B., et al. "Fasting Insulin and Apolipoprotein B Levels and Low Density Lipoprotein Particle Size as Risk Factors for Ischemic Heart Disease," *Journal of the American Medical Association*, 279, 1998, pp. 1955–1961.

50. Lee, B.M., and Wolever, T.M.S., "Effect of Glucose, Sucrose and Fructose on Plasma Glucose and Insulin Responses in Normal Humans: Comparisons with White Bread," *European Journal of Clinical Nutrition*, 52, 1998, pp. 924–928.

51. Facchini, F.S., et al. "Insulin Resistance as a Predictor of Age-Related Disease," *Journal of Clinical Endocrinology and Metabolism*, 86(8), 2001, pp. 3574–3578.

52. Zavaroni, I., et al. "Hyperinsulinemia in a Normal Population as a Predictor of Non-Insulin-Dependent Diabetes Mellitus, Hypertension and Coronary Heart Disease: The Barille Factory Revisited," *Metabolism*, 48(8) 1999, pp. 989–994.

53. Meigs, J.B., et al. "Hyperinsulinemia, Hyperglycemia, and Impaired Homeostasis: The Framingham Offspring Study," *Journal of the American Medical Association*, 283(2), 2000, pp. 221–228.

54. Raynaud, E., et al. "Relationships Between Fibrinogen and Insulin Resistance," *Atherosclerosis*, 150, 2000, pp. 365–370.

55. Durrington, P.N. "Triglycerides Are More Important in Atherosclerosis than Epidemiology has Suggested," *Atherosclerosis*, 141(Supplement 1), 1998, pp. S57–S62.

56. Cleland, S.J., et al. "Insulin as a Vascular Hormone: Implications for the Pathophysiology of Cardiovascular Disease," *Clinical and Experimental Pharmacology and Physiology*, 25, 1998, pp. 175–184.

57. Kim, Young-In. "Diet, Lifestyle, and Colorectal Cancer: Is Hyperinsulinemia the Missing Link?" *Nutrition Reviews*, 56(9), 1998, pp. 275–279.

58. Yu, H., and Rohan, T. "Role of the Insulin-Like Growth Factor Family in Cancer Development and Progression," *Journal of the National Cancer Institute*, 92(18), 2000, pp. 1472–1489.

59. Kaaks, R., et al. "Serum C-Peptide, Insulin-Like Growth Factor (IGF)-I, IGF-Binding Proteins, and Colorectal Cancer Risk in Women," *Journal of the National Cancer Institute*, 92(19), 2000, pp. 1592–1600.

60. Song, E. Y., et al. "Diabetes but not Obesity Is a Prognostic Factor for Disease-Free Survival in Women with Stage I, II, or III Breast Carcinoma Receiving Tamoxifen," program and abstracts of the 23rd Annual San Antonio Breast Cancer Symposium; abstract #120, San Antonio, Texas, December 6–9, 2000.

61. Goodwin, P. J., et al. "Prognostic Effects of Circulating Insulin-Like Growth Factor Binding Proteins (IGFBPS) 1 and 3 in Operable Breast Cancer," program and abstracts of the 23rd Annual San Antonio Breast Cancer Symposium; abstract #118, San Antonio, Texas, December 6–9, 2000.

62. Franceschi, S., et al. "Intake of Macronutrients and Risk of Breast Cancer," *Lancet*, 347, 1996, pp. 1351–1356.

63. Nestler, J., et al. "Ovulatory and Metabolic Effects of D-Chiro-Inositol in the Polycystic Ovary Syndrome," *New England Journal of Medicine*, 340, 1999, pp. 1314–1320.

64. Davison, R. M. "New Approaches to Insulin Resistance in Polycystic Ovarian Syndrome," *Current Opinions in Obstetrics and Gynecology*, 10(3), 1998, pp. 193–198.

65. Legro, R. S., et al. "Prevalence and Predictors of Risk for Type 2 Diabetes Mellitus and Impaired Glucose Tolerance in Polycystic Ovary Syndrome: A Prospective, Controlled Study in 254 Affected Women," *Journal of Clinical Endocrinology and Metabolism*, 84(1), 1999, pp. 165–169.

66. Wolk, A., et al. "A Prospective Study of Association of Monounsaturated Fat and Other Types of Fat with Risk of Breast Cancer," *Archives of Internal Medicine*, 158, 1998, pp. 41–45.

67. Phinney, S. D., et al. "The Human Metabolic Response to Chronic Ketosis Without Caloric Restriction: Physical and Biochemical Adaptation," *Metabolism*, 32(8), 1983, pp. 757–768.

68. Enns, C. W., et al. "Trends in Food and Nutrient Intakes by Adults: NFCS 1977–78, CSFII 1989–91 and CSFII 1994–95," *Family Economics and Nutrition Review*, 10(4), 1997, pp. 2–15.

69. See bibliography to Shafrir, E., "Effect of Sucrose and Fructose on Carbohydrate and Lipid Metabolism and the Resulting Consequences," in Reitner, R., ed., *Regulation of Carbohydrate Metabolism*, Vol. II, Boca Raton, Florida, CRC Press, 1985.

70. Dolnick, E. "Le Paradoxe Francais," *Hippocrates*. May/June 1990, pp. 37–43.

Chapter 5

1. Liu, S., and Manson, J.E. "Dietary Carbohydrates, Physical Inactivity, Obesity, and the 'Metabolic Syndrome' as Predictors of Coronary Heart Disease," *Current Opinion in Lipidology*, 12(4), 2001, pp. 395–404.

2. Meigs, J.B., et al. "Hyperinsulinemia, Hyperglycemia, and Impaired Homeostasis: The Framingham Offspring Study," *Journal of the American Medical Association*, 283(2), 2000, pp. 221–228.

3. Pyorala, M., et al. "Insulin Resistance Syndrome Predicts the Risk of Coronary Heart Disease and Stroke in Healthy Middle-Aged Men: The 22-Year Follow-Up Results of the Helsinki Policeman Study," *Arteriosclerosis Thrombosis and Vascular Biology*, 20(2), 1998, pp. 538–544.

4. Jiang, X., et al. "Association of Fasting Insulin Level with Serum Lipid and Lipoprotein Levels in Children, Adolescents, and Young Adults: The Bogalusa Heart Study," *Archives of Internal Medicine*, 155, 1995, pp. 190–196.

5. Nobels, F., et al. "Weight Reduction with a High Protein, Low Carbohydrate, Caloric Restricted Diet: Effects on Blood Pressure, Glucose and Insulin Levels," *Netherlands Journal of Medicine*, 35(5–6), 1989, pp. 295–302.

6. Abbasi, F., et al. "High Carbohydrate Diets, Triglyceride Rich Lipoproteins, and Coronary Heart Disease Risk," *American Journal of Cardiology*, 85, 2000, pp. 45–48.

7. Assman, G., et al. "The Emergence of Triglycerides as a Significant Independent Risk Factor in Coronary Artery Disease," *European Heart Journal*, 19(M), 1998, pp. M8–M14.

8. Manninen, V., et al. "Joint Effects of Serum Triglyceride and LDL Cholesterol and HDL Cholesterol Concentrations on Coronary Heart Disease Risk in the Helsinki Heart Study: Implications for Treatment," *Circulation*, 85, 1992, pp. 37–47.

9. Erkkila, A.T., et al. "Dietary Associates of Serum Total, LDL, and HDL Cholesterol and Triglycerides in Patients with Coronary Heart Disease," *Preventive Medicine*, 28 (6), 1999, pp. 558–565.

10. Morris, K., et al. "Glycemic Index, Cardiovascular Disease, and Obesity," *Nutrition Reviews*, 57(9), 1999, pp. 273–276.

11. Miller, M., et al. "Normal Triglyceride Levels and Coronary Artery Disease Events: The Baltimore Coronary Observational Long-Term Study," *American College of Cardiology*, 31(6), 1998, pp. 1252–1257.

12. Hu, F.B., et al. "Dietary Protein and Risk of Ischemic Heart Disease in Women," *American Journal of Clinical Nutrition*, 70, (1999), pp. 221–227.

13. Jeppesen, J., et al. "Triglyceride Concentration and Ischemic Heart Disease: An Eight-Year Follow-Up in the Copenhagen Male Study," *Circulation*, 97(11), 1998, pp. 1029–1036.

14. Stavenow, L., and Kjellstrom, T. "Influence of Serum Triglyceride Levels on the Risk for Myocardial Infarction in 12,510 Middle Aged Males: Interaction with Serum Cholesterol," *Atherosclerosis*, 147, 1999, pp. 243–247.

15. Miller, M. "Is Hypertriglyceridaemia an Independent Risk Factor for Coronary Heart Disease? The Epidemiological Evidence," *European Heart Journal*, 19 supplement H, 1998, pp. H18–H22.

16. Reaven, G.M., et al. "Hypertension Is a Disease of Carbohydrate and Lipoprotein Metabolism," *American Journal of Medicine*, 87(supplement 6A), 1989, pp. 2S–6S.

17. McPhillips, J.B., et al. "Cardiovascular Disease Risk Factors Prior to the Diagnosis of Impaired Glucose Tolerance and Non-Insulin-Dependent Diabetes Mellitus in a Community of Older Adults," *American Journal of Epidemiology*, 131(3), 1990, pp. 443–453.

18. Wu, J.T. "Review of Diabetes: Identification of Markers for Early Detection, Glycemic Control, and Monitoring Clinical Complications," *Journal of Clinical Laboratory Analysis*, 7(5), 1993, pp. 293–300.

19. Parks, E., and Hellerstein, M. "Carbohydrate-Induced Hypertriacylglycerolemia: Historical Perspective and Review of Biological Mechanisms," *American Journal of Clinical Nutrition*, 7, 2000, pp. 412–433.

20. McLaughlin, T., et al. "Carbohydrate-Induced Hypertriglyceridemia: An Insight into the Link Between Plasma Insulin and Triglyceride Concentrations," *Journal of Clinical Endocrinology and Metabolism*, 85(9), 2000, pp. 3085–3088.

21. Song, E.Y., et al. "Diabetes but not Obesity Is a Prognostic Factor for Disease-Free Survival in Women with Stage I, II, or III Breast Carcinoma Receiving Tamoxifen," program and abstracts of the 23rd Annual San Antonio Breast Cancer Symposium; abstract #120, San Antonio, Texas, December 6–9, 2000.

22. Goodwin, P.J., et al. "Prognostic Effects of Circulating Insulin-Like Growth Factor Binding Proteins (IGFBPS) 1 and 3 in Operable Breast Cancer," program and abstracts of the 23rd Annual San Antonio Breast Cancer Symposium; abstract #118, San Antonio, Texas, December 6–9, 2000.

23. Franceschi, S., et al. "Intake of Macronutrients and Risk of Breast Cancer," *Lancet*, 347, 1996, pp. 1351–1356.

24. Nestler, J., et al. "Ovulatory and Metabolic Effects of D-Chiro-Inositol in the Polycystic Ovary Syndrome," *New England Journal of Medicine*, 340, 1999, pp. 1314–1320.

25. Davison, R.M. "New Approaches to Insulin Resistance in Polycystic Ovarian Syndrome," *Current Opinions in Obstetrics and Gynecology*, 10(3), 1998, pp. 193–198.

26. Wolk, A., et al. "A Prospective Study of the Association of Monounsaturated Fat and Other Types of Fat with Risk of Breast Cancer," *Archives of Internal Medicine*, 158, 1998, pp. 41–45.

27. Legro, R.S., et al. "Prevalence and Predictors of Risk for Type 2 Diabetes Mellitus and Impaired Glucose Tolerance in Polycystic Ovary Syndrome: A Prospective, Controlled Study in 254 Affected Women," *Journal of Clinical Endocrinology and Metabolism*, 84(1), 1999, pp. 165–169.

28. Balkau, B., et al. "High Blood Glucose Concentration Is a Risk Factor for Mortality in Middle-Aged Non-Diabetic Men: 20-Year Follow-Up in the Whitehall Study, the Paris Prospective Study, and the Helsinki Policeman Study," *Diabetes Care*, 3, 1998, pp. 360–367.

29. See reference #4.

Chapter 6

1. Reaven, G. "Syndrome X," *Current Treatment Options in Cardiovascular Medicine*, 3(4), 2001, pp. 323–332.

2. Fujita, Y., et al. "Basal and Post-Protein Insulin and Glucagon Levels During a High and Low Carbohydrate Intake and Their Relationships to Plasma Triglycerides," *Diabetes*, 24(60), 1975, pp. 552–558.

3. Hilton, A.D., and Hursh, T.A. "Type 2 Diabetes in an Aviator, Protein Diet vs. Traditional Diet: Case Report," *Aviation, Space and Environmental Medicine*, 72(3), 2001, pp. 219–220.

4. Young, C., et al. "Effect on Body Composition and Other Parameters in Obese Young Men of Carbohydrate Level of Reduction Diet," *American Journal of Clinical Nutrition*, 24, 1971, pp. 290–296.

5. Golay, A., et al. "Weight-Loss with Low or High Carbohydrate Diet?," *International Journal of Obesity and Related Metabolic Disorders*, 20(12), 1996, pp. 1067–1072.

6. Benoit, F.L., et al. "Changes in Body Composition During Weight Reduction in Obesity: Balance Studies Comparing Effects of Fasting and a Ketogenic Diet," *Annals of Internal Medicine*, 63, 1965, pp. 604–612.

7. Phinney, S.D., et al. "Capacity for Moderate Exercise in Obese Subjects After Adaptation to a Hypocaloric, Ketogenic Diet," *Journal of Clinical Investigation*, 66(5), 1980, pp. 1152–1161.

8. Willi, S.M., et al. "The Effects of a High-Protein, Low-Fat Ketogenic Diet on Adolescents with Morbid Obesity: Body Composition, Blood Chemistries, and Sleep Abnormalities," *Pediatrics*, 101(1), 1998, pp. 61–67.

9. Sharman, M.J., et al. "Fasting and Postprandial Lipoprotein Responses to a Ketogenic Diet," abstract presentation at American College of Sports Medicine, June 2001.

10. Phinney, S.D., et al. "The Human Metabolic Response to Chronic Ketosis Without Caloric Restriction: Preservation of Submaximal Exercise Capability with Reduced Carbohydrate Oxidation," *Metabolism*, 32(8), 1983, pp. 769–776.

11. Sondike, S., et al. "The Ketogenic Diet Increases Weight Loss but not Cardiovascular Risk: A Randomized Controlled Trial," *Journal of Adolescent Health*, 26, 2000, p. 91.

12. Phinney, S.D., et al. "The Human Metabolic Response to Chronic Ketosis Without Caloric Restriction: Physical and Biochemical Adaptation," *Metabolism*, 32(8), 1983, pp. 757–768.

13. Heaney, R.P. "Dietary Protein and Phosphorous Do Not Affect Calcium Absorption," *American Journal of Clinical Nutrition*, 72(3), 2000, pp. 758–761.

14. Heaney, R.P. "Excess Dietary Protein May not Adversely Affect Bone," *Nutrition*, 8(6), 1998, pp. 1054–1057.

15. Spencer, H., et al. "Do Protein and Phosphorus Cause Calcium Loss?" *Journal of Nutrition*, 118(6), 1988, pp. 657–660.

16. Moriguti, J.C., et al. "Urinary Calcium Loss in Elderly Men on a Vegetable: Animal (1:1) High-Protein Diet," *Gerontology*, 45(5), 1999, pp. 274–278.

17. Spencer, H., et al. "Effect of a High Protein (Meat) Intake on Calcium Metabolism in Man," *American Journal of Clinical Nutrition*, 31, 1978, pp. 2167–2180.

18. Spencer, H., and Kramer, L. "Osteoporosis, Calcium Requirement, and Factors Causing Calcium Loss," *Clinical Geriatric Medicine*, 3(2), 1987, pp. 389–402.

19. Spencer, H., et al. "Further Studies of the Effect of a High Protein Diet as Meat on Calcium Metabolism," *American Journal of Clinical Nutrition*, 37(6), 1983, pp. 924–929.

20. Lausen, B. "No Evidence for Dietary Protein and Dietary Salt as Main Factors of Calcium Excretion in Healthy Children and Adolescents," *American Journal of Clinical Nutrition*, 67(3), 1999, pp. 742–743.

Chapter 7

1. Kekwick, A., and Pawan, L.S. "Calorie Intake in Relation to Body Weight Changes in the Obese," *Lancet*, 1956, pp. 155–161.

2. Kekwick, A., and Pawan, L.S. "Metabolic Study in Human Obesity with Isocaloric Diets High in Fat, Protein or Carbohydrate," *Metabolism*, 1957, pp. 447–460.

3. Benoit, F.L., et al. "Changes in Body Composition During Weight Reduction in Obesity: Balance Studies Comparing Effects of Fasting and a Ketogenic Diet," *Annals of Internal Medicine*, 63, 1965, pp. 604–612.

4. Young, C., et al. "Effect on Body Composition and Other Parameters in Obese Young Men of Carbohydrate Level of Reduction Diet," *American Journal of Clinical Nutrition*, 24, 1971, pp. 290–296.

5. Rabast, U., et al. "Comparative Studies in Obese Subjects Fed Carbohydrate-Restricted and High Carbohydrate 1,000 Calorie Formula Diets," *Nutrition and Metabolism*, 22 (1978), pp. 269–277.

6. Lean, M.E., et al. "Weight Loss with High and Low Carbohydrate 1200 Kcal Diets in Free Living Women," *European Journal of Clinical Nutrition*, 51(4), 1997, pp. 243–248.

7. Skov, A.R., et al. "Randomized Trial on Protein vs. Carbohydrate in *Ad Libitum* Fat Reduced Diet for the Treatment of Obesity," *International Journal of Obesity*, 23, 1999, pp. 528–536.

8. Golay, A., et al. "Similar Weight Loss with Low or High-Carbohydrate Diets," *American Journal of Clinical Nutrition*, 63(2), 1996, pp. 174–178.

9. Golay, A., et al. "Weight-Loss with Low or High Carbohydrate Diet?" *International Journal of Obesity and Related Metabolic Disorders*, 20(12), 1996, pp. 1067–1072.

10. Sondike, S., et al. "The Ketogenic Diet Increases Weight Loss but not Cardiovascular Risk: A Randomized Controlled Trial," *Journal of Adolescent Health*, 26, 2000, p. 91.

Chapter 8

1. Chandalia, M., et al. "Beneficial Effects of High Fibre Intake in Patients with Type 2 Diabetes Mellitus," *New England Journal of Medicine*, 342, 2000, pp. 1392–1398.

2. Liu, S., et al. "A Prospective Study of Dietary Glycemic Load, Carbohydrate Intake, and Risk of Coronary Heart Disease in U.S. Women," *American Journal of Clinical Nutrition*, 71, 2000, pp. 1455–1461.

3. Franceschi, S., et al. "Dietary Glycemic Load and Colorectal Cancer Risk," *Annals of Oncology*, 12(2), 2001, pp. 173–178.

4. Song, E.Y., et al. "Diabetes but not Obesity Is a Prognostic Factor for Disease-Free Survival in Women with Stage I, II, or III Breast Carcinoma

Receiving Tamoxifen," program and abstracts of the 23rd Annual San Antonio Breast Cancer Symposium; abstract #120, San Antonio, Texas, December 6–9, 2000.

5. Goodwin, P.J., et al. "Prognostic Effects of Circulating Insulin-Like Growth Factor Binding Proteins (IGFBPS) 1 and 3 in Operable Breast Cancer," program and abstracts of the 23rd Annual San Antonio Breast Cancer Symposium; abstract #118, San Antonio, Texas, December 6–9, 2000.

6. Davison, R.M. "New Approaches to Insulin Resistance in Polycystic Ovarian Syndrome," *Current Opinions in Obstetrics and Gynecology*, 10(3), 1998, pp. 193–198.

7. Nestler, J., et al. "Ovulatory and Metabolic Effects of D-Chiro-Inositol in the Polycystic Ovary Syndrome," *New England Journal of Medicine*, 340, 1999, pp. 1314–1320.

8. Hu, F.B., et al. "Frequent Nut Consumption and Risk of Coronary Heart Disease in Women: Prospective Cohort Study," *British Medical Journal*, 317(7169), 1998, pp. 1341–1345.

9. Fraser, G.E., "Nut Consumption, Lipids, and Risk of a Coronary Event," *Clinical Cardiology*, 22 (7 Supplement), 1999, pp. III11–III15.

10. Edwards, K., et al. "Effect of Pistachio Nuts on Serum Lipids in Patients with Moderate Hypercholesterolemia," *Journal of the American College of Nutrition,* 18(3), 1999, pp. 229–232.

11. Prior, R.L., et al. "Antioxidant Capacity of Tea and Common Vegetables," *Journal of Agriculture and Food Chemistry*, 44, 1996, pp. 3426–3431.

12. Wang, H.; Cao, G.; and Prior, R.L. "Total Antioxidant Capacity of Fruits," *Journal of Agriculture and Food Chemistry*, 44, 1996, pp. 701–705.

13. Prior, R.L., et al. "Antioxidant Capacity as Influenced by Total Phenolic and Anthocyanin Content, Maturity and Variety of *Vaccinium* Species," *Journal of Agriculture and Food Chemistry*, 46, 1998, pp. 2686–2693.

14. Steinmetz, K.A., and Potter, J.D. "Vegetables, Fruit, and Cancer Prevention: A Review," *Journal of the American Dietetic Association*, 96, 1996, pp. 1027–1039.

Chapter 9

1. Phinney, S.D., et al. "The Human Metabolic Response to Chronic Ketosis Without Caloric Restriction: Physical and Biochemical Adaptation," *Metabolism*, 32(8), 1983, pp. 757–768.

2. Westman, E., et al. "Effect of a Very Low Carbohydrate Diet and Nutritional Supplements on Serum Lipids in Mildly Overweight Individuals,"

abstract presentation at Southern Regional Society General Internal Medicine, February 18, 2000.

3. Hoffer, L.J. "Metabolic Consequences of Starvation" in Shils, M.E., et al. (editors), *Modern Nutrition in Health and Disease*, Lippincott Williams & Wilkens, Baltimore, 9th edition, 1999, pp. 645–665.

4. Sharman, M.J., et al. "Fasting and Postprandial Lipoprotein Responses to a Ketogenic Diet," abstract presentation at American College of Sports Medicine, June 2001.

5. See reference #1.

6. Spencer, H., et al. "Do Protein and Phosphorus Cause Calcium Loss?," *Journal of Nutrition*, 118(6), 1988, pp. 657–660.

7. Heaney, R.P. "Excess Dietary Protein May not Adversely Affect Bone," *Journal of Nutrition*, 128(6), 1998, pp. 1054–1057.

8. Heaney, R.P. "Dietary Protein and Phosphorous Do not Affect Calcium Absorption," *American Journal of Clinical Nutrition*, 72(3), 2000, pp. 758–761.

9. Moriguti, J.C., et al. "Urinary Calcium Loss in Elderly Men on a Vegetable: Animal (1:1) High-Protein Diet," *Gerontology*, 45(5), 1999, pp. 274–278.

10. Spencer, H., and Kramer, L. "Osteoporosis, Calcium Requirement, and Factors Causing Calcium Loss," *Clinics in Geriatric Medicine*, 3(2), 1987, pp. 389–402.

11. Spencer, H., et al. "Effect of a High Protein (Meat) Intake on Calcium Metabolism in Man," *American Journal of Clinical Nutrition*, 31, 1978, pp. 2167–2180.

12. Lausen, B. "No Evidence for Dietary Protein and Dietary Salt as Main Factors of Calcium Excretion in Healthy Children and Adolescents," *American Journal of Clinical Nutrition*, 67(3), 1999, pp. 742–743.

13. See reference #1.

14. Skov, A.R., et al. "Changes in Renal Function During Weight Loss Induced by High vs. Low-Protein, Low-Fat Diets in Overweight Subjects," *International Journal of Obesity*, 23, 1999, pp. 1170–1177.

15. Bellomo, R., et al. "A Prospective Comparative Study of Moderate Versus High-Protein Intake for Critically Ill Patients with Acute Renal Failure," *Renal Failure*, 20(3), 1998, pp. 545–547.

16. Blum, M., et al. "Protein Intake and Kidney Function in Humans: Its Effect on Normal Aging," *Archives of Internal Medicine*, 149(1), 1989, pp. 211–212.

17. Newbold, H.L. "Reducing the Serum Cholesterol Level with a Diet High in Animal Fat," *Southern Medical Journal*, 81(1), 1988, pp. 61–63.

18. Wolfe, B.M. "Potential Role of Raising Dietary Protein Intake for Reducing Risk of Atherosclerosis," *Canadian Journal of Cardiology,* 11(Supplement G), 1995, pp. 127G–131G.

19. Gillman, M.W., et al. "Inverse Association of Dietary Fat with Development of Ischemic Stroke in Men," *Journal of The American Medical Association,* 278(24), 1997, pp. 2145–2150.

20. Cerami, A., et al, "Protein Glycosylation and the Pathogenesis of Atherosclerosis," *Metabolism,* 34(12 Supplement 1), 1985, pp. 37–42.

21. Cerami, A., et al "Role of Nonenzymatic Glycosylation in Atherogenesis," *Journal of Cellular Biochemistry,* 30(2), 1986, pp. 111–120.

22. Nelson, G., et al. "Low-Fat Diets Do not Lower Plasma Cholesterol Levels in Healthy Men Compared to High-Fat Diets with Similar Fatty Acid Composition at Constant Caloric Intake," *Lipids,* 30, 1995, pp. 969–976.

23. Reaven, G.M., et al. "Hypertension Is a Disease of Carbohydrate and Lipoprotein Metabolism," *American Journal of Medicine,* 87 (supplement 6A), 1989, pp. 2S–6S.

24. Gaziano, J.M., et al. "Fasting Triglycerides, High-Density Lipoprotein, and Risk of Myocardial Infarction," *Circulation,* 96(8), 1997, pp. 2520–2525.

25. Austin, M.A., et al. "Hypertriglyceridemia as a Cardiovascular Risk Factor," *American Journal of Cardiology,* 81(4A), 1998, pp. 7B–12B.

26. Pieke, B., et al. "Treatment of Hypertriglyceridemia by Two Diets Rich Either in Unsaturated Fatty Acids or in Carbohydrates: Effects on Lipoprotein Subclasses, Lipolytic Enzymes, Lipid Transfer Proteins, Insulin and Leptin," *International Journal of Obesity,* 24(10), 2000, pp. 1286–96.

27. Abbasi, F., et al. "High Carbohydrate Diets, Triglyceride Rich Lipoproteins, and Coronary Heart Disease Risk," *American Journal of Cardiology,* 85, 2000, pp. 45–48.

28. Stavenow, L., and Kjellstrom, T. "Influence of Serum Triglyceride Levels on the Risk for Myocardial Infarction in 12,510 Middle Aged Males: Interaction with Serum Cholesterol," *Atherosclerosis,* 147, 1999, pp. 243–247.

29. Sondike, S., et al. "The Ketogenic Diet Increases Weight Loss but not Cardiovascular Risk: A Randomized Controlled Trial," *Journal of Adolescent Health,* 26, 2000, p. 91.

30. Young, C., et al. "Effect on Body Composition and Other Parameters in Obese Young Men of Carbohydrate Level of Reduction Diet," *American Journal of Clinical Nutrition,* 24, 1971, pp. 290–296.

31. Spirt, B.A., et al. "Gallstone Formation in Obese Women Treated by a Low-Calorie Diet," *International Journal of Obesity,* 19, 1995, p. 595.

32. See reference #7.

33. See reference #4.

34. Gillman, M. W., et al. "Inverse Association of Dietary Fat with Development of Ischemic Stroke in Men," *Journal of the American Medical Association*, 278(24), 1997, pp. 2145–2150.

35. See references #24–28.

36. See reference #7.

Chapter 10

1. Gaziano, J. M., et al. "Fasting Triglycerides, High-Density Lipoprotein, and Risk of Myocardial Infarction," *Circulation*, 96(8), 1997, pp. 2520–2525.

2. Westman, E., et al. "Effect of a Very Low Carbohydrate Diet and Nutritional Supplements on Serum Lipids in Mildly Overweight Individuals," abstract presentation at Southern Regional Society General Internal Medicine, February 18, 2000.

3. Sondike, S., et al. "The Ketogenic Diet Increases Weight Loss but not Cardiovascular Risk: A Randomized Controlled Trial," *Journal of Adolescent Health*, 26, 2000, p. 91.

4. Dreon, D., et al. "Change in Dietary Saturated Fat Intake Is Correlated with Change in Mass of Large Low-Density-Lipoprotein Particles in Men," *American Journal of Clinical Nutrition*, 67, 1998, pp. 828–836.

5. Phinney, S. D., et al. "The Human Metabolic Response to Chronic Ketosis Without Caloric Restriction: Physical and Biochemical Adaptation," *Metabolism*, 32(8), 1983, pp. 757–768.

6. Skov, A. R., et al. "Randomized Trial on Protein vs. Carbohydrate in *Ad Libitum* Fat Reduced Diet for the Treatment of Obesity," *International Journal of Obesity and Related Metabolic Disorders*, 23, 1999, pp. 528–536.

7. Dessein, P. H., and Stanwix, A. E. "Beneficial Effects of Weight Loss Associated with Moderate Calorie/Carbohydrate Restriction, and Increased Proportional Intake of Protein and Unsaturated Fat on Serum Urate and Lipoprotein Levels in Gout: A Pilot Study," *Annals of Rheumatoid Disorders*, 59 (7), 2000, pp. 539–543.

8. Mokdad, A. H., et al. "Diabetes Trends in the U.S.:1990–98," *Diabetes Care*, 23(9), 2000, pp. 1278–1283.

Chapter 14

1. Jeppesen, J., et al. "Triglyceride Concentration and Ischemic Heart Disease: An Eight-Year Follow-Up in the Copenhagen Male Study," *Circulation*, 97(11), 1998, pp. 1029–1036.

Chapter 15

1. Bischoff, S.C., et al. "Allergy and the Gut," *International Archives of Allergy Immunology*, 121(4), 2000, pp. 270–283.

2. Sampson, H.A. "Food Allergy, Part I: Immunopathogenesis and Clinical Disorders," *Journal of Allergy and Clinical Immunology*, 103(5), 1999, pp. 717–728.

3. Astrup, A., et al. "Low Resting Metabolic Rate in Subjects Predisposed to Obesity: A Role for Thyroid Function," *American Journal of Clinical Nutrition*, 63(6), 1996, pp. 879–883.

4. Kerr, D., et al. "Effects of Caffeine on the Recognition of and Responses to Hypoglycemia in Humans," *Annals of Internal Medicine*, 119 (8), 1993, pp. 799–804.

Chapter 17

1. Katan, M.B., et al. "Should a Low-Fat, High Carbohydrate Diet Be Recommended for Everyone? Beyond Low-Fat Diets," *New England Journal of Medicine*, 337, 1997, pp. 563–566.

2. "Methods for Voluntary Weight Loss and Control," NIH Technology Assessment Conference Panel, Consensus Development Conference, 30 March to 1 April 1992, *Annals of Internal Medicine*, 119 (7 part 2), 1993, pp. 764–770.

Chapter 18

1. Sharman, M.J., et al. "Fasting and Postprandial Lipoprotein Responses to a Ketogenic Diet," abstract presentation at American College of Sports Medicine, June 2001.

2. Phinney, S.D., et al. "The Human Metabolic Response to Chronic Ketosis Without Caloric Restriction: Physical and Biochemical Adaptation," *Metabolism*, 32(8), 1983, pp. 757–768.

3. Langfort, J., et al. "Effect of Low-Carbohydrate-Ketogenic Diet on Metabolic and Hormonal Responses to Graded Exercise in Men," *Journal of Physiology and Pharmacology*, 47(2), 1996, pp. 361–371.

4. Hoffer, L.J. "Metabolic Consequences of Starvation" in Shils, M.E., et al. (editors), *Modern Nutrition in Health and Disease*, Lippincott Williams & Wilkens, Baltimore, 9th edition, 1999, pp. 645–665.

5. Kasper, H., et al. "Response of Body Weight to a Low Carbohydrate, High Fat Diet in Normal Obese Subjects," *American Journal of Clinical Nutrition*, 26, 1973, pp. 197–204.

Chapter 20

1. Cusin, I., et al. "Hyperinsulinemia and Its Impact on Obesity and Insulin Resistance," *International Journal of Obesity and Related Metabolic Disorders*, 16(supplement 4), 1992, pp. S1–S11.

2. Holt, S.H., and Miller, J.B. "Increased Insulin Response to Ingested Foods Are Associated with Lessened Satiety," *Appetite*, 24, 1995, pp. 43–54.

3. Parks, E., and Hellerstein, M. "Carbohydrate-Induced Hypertriacyl-glycerolemia: Historical Perspective and Review of Biological Mechanisms," *American Journal of Clinical Nutrition*, 7, 2000, pp. 412–433.

4. Sigal, RJ., et al. "Acute Post Challenge Hyperinsulinemia Predicts Weight Gain: A Prospective Study," *Diabetes*, 46, 1997, pp. 1025–1029.

5. Rebouche, C.J. "Carnitine" in Shils, M.E., et al. (editors), *Modern Nutrition in Health and Disease*, Lippincott Williams & Wilkins, Baltimore, 9th edition, 1999, p. 505.

6. Carter, A.L., et al. "Biosynthesis and Metabolism of Carnitine," *Journal of Child Neurology*, 10(supplement 2), 1995, pp. S3–S7.

7. Hacckel, R., et al. "Carnitine: Metabolism, Function and Clinical Application," *Journal of Clinical Chemistry and Clinical Biochemistry*, 28(5), 1990, pp. 291–295.

8. Lenaz, G., et al. "Mitochondrial Bioenergetics in Aging," *Biochimica et Biophysica Acta*, 1459(2–3), 2000, pp. 397–404.

9. Rajala, U., et al. "Antihypertensive Drugs as Predictors of Type 2 Diabetes Among Subjects with Impaired Glucose Tolerance," *Diabetes Research and Clinical Practice*, 50(3), 2000, pp. 231–239.

10. Lewis, P.J., et al. "Deterioration of Glucose Tolerance in Hypertensive Patients on Prolonged Diuretic Treatment," *Lancet*, 1 (7959), 1976, pp. 564–566.

11. Amery, A., et al. "Glucose Intolerance During Diuretic Therapy: Results of Trial by European Working Party on Hypertension in the Elderly," *Lancet*, 1(8066), 1978, pp. 681–683.

Chapter 22

1. Murray, C. J. L., and Lopez, A. D. *Global Burden of Disease: A Comprehensive Assessment of Mortality and Disability from Diseases, Injuries, and Risk Factors in 1990 and Projected*, Harvard School of Public Health, Boston, 1996, pp. 309–310.

2. Kayman, S., et al. "Maintenance and Relapse After Weight Loss in Women: Behavioral Aspects," *American Journal of Clinical Nutrition*, 52(5), 1990, pp. 800–807.

3. Lee, I. M., and Skerrett, P. J. "Physical Activity and All-Cause Mortality: What is the Dose-Response Relation?," *Medical Science and Sports Exercise*, 33(Supplement 6), 2001, pp. S459–471, and discussion pp. S493–494.

4. Hassmen, P., et al. "Physical Exercise and Psychological Well-Being: A Population Study in Finland," *Preventive Medicine*, 30(1), 2000, pp. 17–25.

5. Hakim, A. A., et al. "Effects of Walking on Coronary Heart Disease in Elderly Men: The Honolulu Heart Program," *Circulation*, 100(1), 1999, pp. 9–13.

6. *Physical Activity and Health: A Report of The Surgeon General, U.S. Department of Health and Human Services*, Centers for Disease Control and Prevention, National Center for Chronic Disease Prevention and Health Promotion, July 1996.

7. Paffenbarger, R. *LifeFit: An Effective Exercise Program for Optimal Health and a Longer Life*, Human Kinetics, Champaign, Illinois, 1996.

8. Lambert, E. V., et al. "Enhanced Endurance in Trained Cyclists During Moderate Intensity Exercise Following 2 Weeks Adaptation to a High Fat Diet," *European Journal of Applied Physiology and Occupational Physiology*, 69 (4), 1994, pp. 287–293.

9. Leddy, J., et al. "Effect of a High or a Low Fat Diet on Cardiovascular Risk Factors in Male and Female Runners," *Medical Science and Sports Exercise*, 29, 1997, pp. 17–25.

10. Muoio, D. M., et al. "Effect of Dietary Fat on Metabolic Adjustments to VO_2 and Endurance in Runners," *Medical Science and Sports Exercise*, 26, 1994, pp. 81–88.

Chapter 23

1. Evan, G. W. "The Effects of Chromium Picolinate on Insulin Controlled Parameters in Humans," *International Journal of Biosocial Medical Research*, 11, 1989, pp. 163–180.

2. Cattin, L., et al. "Treatment of Hypercholesterolemia with Pantethine and Fenofibrate: An Open Randomized Study on 43 Subjects," *Current Theories in Research*, 38(3), 1985, pp. 386–395.

3. Coggeshall, J. C., et al. "Biotin Status and Plasma Glucose in Diabetics," *Annals of New York Academy of Science*, 447, 1985, pp. 389–392.

4. Ferrari, R., et al. "The Metabolic Effects of L-Carnitine in Angina Pectoris," *International Journal of Cardiology*, 5, 1984, p. 213.

5. Van Gall, L., et al. "Exploratory Study of Coenzyme Q_{10} in Obesity" in Folkers, K., and Yamamura, Y. (editors), *Biomedical and Clinical Aspects of Coenzyme Q_{10}*, Elsevier Science Publishers, Amsterdam, 4th Edition, 1984, pp. 369–373.

6. Azuma, J., et al. "Therapeutic Effect of Taurine in Congestive Heart Failure: A Double Blind Crossover Trial," *Clinical Cardiology*, 8, 1985, pp. 276–282.

7. Ellis, F. R., and Nassar, S. "A Pilot Study of Vitamin B_{12} in the Treatment of Tiredness," *British Journal of Nutrition*, 30, 1973, pp. 277–283.

8. Jamal, C. A., et al. "Gamma-Linolenic Acid Diabetic Neuropathy," *Lancet*, 1, 1986, p. 1098.

9. Ceriello, A., et al. "Hypomagnesemia in Relation to Diabetic Retinopathy," *Diabetes Care*, 5, 1982, pp. 558–559.

10. Cohen, L. "Magnesium and Hypertension," *Magnesium Bulletin*, 8, 1986, pp. 1847–1849.

11. Norris, P. G., et al. "Effect of Dietary Supplementation with Fish Oil on Systolic Blood Pressure in Mild Essential Hypertension," *British Medical Journal*, 293, 1986, p. 104.

12. Kosolcharoen, P., et al. "Improved Exercise Tolerance After Administration of Carnitine," *Current Theories in Research*, 1981, pp. 753–764.

13. Haeger, K. "Long-Time Treatment of Intermittent Claudication with Vitamin E," *American Journal of Clinical Nutrition*, 27(10), 1974, pp. 1179–1181.

14. Kamikawa, T., et al. "Effects of Coenzyme Q_{10} on Exercise Tolerance in Chronic Stable Angina Pectoris," *American Journal of Cardiology*, 56, 1985, p. 247.

15. Taussig, S. J., and Nieper, H. A. "Bromelain: Its Use in Prevention and Treatment of Cardiovascular Disease: Present Status," *Journal of the International Academy of Preventive Medicine*, 6(1), 1979, pp. 139–151.

Chapter 24

1. Bernstein, G. "Letter to *The New York Times*," August 16, 2001.

2. Cleave, T. L. *Saccharine Disease: The Master Disease of Our Time*, Keats Publishing, New Canaan, Connecticut, 1978.

3. "Global Burden of Diabetes," press release, World Health Organization/63 September 14, 1998.
http://www.who.int/inf-pr-1998/en/pr98-63.html

4. "Economic Consequences of Diabetes Mellitus in the U.S. in 1997," American Diabetes Association, *Diabetes Care*, 21(2), 1998, pp. 296–309.

5. "Type 2 Diabetes in Children and Adolescents," American Diabetes Association, *Diabetes Care*, 23(3), 2000, pp. 381–389.

6. Publications and Products: National Diabetes Fact Sheet Centers for Disease Control Program, 1998.
http://www.cdc.gov/diabetes/pubs/facts98.htm

7. American Podiatric Medical Association e-Foot Faqs, "Diabetes and Feet: Frequently Asked Questions."
http://www.apma.org/faqsdiab.html

8. Atkins Diet Study, Roper Starch Worldwide Survey, #CN0216. November 1999.

9. Harris, M. I., et al. "Prevalence of Diabetes, Impaired Fasting Glucose Tolerance in U.S. Adults," *Diabetes Care*, 21(4), 1998, pp. 518–524.

10. DeFronzo, R. A., et al. "Pathogenesis of NIDDM: A Balanced Overview," *Diabetes Care*, 15(3), 1992, pp. 318–368.

11. Garg, A., et al. "Comparison of Effects of High and Low Carbohydrate Diets on Plasma Lipoproteins and Insulin Sensitivity in Patients with Mild NIDDM," *Diabetes*, 41(10), 1999, pp. 1278–1285.

12. Campbell, L., et al. "The High Monounsaturated Fat Diet as a Practical Alternative for NIDDM," *Diabetes Care*, 17(3), 1994, pp. 177–182.

13. Gumbiner, B., et al. "Effects of Diet Composition and Ketosis on Glycemia During Very-Low-Energy-Diet Therapy in Obese Patients with Non-Insulin-Dependent Diabetes Mellitus," *American Journal of Clinical Nutrition*, 63, 1996, pp. 110–115.

14. Gutierrez, M., et al. "Utility of a Short-Term 25% Carbohydrate Diet on Improving Glycemic Control in Type 2 Diabetes Mellitus," *Journal of the American College of Nutrition*, 17(6), 1998, pp. 595–600.

15. Goldwasser, I., et al. "Insulin-Like Effects of Vanadium: Basic and Clinical Implications," *Journal of Inorganic Biochemistry*, 80(1–2), 2000, pp. 21–25.

16. Verma, S., et al. "Nutritional Factors That Can Favorably Influence the Glucose/Insulin System: Vanadium," *Journal of the American College of Nutrition*, 17(1), 1998, pp. 11–18.

17. Thompson, K. H. "Vanadium and Diabetes," *BioFactors*, 10(1), 1999, pp. 43–51.

18. Anderson, R. A., et al. "Potential Antioxidant Effects of Zinc and Chromium Supplements in People with Type 2 Diabetes Mellitus," *Journal of the American College of Nutrition*, 20(3), 2001, pp. 212–218.

19. Cerami, A. "Hypothesis: Glucose as a Mediator of Aging," *Journal of the American Geriatric Society*, 33(9), 1985, pp. 626–634.

20. Lyons, T. J. "Glycation and Oxidation: A Role in the Pathogenesis of Atherosclerosis," *American Journal of Cardiology*, 71(6), 1993, pp. 26B–31B.

Chapter 26

1. Walker-Smith, J. A., et al. "The Spectrum of Gastrointestinal Allergies to Food," *Annals of Allergy*, 53(6 part. 2), 1984, pp. 629–636.

2. Egger, J., et al. "Is Migraine Food Allergy? A Double-Blind Trial of Oligoantigenic Diet Treatment," *Lancet*, 1994, pp. 719–721.

3. Sampson, H. A. "Disease of the Gastrointestinal Tract of Children Caused by Immune Reactions to Foods," *Monographs in Allergy*, 32 (1996), pp. 36–48.

Chapter 27

1. Kaplan, N. M. "The Deadly Quartet: Upper-Body Obesity, Glucose Intolerance, Hypertriglyceridemia, and Hypertension," *Archives of Internal Medicine*, 149, 1989, pp. 1514–1520.

2. "What Is Obesity?," American Obesity Association, *http://www. obesity.org*. Accessed September 2001.

3. *National Health and Nutrition Examination Survey III (NHANES III)*, 1988–94. CDC/NCHS and the American Heart Association.

4. Rocchini, A. P. "Proceedings of the Council for High Blood Pressure Research, 1990: Insulin Resistance and Blood Pressure Regulation in Obese and Nonobese Subjects: Special Lecture," *Hypertension*, 17(6 part 2), 1991, pp. 837–842.

5. Reaven, G. M., et al. "Hypertension as a Disease of Carbohydrate and Lipoprotein Metabolism,"*American Journal of Medicine*, 87 (supplement 6A),1989, pp. S2–S6.

6. Reaven, G. M., et al. "Banting Lecture 1988. The Role of Insulin Resistance in Human Disease," *Diabetes*, 37(12), 1988, pp. 1595–1607.

7. Assman, G., and Schulte, H. "Relation of High-Density Lipoprotein Cholesterol and Triglycerides to Incidence of Atherosclerotic Coronary

Artery Disease (The PROCAM Experience): Prospective Cardiovascular Munster Study," *American Journal of Cardiology*, 70(7), 1992, pp. 733–737.

8. Gaziano, J. M., et al. "Fasting Triglycerides, High-Density Lipoprotein, and Risk of Myocardial Infarction," *Circulation*, 96(8), 1997, pp. 2520–2525.

9. Castelli, W. P. *Medical Tribune*, 33(2), 1992.

10. Manninen, V., et al. "Joint Effects of Serum Triglyceride and LDL Cholesterol and HDL Cholesterol Concentrations on Coronary Heart Disease Risk in the Helsinki Heart Study: Implications for Treatment," *Circulation*, 85(1), 1992, pp. 37–45.

11. Lichtenstein, M. J., et al. "Sex Hormones, Insulin, Lipids and Prevalent Ischemic Heart Disease," *American Journal of Epidemiology*, 126(4), 1987, pp. 647–657.

12. Pyorala, K., et al. "Plasma Insulin as Coronary Heart Disease Risk Factor: Relationship to Other Risk Factors and Predictive Value during 9½-Year Follow Up of the Helsinki Policeman Study Population," *Acta Medicina Scandvica. Supplementum*, 701, 1985, pp. 38–52.

13. Fontbonne, A., et al. "Coronary Heart Disease Mortality Risk: Plasma Insulin Level Is a More Sensitive Marker Than Hypertension or Abnormal Glucose Tolerance in Overweight Males. The Paris Prospective Study," *International Journal of Obesity*, 12(6), 1988, pp. 557–565.

14. Despres, J. P., et al. "Hyperinsulinemia as an Independent Risk Factor for Ischemic Heart Disease," *New England Journal of Medicine*, 334(15), 1996, pp. 952–957.

15. "2001 Heart and Stroke Statistical Update, Cardiovascular Diseases," American Heart Association.
http://www.americanheart.org/statistics/cvd.html

16. Willett, W. C., et al. "Intake of Trans Fatty Acids and Risk of Coronary Heart Disease Among Women," *Lancet*, 341(8845), 1993, pp. 581–585.

17. Mensink, R. P., et al. "Effects of Dietary Cis and Trans Fatty Acids on Serum Lipoprotein [A] Levels in Humans," *Journal of Lipid Research*, 33(10), 1992, pp. 1493–1501.

18. Wolfe, B. M., and Giovannetti, P. M. "Short-Term Effects of Substituting Protein for Carbohydrate in the Diets of Moderately Hypercholesterolemic Human Subjects," *Metabolism: Clinical and Experimental*, 40(4), 1991, pp. 338–343.

19. Stamler, J., et al. "Inverse Relation of Dietary Protein Markers with Blood Pressure: Findings for 10,020 Men and Women in the INTERSALT Study. INTERSALT Cooperative Research Group. International Study of Salt and Blood Pressure," *Circulation*, 94(7), 1996, pp. 1629–1634.

20. Gillman, M. W., et al. "Inverse Association of Dietary Fat with Development of Ischemic Stroke in Men," *Journal of the American Medical Association*, 278(24), 1997, pp. 2145–2150.

21. Austin, M. A., et al. "Hypertriglyceridemia as a Cardiovascular Risk Factor," *American Journal of Cardiology*, 81(4A), 1998, pp. 7B–12B.

22. Hu, F. B., et al. "Dietary Protein and Risk of Ischemic Heart Disease in Women," *American Journal of Clinical Nutrition*, 70(2), 1999, pp. 221–227.

23. Ridker, P. M., et al. "C-Reactive Protein and Other Markers of Inflammation in the Prediction of Cardiovascular Disease in Women," *New England Journal of Medicine*, 342(12), 2000, pp. 836–843.

24. Keys, A., et al. *Epidemiological Studies Relating to CHD: Characteristics of Men 40–59 in Seven Countries*, Tampire, Hameen Kirjataino Oy, 1966, p. 337.

25. Yudkin, J., and Carey, M. "The Treatment of Obesity by the High-Fat Diet: The Inevitability of Calories," *Lancet*, 1960, pp. 939–941.

26. Cleave, T. L. *Saccharine Disease: The Master Disease of Our Time*, Keats Publishing, New Canaan, Connecticut, 1975.

Chapter 28

1. "Prevalance of Overweight Among Children and Adolescents: United States, 1999," National Center for Health Statistics, HealthE-Stats from the Centers for Disease Control and Prevention.
http://www.cdc.gov/nchs/products/pubs/pubd/hestats/overwght99.htm

Index